Horizons in Medicine

.... *number* **17**

Edited by
Dorian Haskard

Professor of Rheumatology,
Eric Bywaters Centre for Vascular Inflammation,
British Heart Foundation Cardiovascular Medicine Unit,
Imperial College, London

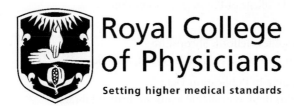

Royal College
of Physicians
Setting higher medical standards

Acknowledgement

The Royal College of Physicians acknowledges the contribution of The Lavenham Press towards the cost of printing this book.

The Royal College of Physicians of London

The Royal College of Physicians plays a leading role in the delivery of high quality patient care by setting standards of medical practice and promoting clinical excellence. We provide physicians in the UK and overseas with education, training and support throughout their careers. As an independent body representing over 20,000 Fellows and Members worldwide, we advise and work with government, the public, patients and other professions to improve health and healthcare.

Citation of this book: Royal College of Physicians. *Horizons in medicine*, volume 17. London: RCP, 2005.

Front cover photograph:
ZEPHYR/SCIENCE PHOTO LIBRARY
Chest blood vessels, MRA scan

Royal College of Physicians of London
11 St Andrews Place, London NW1 4LE

Registered Charity No. 210508

Typeset by Dan-Set Graphics, Telford, Shropshire
Printed in Great Britain by The Lavenham Press Ltd, Suffolk

British Library Cataloguing in Publication Data
A catalogue record of this book is available from the British Library

Editor's introduction

This volume of *Horizons in Medicine* represents the talks given at the 2005 Advanced Medicine Conference. As the conference organiser, I was set the task of arranging a programme highlighting clinical advances of interest to a general medical audience, encompassing a broad range of specialisations. The conference attracted an outstanding series of lectures, documented in the chapters herein. Many of the contributions highlight the major advances that have emerged through molecular and clinical research. Others provide fresh insights into clinically challenging problems, such as headache and fibromyalgia.

Key themes of the conference were the molecular classification of disease (such as the cardiomyopathies and endocrine cancer syndromes), advances in imaging technology, and the successful application of monoclonal antibody and other biological therapies to the treatment of inflammatory diseases (rheumatoid arthritis, systemic lupus erythematosus, Crohn's disease, psoriasis).

Particular highlights were the two named college lectures. In the Lumleian Lecture, Professor Steve R Bloom outlined advances in obesity, focusing on new insights into satiety that have major therapeutic promise. Professor David Lomas used the Croonian Lecture to discuss the molecular basis of disorders of serine proteinase inhibitors ('serpinopathies'), the clinical manifestations of which range from cirrhosis and emphysema to dementia.

Throughout the conference, I was struck by the overwhelming desire of physicians to achieve clinical excellence and by the immense resource that exists in the United Kingdom for improving patient care through clinical research. There is a pressing need to foster and maintain an environment that allows the translation of basic research into clinical evaluation and then into clinical practice. We are living in exciting times, with all the efforts of molecular research over the last two decades now offering real prospects for the benefit of patients.

DORIAN HASKARD
September 2005

Contributors

STEVE R BLOOM, *Professor of Medicine, Department of Metabolic Medicine, Imperial College, Hammersmith Hospital, Du Cane Road, London W12 0NN*

MARIETTA CHARAKIDA, *Research Fellow, Vascular Physiology Unit, 30 Guilford Street, London WC1N 1EH*

OWAIS CHAUDHRI, *Clinical Research Fellow, Department of Metabolic Medicine, Imperial College, Hammersmith Hospital, Du Cane Road, London W12 0NN*

SRIJITA SEN-CHOWDHRY, *Research Fellow, The Heart Hospital, 16–18 Westmoreland Street, London W1G 8PH*

PAUL J CICLITIRA, *Professor of Gastroenterology, Department of Gastroenterology (GKT), The Rayne Institute, 4th Floor, Lambeth Wing, St Thomas' Hospital, London SE1 7EH*

JOHN E DEANFIELD, *Professor of Cardiology, Vascular Physiology Unit, Institute of Child Health, 30 Guilford Street, London WC1N 1EH*

MICHAEL DOHERTY, *Professor of Rheumatology, University of Nottingham, Academic Rheumatology, Clinical Sciences Building, City Hospital, Nottingham NG5 1PB*

PAUL DURRINGTON, *Professor of Medicine, University of Manchester, Division of Cardiovascular and Endocrine Science, Department of Medicine, Manchester Royal Infirmary, Oxford Road, Manchester M13 9WL*

FARIDA FORTUNE, *Professor of Medicine in Relation to Oral Health, Barts and the London Queen Mary's School of Medicine and Dentistry, University of London, Turner Street, London E1 2AD*

J SIMON R GIBBS, *Senior Lecturer in Cardiology, Imperial College London; Honorary Consultant Cardiologist, Department of Cardiology, Hammersmith Hospital, Du Cane Road, London W12 0HS*

PETER J GOADSBY, *Professor of Clinical Neurology, Headache Group, Institute of Neurology, University College London, Queen Square, London WC1N 3BG*

CHRISTOPHER EM GRIFFITHS, *Professor of Dermatology, Dermatology Centre, Irving Building, Hope Hospital, Salford, Manchester M6 8HD*

DORIAN HASKARD, *Professor of Rheumatology, Eric Bywaters Centre for Vascular Inflammation, British Heart Foundation Cardiovascular Medicine Unit, Imperial College, Hammersmith Campus, Du Cane Road, London W12 0NN*

JOHN HAWK, *Professor of Dermatological Photobiology, St John's Institute of Dermatology, St Thomas' Hospital, London SE1 7EH*

DAVID ISENBERG, *Professor of Rheumatology, Arthritis Research Campaign, Centre for Rheumatology, University College London, Arthur Stanley House, 40–50 Tottenham Street, London W1T 4NJ*

DAVID EJ JONES, *Professor of Liver Immunology, School of Clinical Medical Sciences, University of Newcastle, 4th Floor William Leech Building, Medical School, Framlington Place, Newcastle-upon-Tyne NE2 4HH*

ANDREW KEAT, *Consultant Physician, Arthritis Centre, Northwick Park Hospital, Watford Road, Harrow, Middlesex HA1 3UJ*

DAVID A LOMAS, *Professor of Respiratory Biology/Honorary Consultant Physician, Department of Medicine, University of Cambridge, Cambridge Institute for Medical Research, Wellcome Trust/MRC Building, Hills Road, Cambridge CB2 2XY*

LINDA M LUXON, *Professor of Audiological Medicine, Academic Unit of Audiological Medicine, Institute of Child Health, University College London, 30 Guilford Street, London WC1N 1EH; Consultant Physician in Neuro-otology, National Hospital for Neurology and Neurosurgery, Queen Square, London WC1N 3BG*

NIAMH M MARTIN, *Specialist Registrar in Diabetes and Endocrinology, Endocrine Unit, Hammermsith Hospital, Du Cane Road, London W12 0NN*

WILLIAM J MCKENNA, *Professor of Cardiology, University College London, The Heart Hospital, 16–18 Westmoreland Street, London W1G 8PH*

JOHN JV MCMURRAY, *Professor of Medical Cardiology, Department of Cardiology, Western Infirmary, Glasgow G11 6NT*

RACHEL J MIDDLETON, *Specialist Registrar in Nephrology, Department of Renal Medicine, Hope Hospital, Stott Lane, Salford M6 8HD*

DAVID H MILLER, *Professor of Clinical Neurology, Department of Neuroinflammation, Institute of Neurology, University College London, London WC1N 3BG*

NIKOLAI V NAOUMOV, *Reader in Hepatology/Honorary Consultant Physician, Institute of Hepatology, University College London, 69–75 Chenies Mews, London WC1E 6HX*

STEFAN NEUBAUER, *Professor of Cardiovascular Medicine, Clinical Director, University of Oxford Centre for Clinical Magnetic Resonance Research, Department of Cardiovascular Medicine, John Radcliffe Hospital ORH Trust, Headley Way, Oxford OX3 9DU*

JULIA L NEWTON, *Senior Lecturer in Cardiovascular Medicine, School of Clinical Medical Sciences, University of Newcastle, 4th Floor William Leech Building, Medical School, Framlington Place, Newcastle-upon-Tyne NE2 4HH*

PETROS NIHOYANNOPOULOS, *Consultant Cardiologist, Echocardiography, Hammersmith Hospital, Du Cane Road, London W12 0HS*

DONAL J O'DONOGHUE, *Consultant Nephrologist, Department of Renal Medicine, Hope Hospital, Stott Lane, Salford M6 8HD*

L PETER ORMEROD, *Professor of Respiratory Medicine, Consultant Chest Physician, Blackburn Royal Infirmary, Blackburn, Lancashire BB2 3LR; Lancashire Postgraduate School of Medicine and Health, University of Central Lancashire, Preston PR1 2HE*

DUNCAN PORTER, *Consultant Rheumatologist, Gartnavel General Hospital, 1053 Great Western Rd, Glasgow G12 0YN*

DOUGLAS S ROBINSON, *Reader and Honorary Consultant Physician, Departments of Allergy and Clinical Immunology and Leukocyte Biology, National Heart and Lung Institute, Faculty of Medicine, Imperial College London, Exhibition Road, London SW7 2AZ*

ANAND SAGGAR, *Consultant in Clinical Genetics, St George's Medical School, University of London, Cranmer Terrace, London SW17 0RE*

PAUL G SHIELS, *Senior Lecturer in Surgery, University of Glasgow, Division of Cancer, Sciences and Molecular Pathology, Dept. Surgery, Western Infirmary Glasgow, 44 Church St, Glasgow G11 6NT*

CLAIRE SHOVLIN, *Senior Lecturer, BHF Cardiovascular Medicine Unit, National Heart and Lung Institute, Imperial College, and Honorary Consultant in Respiratory Medicine, Hammersmith Hospital, Du Cane Road, London W12 0NN*

GAVIN SPICKETT, *Consultant Clinical Immunologist, Regional Department of Immunology, Royal Victoria Infirmary, Newcastle-upon-Tyne NE1 4LP*

RAJESH V THAKKER, *May Professor of Medicine, Academic Endocrine Unit, Nuffield Department of Clinical Medicine, Oxford Centre for Diabetes, Endocrinology and Metabolism (OCDEM), University of, Oxford, Churchill Hospital, Headington, Oxford OX3 7LJ*

JANE WARDLE, *Professor of Clinical Psychology, Director, Cancer Research UK, Health Behaviour Unit, Department of Epidemiology and Public Health, University College London, Gower Street, London WC1E 6BT*

ANTHONY N WARRENS, *Senior Lecturer and Honorary Consultant Physician in Renal Medicine and Immunology, Department of Immunology, Division of Medicine, Imperial College London, Hammersmith Hospital, Du Cane Road, London W12 0HS*

MICHAEL WILKS, *Chairman of Representative Body/Chairman of Medical Ethics Committee, Medical Ethics Department, British Medical Association, BMA House, Tavistock Square, London WC1H 9JP*

GRAHAM R WILLIAMS, *Professor of Endocrinology and Honorary Consultant Physician, Molecular Endocrinology Group, Division of Medicine and MRC Clinical Sciences Centre, Hammersmith Hospital, Du Cane Road, London W12 0NN*

KATIE WYNNE, *Clinical Research Fellow, Department of Metabolic Medicine, Imperial College, Hammersmith Hospital, Du Cane Road, London W12 0NN*

Contents

RHEUMATOLOGY

ENDOCRINOLOGY

TRANSPLANTATION

RENAL

The ear and the mouth in general medicine

Medicine of the ear

Linda M Luxon

□ INTRODUCTION

For doctors, the ear is dismissed as an unimportant organ buried deep in the temporal bone of the skull, which provides little relevant information about systemic disease. Indeed, disorders of the ear are considered to fall entirely within the domain of our surgical colleagues. Recent advances in genetics, public health, diagnostic techniques, the understanding of the pathophysiology of the auditory and vestibular system and therapeutics, however, has lead to a very significant change in the type and prevalence of hearing and balance disorders – most of which do not have a surgical solution. Thus, although the eye commonly is referred to as the 'window to the body' in disease, the ear perhaps should be considered a mirror that reflects a plethora of medical disorders. The importance of the ear to doctors lies in the prevalence and disability attributable to pathology in this organ.

The ear is unique in that it serves two sensory systems: hearing and balance. The membranous labyrinth is comprised anteriorly of the cochlea and posteriorly of the vestibular apparatus, which comprises two otolithic organs (the saccule and utricle) to sense linear acceleration and the cristae of the semicircular canals (which lie in each of the three planes of space) to sense angular acceleration (Fig 1). The anatomy of the cochlea and vestibular receptors are similar, with hair cells surmounted by a gelatinous mass, into which the hairs of the hair cells are embedded. Mechanical energy in the form of sound pressure waves or movement causes the hairs of the hair cells to bend, and this is the fundamental process by which energy is transduced into electrical activity within the central nervous system to provide auditory and vestibular information.

□ HEARING

Hearing loss is the most common sensory disability worldwide. The World Health Organization estimates that 250 million people worldwide have a disabling hearing impairment. In the United Kingdom, the National Study of Hearing identified that approximately 8.6 million (that is, 17% of the population) had significant hearing loss, while approximately 3 million have moderate loss and 150,000 profound hearing impairment.[1] In this latter group, 90% develop impaired hearing during adult life and the remaining 10% are born with profound loss of hearing. Identification of this latter group (one in 1,000 neonates) is important to ensure appropriate habilitation that allows optimal language development and

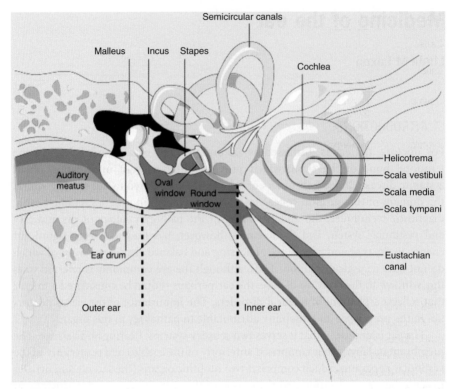

Fig 1 The ear.

occupational opportunities. In the United Kingdom, universal screening of neonatal hearing with transient otoacoustic emissions has been introduced as government policy to enable prompt and timely provision of family-friendly interventions.

During the last 50 years, the causes of hearing loss have been defined clearly (Table 1), although the prevalence of different disorders has changed dramatically as a result of improved public health and the introduction of antibiotic and vaccination programmes for infectious diseases such as rubella, mumps and measles, which prenatally or postnatally may cause significant hearing loss. Our understanding of the genetic factors, which underpin about half of all cases of congenital hearing loss, is increasing rapidly, with 50 loci for autosomal-recessive hearing loss and 54 loci for autosomal-dominant hearing loss now recognised, in addition to mitochondrial mutations and syndromic conditions, such as Waardenburg, Pendred and Jervell Lange-Neilson syndromes, with which hearing loss is associated.[2] Genetic advances are such that genetic engineering to alleviate hearing loss is now a realistic possibility.

Importantly, we now recognise that although a genetic predisposition to degeneration of the cochlea may exist, presbyacusis represents the accumulation of a number of toxic insults upon the cochlea over a lifetime.

In the developed world, prevention of hearing impairment has resulted in significantly fewer people being rendered profoundly deaf, and has altered the

Table 1 Causes of sensorineural hearing loss.

Cause	Type	Cause	Type
Genetic	Non-syndromal	Infection	Bacterial
	Syndromal		Viral
Trauma	Physical		Fungal
	Barotrauma	Iatrogenic	Drugs
	Acoustic trauma		Surgical
Vascular	Malformation		Organic chemicals
	Cardiovascular	Degenerative	Cochlear
	Cerebrovascular		Neuropathy
Autoimmune	Isolated inner ear		Neurological
	Systemic, eg systemic lupus erythematosus, Polyarteritis nodosa		

historical perspective of ear disease, characterised by a preponderance of chronic middle ear disease needing operative intervention.

Excessive noise that causes damage to the inner ear is controlled by legislation that places an obligation upon both employee and employer, limiting noise emissions and enforcing noise protection. Systemic disorders, such as diabetes and vascular disease, are treated routinely, thus limiting auditory and vestibular involvement. Ototoxic drugs are available only on prescription, and, therefore, the aminoglycosides cannot be given indiscriminantly to babies and young children with trivial infections – a common problem in the developing world. Indeed, in the developing world, large numbers of children and young people become deaf unnecessarily. The World Health Organization has established an active hearing intervention programme to try to solve the low priority of prevention or mitigation of hearing impairment in national and international political agendas. Interestingly, despite improvements in the developed world, ear disease remains an area poorly represented in terms of research activity. A study conducted by the Royal National Institute of the Deaf showed the number of Medline articles published between the beginning of 1995 and the middle of 2000 were threefold less for ear disease than eye disease and some 10-fold less than for cardiovascular disease (King A, personal communication, 2000).

□ BALANCE

Humans have developed a very sophisticated mechanism for maintaining balance, which relies on vision, proprioception and vestibular signals. These sensory inputs pass into the central nervous system, where they are integrated and modulated with activity from the cerebellum, pyramidal system, reticular formation and cerebral cortex to provide mechanisms to control eye movement, the vestibulo-ocular reflex, and posture and gait through the vestibulo-spinal reflexes and to enable perception of motion (Fig 2).

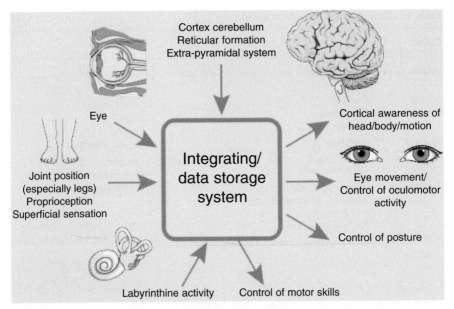

Cortex cerebellum
Reticular formation
Extra-pyramidal system

Eye

Cortical awareness of
head/body/motion

Joint position
(especially legs)
Proprioception
Superficial sensation

Integrating/
data storage
system

Eye movement/
Control of oculomotor
activity

Control of posture

Labyrinthine activity   Control of motor skills

Fig 2 Mechanism for maintaining balance in man.

Not surprisingly, pathology in many different systems of the body may affect balance (Table 2).[3] Patients may present in a range of medical and surgical clinics, including general medicine, cardiology, renal medicine, endocrinology, ophthalmology, geriatrics, neurology, haematology, rheumatology, orthopaedics and psychological medicine. Most doctors confronted with a dizzy patient feel a sense of despair, partly because of the plethora of conditions that may give rise to this symptom and partly because they do not have a simple diagnostic strategy with which to approach the patient. In this context, an understanding of the mechanisms of vertigo and dizziness is helpful.

Mechanisms of vertigo

Medical

The vestibular nuclei are supplied by penetrating branches of the anterior inferior cerebellar artery, which arises from the vertebrobasilar system. The labyrinth is supplied by an end artery that arises from the same system. The blood supply to the vestibular system thus may be compromised in the tiny penetrating vessels of the brainstem or in the labyrinthine artery, anterior inferior cerebellar artery, basilar artery or vertebral artery. The vestibular nuclei occupy an area within the lateral zone of the brainstem that is the area most likely to be affected by a reduction of blood flow in the main basilar artery. Not surprisingly, therefore, presyncope – that is, diffuse cerebral ischemia associated with hypotension or cardiac dysrhythmias – may well present with dizziness.

Hypoglycaemia may occur in patients with poor diabetic control, insulinoma or elevated catecholamines and may precipitate dizziness. Many drugs may produce

Table 2 Causes of balance disorder. Reproduced from Ref 3 with permission of John Wiley and Sons Ltd.

Body system	Example
GENERAL MEDICAL	
Haematological	Anaemia
	Hyperviscosity
	Miscellaneous
Cardiovascular	Postural hypotension
	Carotid sinus syndrome
	Dysrhythmias, eg sick sinus syndrome and mitral leaflet prolapse syndrome
	Mechanical dysfunction, eg ventricular hypokinesis and aortic stenosis
Metabolic	Hypoglycaemia
	Hyperventilation
NEUROLOGICAL	
Supratentorial	Epilepsy
	Syncope
	Psychogenic
Infratentorial	Multiple sclerosis
	Vertebro-basilar insufficiency,
	eg subclavian steal syndrome, Wallenberg's syndrome, anterior inferior cerebellar artery syndrome
	Infective disorders,
	eg Ramsay Hunt, neurosyphilis, tuberculosis
	Degenerative disorders, including neuropathy
	Tumours, including acoustic neuroma
	Foramen magnum abnormalities
OTOLOGICAL	Menière's syndrome
	Post-traumatic syndrome
	Positional nystagmus
	Vestibular neuronitis
	Infection
	Otosclerosis and Paget's disease
	Vascular accidents
	Tumours
	Autoimmune disorders
	Drug intoxication
MISCELLANEOUS	
Ocular or visual	
Orthopaedic, including cervical	
Multisensory dizziness syndrome	

dizziness through a variety of mechanisms, including depression of the central nervous system, cardiovascular effects, cerebellar toxicity, changes in the specific gravity of the cupula and ototoxicity.

Vestibular

'Vertigo' (an illusion of movement) is the result of asymmetrical vestibular input. Stimulation of the vestibular apparatus – for example, on a roundabout – gives rise to physiological vertigo. Under normal circumstances, the identical vestibular receptors in each labyrinth – for example, the cristae of the horizontal semicircular canals – are paired in the upright resting position. Equal neural activity is generated spontaneously from each labyrinth and passes into the central nervous system, where it is 'monitored'. When the head turns to the right in the horizontal plane, an increase in activity occurs in the right horizontal canal with a concomitant decrease in activity in the left horizontal canal. This asymmetry of information provides the stimulus for a corrective eye movement through the vestibulo-ocular reflex and appropriate adjustment of the neck and limb muscles maintains balance and a perception of motion to the right. Conversely, if the head turns to the left, an increase in activity occurs in the left horizontal semicircular canal, with a decrease in activity in the right semi-circular canal. Thus, asymmetry of neural information provides the stimulus for vestibular activity.

If pathology alters vestibular input on one side, such that an imbalance in tonic vestibular signals is generated, this is perceived as motion – that is, vertigo – and often is accompanied by the clinical signs of nystagmus generated by the vestibulo-ocular reflex and a tendency to veer to the affected side as a result of vestibulo-spinal inputs. In older patients, two or more of the sensory inputs for balance may be impaired; although the brain can compensate for such changes by means of cerebral plasticity in a young adult, increasing age and increasing dysfunction in both sensory systems, together with a reduction in integrating and modulating cerebral activity, makes efficient adaptation and compensation less likely. Older patients with cataracts, arthritis and mild vestibular dysfunction thus constantly may feel disorientated; this is known as the multisensory dizziness syndrome.

Vertigo also may be the result of a mismatch of visual and vestibular signals. A common example is an older patient who wears bifocal glasses and thus alters their visual input as a result of altering focal distance, which makes them feel disorientated. Many young people with a peripheral vestibular deficit will feel extremely disorientated by movement in the visual surround[4] – perhaps more markedly than by physical movement of the head or body. This situation is explained by the mismatch hypothesis of vertigo.[5] Voluntary movement generates vestibular visual and proprioceptive inputs, but, simultaneously, the brain activates a databank of 'expected' signals that have been learned over many years of carrying out similar movements. When the 'expected' sensory inputs match the received afferent inputs, balance is subconscious, and the appropriate perception of motion (the corrective generation of eye and body movements) occurs. However, when a mismatch occurs – for example, the visual signal does not match with the expected vestibular and proprioceptive signal, a mismatch of sensory information gives rise to a perception of disorienetation and disequilibrium (Fig 3).

Neurological causation

The final group of mechanisms of dizziness and vertigo is associated with neurological disorders. Psychophysiological dysfunction occurs when central integration of the sensory inputs required for balance is impaired, as may happen in

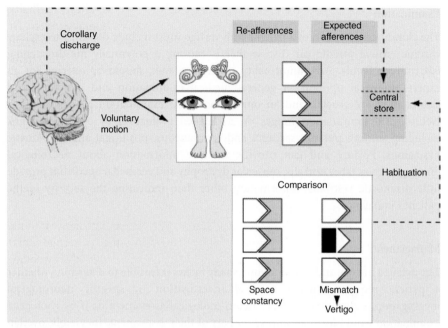

Fig 3 Mismatch hypothesis. Reproduced from Ref 5 with permission of Springer Science and Business Media.

aged brains or in patients with diffused cerebrovascular disease. Dysequilibrium and ataxia in association with disorientation are seen commonly in patients with loss of neurological functions, such as loss of vibration sense, proprioceptive sense, cerebellar function or motor function.

☐ DIAGNOSTIC STRATEGY

History

A detailed clinical history, as in every branch of medicine, is crucial to the diagnosis of vertigo, but three specific areas of questioning frequently are invaluable in establishing a neurological diagnosis. The *character* of the symptom is helpful. Dizziness is a lay term applied to any sense of disorientation and is common in many general conditions, while vertigo implies a specific sense of motion that is not generated by an external stimulus and is a cardinal symptom of disordered vestibular function. In addition, *the time course* of the illness, together with the duration of episodes of vertigo and interval symptoms, is the key to differential diagnosis. Finally, temporally related *associated symptoms* are important. The auditory and vestibular systems are related intimately in the labyrinth and eighth nerve, so specific questioning should include cochlear symptoms that may be overlooked, particularly by older patients who expect to get hard of hearing as they become older. Cardiovascular and neurological symptoms also are of great diagnostic importance.

Examination

The clinical examination of a patient with vertigo must include otoscopy to exclude chronic erosive middle ear disease that is causing a potentially life-threatening labyrinthine fistula. Any abnormality, other than wax, should be referred for an expert otological opinion. A general medical examination and a neurological examination are crucial, and an ophthalmological examination also is of value. Neurological examination hinges on a detailed evaluation of eye movements, including smooth pursuit, saccades and spontaneous, positional and optokinetic nystagmus. Posture and gait provide valuable information about neurological diseases, such as tabes dorsalis, muscular dystrophy and cerebellar ataxia but provide little diagnostic vestibular information other than indicating the severity of the patient's imbalance.

Management

The detailed history and examination usually makes it feasible to determine whether a patient requires further medical investigation or specific neurological investigation, rather than primary neuro-otological assessment or if psychological examination would form an important part of their assessment. Inevitably, overlap exists between these three groups of patients, as patients with diabetes mellitus, cardiovascular disease or autoimmune disorders may have systemic pathology while also experiencing neuro-otological symptoms. Similarly, many neurological conditions involve the labyrinth and may need auditory and vestibular management in addition to neurological management.[6]

As a general rule, patients with acute vertigo that has not improved substantially within six weeks or who present with other neurological symptoms and signs need specialist referral for diagnosis and appropriate management.

Most patients with vestibular disorders will fall into two groups:

- □ patients with a specific diagnosis that needs medical treatment, such as Menière's disease, or surgical treatment, such as vestibular schwannoma

- □ patients with no clear aetiological diagnosis but whose standard vestibular tests show evidence of a peripheral vestibular disorder. In these patients, acute vertigo needs treatment with reassurance, antiemetics and vestibular sedatives, although these latter drugs should be discontinued as soon as possible to ensure optimal vestibular compensation in the long term.

A group of patients with peripheral labyrinthine disease, however, present with chronic vertigo that may be constant or recurrent as a result of failure of vestibular compensation, which is dependent upon cerebral plasticity (Fig 4).[7] These patients require management with rehabilitation physiotherapy and, not infrequently, psychological support. Vestibular sedatives are contraindicated as they delay vestibular compensation. A small proportion of these patients will fail medical management and may need surgical intervention with therapeutic or destructive procedures.

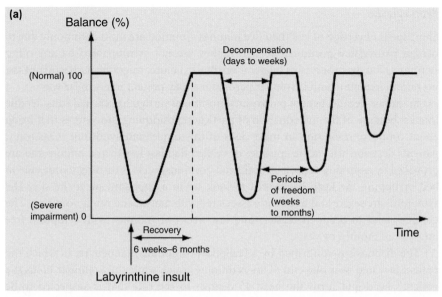

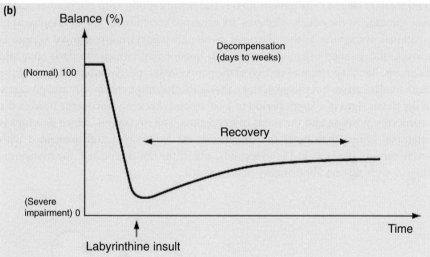

Fig 4 Diagrammatic representation of patients with peripheral vestibular pathology and recurrent decompensation (a) and failure of compensation (b). Reproduced from Ref 7 with permission of John Wiley and Sons Ltd.

Common causes of vertigo

In a tertiary balance clinic, about one quarter of patients have no vestibular abnormality, as their dizziness is due to non-vestibular mechanisms. About three quarters of patients have a vestibular disorder, however, with the most common cases being the result of uncompensated peripheral vestibular disorder secondary to viral infection (vestibular neuritis), ischaemia, trauma, migraine and benign paroxysmal positional vertigo. Duration of the symptoms provides a helpful diagnostic classification.

Short episodes

Short spells of vertigo of less than five minutes' duration are most commonly due to benign paroxysmal positional vertigo if they are not accompanied by any other symptom. Rarely, progressive bilateral vestibular failure, migraine, ischaemia of the posterior circulation and vestibular paroxysmia may present in a similar way.

In the last decade, benign paroxysmal positional vertigo has excited considerable interest because of the introduction of particle repositioning procedures that bring about complete resolution in most cases of this unpleasant syndrome. Classically, patients describe brief acute episodes of vertigo that last less than a minute and are provoked by assuming certain critical head positions, such as turning to one side in bed or tipping the head backwards to look up in a cupboard or at the sky. The symptoms are severe and frequently associated with nausea and rarely vomiting. The episodes tend to occur in clusters and last weeks or months, with symptom-free intervals of months or years.

The diagnosis is confirmed by a Hallpike positioning manoeuvre, in which the patient is seated near one end of an examining couch while the examiner holds the patient's head and turns the head 45 degrees to the side that is suspected to be symptomatic (Fig 5). The patient then is laid down rapidly, with the head extended over the edge of the couch. The eyes are observed carefully for the development of positional nystagmus. If the diagnosis of benign paroxysmal positional vertigo is correct, the patient often will resist this manoeuvre, which in itself may aid diagnosis. Benign positional vertigo of the paroxysmal type may affect all three of the semicircular canals, but the posterior canal is affected most commonly and gives rise to the classic signs of a latent period of 2–20 seconds between placing the head in the provocative position and the onset of nystagmus. The nystagmus, which develops is rotational, directed towards the undermost ear (geotropic) and associated with severe vertigo. It adapts in 15–60 seconds, and, if the test is repeated, the nystagmus fatigues such that no abnormality may be noted.

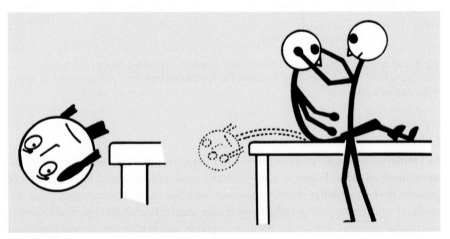

Fig 5 Hallpike test for positional nystagmus.

A variety of different nystagmic characteristics may be observed on positioning the patient in the Hallpike manoeuvre (Table 3). If the characteristic signs of benign paroxysmal positional vertigo are not identified, the patient should be investigated for neurological disease, as the examiner may be observing central positional nystagmus.

Table 3 Characteristics of positional nystagmus.

Characteristic	Benign paroxysmal positional vertigo	Central type nystagmus
Latent period	2–20 seconds	None
Adaptation	Disappears in 50 seconds	Persists
Fatigability	Disappears on repetition	Persists
Vertigo and nausea	Always present and commonly severe	Typically absent
Direction of nystagmus	Geotropic	Variable

Canalithiasis is the pathophysiological mechanism that now has gained widespread acceptance as the theory that best explains the characteristic features of benign paroxysmal positional vertigo. This theory proposes that calcium carbonate crystal debris from the otolith organ forms in the most dependent portion of the posterior semicircular canal. When the patient assumes the critical head position, the clot moves in an ampullofugal direction and has a 'plunger effect' in the narrow posterior semicircular canal. This causes deflection of the cupula and bending of the hairs of the hair cells, with a brief resulting paroxysm of vertigo and nystagmus. The rationale behind the Epley and Semont particle repositioning procedures is that a specific sequence of head movements brings about clearance of the debris, under gravity, from the most dependent part of the semicircular canal into the body of the vestibule. There, the debris no longer interferes with the dynamics of the semicircular canal and the patient is rendered asymptomatic. Most reports in the literature present a cure rate of 70–90% for all particle repositioning procedures, although the condition may recur.

Moderate duration episodes

Episodes of vertigo of less than 24 hours' duration most commonly are the result of migraine, if no associated cochlear symptoms are present, or Menière's disease, if the vertigo is accompanied by hearing loss, aural pressure or fullness and tinnitus.

Migraine is a very common cause of vertigo in specialist clinics, although it frequently is misdiagnosed.[8] Migraine is a clinical diagnosis made on the basis of a number of features. Diagnostic criteria published by the International Headache Society[9] in 1988 classified migraine as:

☐ migraine without aura (formerly known as common migraine);

☐ migraine with aura (formerly known as classic migraine).

Vertigo may occur with both forms of migraine and may assume different presentations, with momentary spells of dizziness, acute episodes of dizziness lasting hours and prolonged instability. The diagnosis is made on the basis of a previous history of migrainous headache or a family history, or both; the presence of space or motion discomfort; frequent presence of phonophobia or photophobia, or both; and rarely fluctuating hearing loss. Commonly, vertigo is associated with nausea and vomiting and the patient may feel tired and frequently is much improved after sleep.[10] The seminal work of Kayan and Hood in 1984 showed that vestibular symptoms and vertigo were significantly more common in patients with migraine than tension headaches.[11] Interestingly, from a neurological perspective, patients with migrainous vertigo commonly show no abnormality on standard vestibular testing despite the severity of their symptoms, whereas patients with vertigo not associated with migraine almost always (94%) show evidence of a peripheral vestibular disorder.[12]

Anti-migrainous prophylaxis is effective for migrainous vertigo and, in cases of diagnostic uncertainty, may constitute a therapeutic trial. Propranolol and pizotofen are the two drugs most commonly used for this condition.

Prolonged episodes

Prolonged episodes of vertigo that last more than 24 hours, with no accompanying symptoms most commonly result from failure of compensation or decompensation from a peripheral vestibular disorder.

Any pathology that affects the labyrinth – for example, viral labyrinthitus, ischaemia, trauma or inflammation – may damage the hair cells of the sensory vestibular epithelium, giving rise to a peripheral vestibular disorder. This may be identified by vestibular tests such as the caloric test or rotation testing. Acute impairment of the vestibular components of the labyrinth gives rise to vertigo, spontaneous vestibular nystagmus directed away from the affected ear and ataxia. In most cases, symptoms abate and the patient becomes asymptomatic without intervention – usually over a period of three or four weeks to several months (Fig 6). The processes that bring about resolution of vestibular symptoms collectively are known as cerebral compensation. They are attributable to cerebral plasticity, in which sensory inputs, vision, proprioception and residual labyrinthine function facilitate recalibration of the dynamic vestibular reflexes to ensure symmetrical compensatory vestibulo-spinal and vestibulo-ocular reflex action during head and body movements and substitution of sensory inputs (vision and proprioception) and motor response strategies.

Although most patients in the community with acute peripheral vestibular pathology recover spontaneously, as many as 50% of patients who present in the tertiary care setting do not recover fully or initially compensate and then 'decompensate'. There are many causes of decompensation (Fig 7); the most common include psychological dysfunction (which is a common correlate of vestibular disorders), impaired neurological function, impaired sensory inputs or fluctuating vestibular activity (it is not possible to compensate for a changing level of vestibular dysfunction). Moreover, any physical or psychological stress factor may

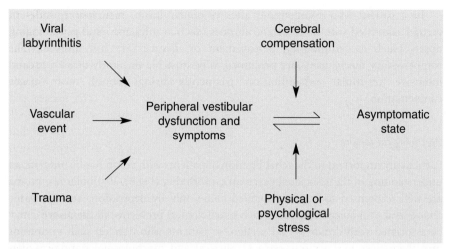

Fig 6 Natural history of peripheral vestibular disorder. Reproduced from Ref 7 with permission of John Wiley and Sons Ltd.

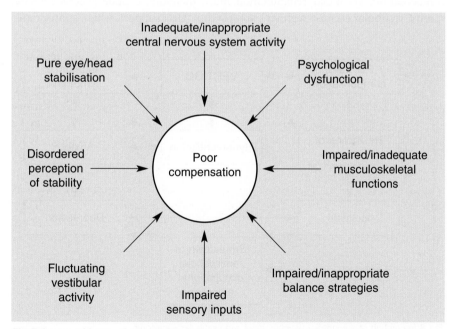

Fig 7 Causes of failure of compensation. Reproduced from Ref 7 with permission of John Wiley and Sons Ltd.

lead to decompensation.[7] An understanding of vestibular compensation, however, is crucial to ensure appropriate vestibular rehabilitation, which depends on repeated stimulation of the sensory inputs and motor activity required for balance to facilitate the compensatory mechanisms that are dependent on the cerebellum and inferior olive.

In a patient who compensates after vestibular insult, recurrent episodes of vertigo associated with intercurrent illnesses (such as influenza) and psychological upsets (such as redundancy, bereavement or divorce) are not unusual. The compensatory mechanisms are presumed to be unstable or poorly developed, and intensive vestibular rehabilitation frequently brings about more stable compensation.

Psychological factors

Particularly important in the rehabilitation of patients with vestibular disorders is an understanding of the associated psychiatric morbidity (Fig 8). Vestibular symptoms are well recognised to be accompanied commonly by depression, anxiety, panic attacks and avoidance behaviour. Such psychological problems, in themselves, may be associated with dizziness and vertigo, so patients who develop such symptoms find themselves in a vicious cycle of physical and psychological symptoms that compound each other.[13] This leads to a reduction in social- and work-related activity, with a reduction in motor activity and a concomitant failure of compensation. Vestibular rehabilitation must, therefore, include general exercise, specific vestibular exercise regimens and psychological support, where appropriate.

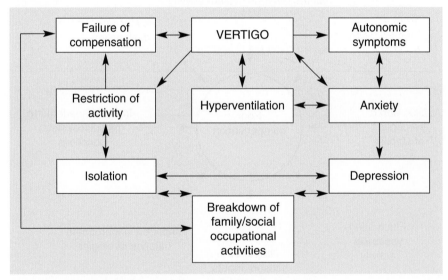

Fig 8 Interaction of autonomic, psychological and vestibular symptoms.

☐ CONCLUSION

Hearing and balance disorders are common in the population and often present at the primary care level and in the tertiary care setting. Patients may present across a range of different disciplines, and a broad diagnostic strategy is needed if the doctor is to establish the correct diagnosis and institute an appropriate and effective management strategy. Although auditory and vestibular pathologies rarely are associated with significant mortality, they do carry a very significant personal, occupational and economic morbidity. Treatment of such disorders is highly effective, so every doctor should have an understanding of these common and debilitating symptoms.

REFERENCES

1 Davis A. *Hearing in adults.* London: Whurr Publishers, 1995.

2 Van Camp G, Smith RJH. *Hereditary hearing loss homepage.* http://dnalab-www.uia.ac.be/dnalab/hhh/ (last accessed 11 Aug 2005).

3 Luxon LM. Balance disorders. In: Kerr AG, ed. *Adult audiology. Scott-Browne's otolaryngology.* London: Butterworths, 1997.

4 Bronstein AM. Vision and vertigo: some visual aspects of vestibular disorders. *J Neurol* 2004;**251**:381–7.

5 Brandt T. *Vertigo: its multisensory syndromes.* London: Springer-Verlag, 1999.

6 Luxon LM. Evaluation and management of the dizzy patient. *J Neurol Neurosurg Psychiatry* 2004;**75**:iv45–52.

7 Luxon, LM. Vestibular compensation. In: Luxon LM, Davies RA, eds. *Handbook of vestibular rehabilitation.* London: Whurr Publishers, 1997:17–29.

8 Davies RA. Disorders of balance. In: Luxon LM, Davies RA, eds. *Handbook of vestibular rehabilitation.* London: Whurr Publishers, 1997:30–40.

9 Stewart J, Tepper MD, Afridi SK, Kaube H *et al.* International classification of headache disorders II. *Cephalalgia* 1988;**8**(Suppl 7):1–96.

10 Neuhauser H, Lempert T. Vertigo and dizziness related to migraine: a diagnostic challenge. *Cephalalgia* 2004;**24**:83–91.

11 Kayan A, Hood JD. Neuro-otological manifestations of migraine. *Brain* 1984;**107**:1123–42.

12 Savundra PA, Carroll JD, Davies RA, Luxon LM. Migraine-associated vertigo. *Cephalalgia* 1997;**17**:505–10.

13 Furman JM, Jacob RG. A clinical taxonomy of dizziness and anxiety in the otoneurological setting. *J Anxiety Disord* 2001;**15**:9–26.

The mouth

Farida Fortune

Oral medicine includes the medical management of diseases specific to the orofacial tissues and oral manifestations of systemic disease.[1]

The mouth may be the first place or major site of systemic disease. Unless a patient volunteers information about oral symptoms, doctors frequently forget to elicit this important diagnostic feature. Similarly, the mouth usually is examined by asking the patient to say 'aah', with only a fragmentary view of the tongue, palate or uvula visualised and none of the information processed consciously.

Examination of the mouth is crucial if a correct diagnosis of an oral lesion is to be made. Extraoral examination of the head and neck, as well as a careful intraoral examination should be made. A mouth map may prove useful for descriptive diagrammatic location of a lesion (Fig 1). The hard and soft tissues should be examined. The whole of the intraoral region should be visualised, including the hard and soft palate, buccal mucosae, tongue (dorsal and ventral surface) and floor of the mouth. Intraoral and extraoral examination of all the salivary glands should be undertaken.

The mouth may be the site of disease or disorders localised to the mouth or systemic disease. Careful examination may help differentiate between systemic or localised disease or help to confirm a diagnosis of a systemic problem, but it equally may help difficult diagnostic problems – for example, the diagnosis of ulcerative colitis and Crohn's disease may sometimes be difficult, but oral lesions are very distinct. Equally, clinical features in the mouth (such as oral ulcerations, which occur in 15–20% of the population) may be an indication of underlying systemic disease in which all systems may be affected. Some causes are:

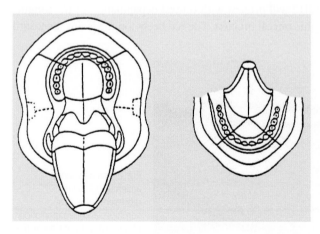

Fig 1 Mouth map. The map or the inside of the mouth helps with the methodical examination and is a useful guide for cataloguing areas that show signs of local oral disease or systemic disorders.

- [ ] haematological disorders

- [ ] infection

- [ ] gastrointestinal disorders

- [ ] respiratory disorders

- [ ] immune-related disorders.

Examples of common and unusual presentations are given below. This is not an exhaustive list, as all systemic diseases may produce oral lesions. Some lesions are seen easily on careful examination, while other lesions are less apparent to the untrained eye.

☐ BLOOD

The mouth is a common site for early signs of haematological disorders:

- [ ] anaemia

- [ ] leukaemia

- [ ] nutritional deficiencies, including deficiencies of iron, vitamin B12 or zinc.

Iron-deficiency anaemia usually presents as an early sign in the mouth. Iron is stored in cytochrome oxidase in the filiform papillae of the tongue; this is a non-essential store, and deficiency results in depapillation and glossitis. It usually is seen in young women in the early years of menstruation or in women with menorrhagia. Glossitis increasingly is becoming common in young menstruating women on 'faddish' diets (Fig 2). The smooth tongue is seen very late, after years of clinical deficiency. When a smooth tongue is apparent, koilinychia and oesophageal web formation are also present.

Deficiency of vitamin B12 will present with central depapillation of the tongue, angular cheilitis and atrophic buccal mucosa. The red beefy tongue is not seen until

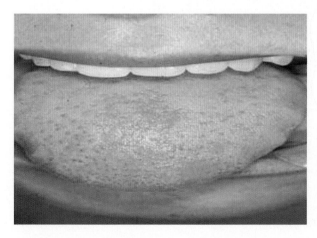

Fig 2 Iron-deficiency anaemia: glossitis represented by oral soreness and depapillation of the filliform papillae at the tip and lateral borders of the tongue. This is the earliest sign of low iron stores.

late and usually is associated with a glove and stocking peripheral neuropathy. Deficiency of zinc gives a railroad pattern of depapillation, with a painful glossitis (Fig 3).

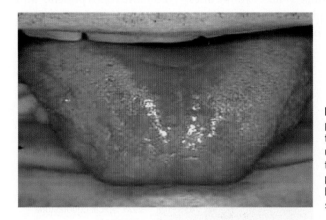

Fig 3 Deficiency of zinc: the patient presented with sore tongue non-healing intra-oral ulcers. The appearance of the tongue shown in this photograph is typical of very low levels of zinc in the serum.

Leukaemia commonly presents early in the mouth. The low levels of haemoglobin result in oral pallor, low platelet counts result in mucosal petechiae or excessive bleeding on toothbrushing (occasionally there may be frank gingival bleeding) and abnormal white cell counts may cause oral infection such as *Candida* (Fig 4).

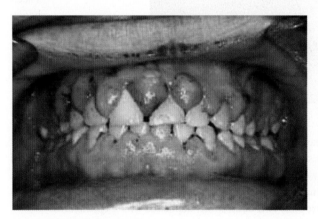

Fig 4 Acute myelomonocytic leukaemia. Typical gingival infiltration with leukaemic cells. The pallor of the mucosa and spontaneous bleeding distinguishes the aetio-pathology from other causes of gingival enlargement, such as calcium-channel blocker or phenytoin drug enlargement.

☐ GUT

Gut disease almost always involves the orofacial region, with the mouth being the area frequently affected. Crohn's disease, ulcerative colitis and coeliac disease easily are differentiated from each other by their distinct characteristics in the mouth.

Careful examination of the mouth may help when it is uncertain whether the patient has Crohn's disease or ulcerative colitis, as the oral changes are characteristic for the individual conditions. Crohn's disease presents with mucosal tag 'cobblestoning' in addition to oral ulcers (Fig 5). Facial swelling results from intra-oral mucosal lesions that extend from the mucosal surface to the skin on the face and may be mistaken for staphylococcal peri-oral infection. Deep biopsy is needed to show the characteristic granuloma. Unlike Crohn's disease, ulcerative colitis presents with persistent deep 'major aphthae' type ulcerations that may occur bilaterally on the lateral surface for up to six weeks at a time (Fig 6).

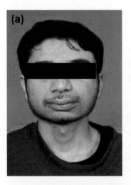 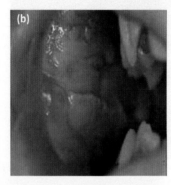

Fig 5 Crohn's disease: (a) facial rash that results from mucosal lesions that extend from the mucosal surface to the external surface of the skin and (b) mucosal lesions show typical cobblestone appearance.

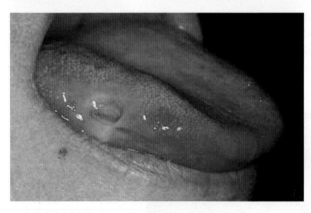

Fig 6 Ulcerative colitis. Bilateral deep persistent ulcers of the tongue – usually present when gut lesions are active.

Lesions in coeliac disease may mimic ulcerative lichen planus or widespread minor aphthous ulcers or have a similar appearance to dermatitis herpetiformis (vesicles and papules on an erythematous base on the tongue, buccal mucosa or palate) (Fig 7). Biopsy that mimics dermatitis herpetiformis will show sub-epithelial vesicles with immunoglobulin A, neutrophils and oesinophils deposited in the epithelium.

☐ LUNGS AND SALIVARY GLANDS

Enlargement of the two submandibular glands, as well as the parotid glands, may be a feature of systemic disease that involves the lungs. Bilateral enlargement of the submandibular glands is an indication to X-ray the lungs in patients with fever or malaise (Fig 8). These glands, along with the lachrymal glands, show increased uptake during gallium scanning of patients with sarcoidosis. Churg-Strauss disease may present in a patient with a history of asthma and recurrent swelling of all or

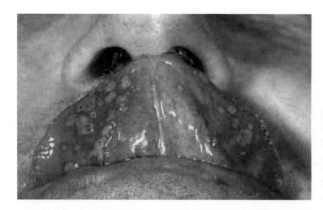

Fig 7 Coeliac disease: this case presented with widespread herpetiform aphthous ulceration non-responsive to local treatment but responsive to a gluten-free diet.

individual salivary glands (Fig 9). Patients frequently have one of the submandibular glands removed before diagnosis. The salivary gland tissues swell secondary to infiltration with oesinophils. Heerfordt-Waldenstrom syndrome is associated with enlarged parotids, fever, anterior uveitis and facial nerve palsy.

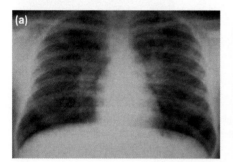
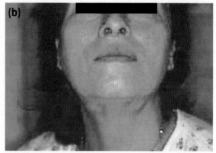

Fig 8 Sarcoidosis: patient presented with intermittent jaundice and enlarged submandibular glands. (a) chest X-ray showing hilar lymphadenopathy and (b) enlarged submandibular glands.

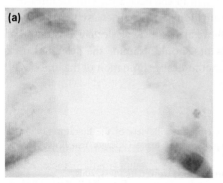
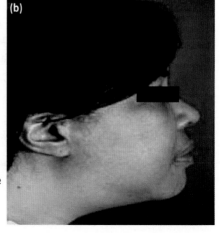

Fig 9 Churg-Strauss disease. (a) 'White out' of the lung with eosinophilic infiltration and (b) enlarged salivary glands and facial tissues with similar eosinophilic infiltration in the same patient.

☐ INFECTION

Infection invariably affects the mouth (Fig 10). Exanthema in childhood almost without exception includes generalised erythema in the mouth. Other infective processes may present with symptoms such as dry or burning mouth or signs of ulceration with or without pain and swelling, keratosis or pigmentation.

Tuberculosis is an increasing clinical problem, and the oral signs seem to have been forgotten or the mouth not examined. Patients often are admitted onto open wards, with persistent ulceration, weight loss and night sweats, with a presumptive diagnosis of oral malignancy.

A similar array of lesions occurs with HIV. New cases not infrequently present with oral lesions as their first presentation of HIV or AIDS. In sub-Saharan Africa, children with oral lesions who are already malnourished are unable to feed because of candidosis, which may be pseudomembranous or erythematous *Candida* and often is not diagnosed (even by local doctors).

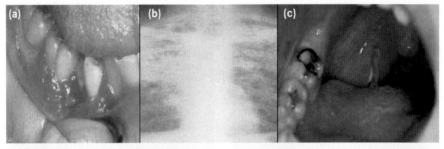

Fig 10 Tuberculosis, oral ulcers: (a) deep non-healing oral ulcer, (b) chest X-ray showing apical lesion typical of tuberculosis, (c) faucal ulcer presenting as a painful, vertically deep ulcer filled with slough.

☐ CONCLUSION

Almost all disease processes can manifest in the head and neck area, with the intra-oral cavity showing signs relating to most nutritional deficiencies, systemic disease processes and drug induced lesions.[2] The above article gives a selective illustration of oral manifestation of systemic disease. Doctors should examine the head and neck area of all patients carefully and perform a methodical examination of the oral cavity.

REFERENCES

1   Eversole LR. Diseases of the oral mucous membranes. Review of the literature 1998. In: Millard HD, Mason DK, eds. *World workshop on oral medicine.* Chicago: Year Book Medical Publishers, 1989.

2   Fortune F. *Human disease for dentistry.* Oxford: Oxford University Press, 2004.

☐ THE EAR IN GENERAL MEDICINE SELF ASSESSMENT QUESTIONS

Ear

1   Hearing loss is:
    (a) The most common sensory disability
    (b) Characterised by gradual social withdrawal
    (c) Usually of a conductive type
    (d) Frequently multifactorial in aetiology in older people
    (e) Most commonly genetic in origin in infancy

2   Vertigo is often the result of:
    (a) Movement of the visual surround
    (b) Migraine
    (c) Acoustic neurinoma
    (d) Vertebrobasilar ischaemia
    (e) Benign positional vertigo

3   Benign positional paroxysmal vertigo is:
    (a) More common in older people
    (b) Often the result of head trauma
    (c) Commonly associated with vomiting
    (d) Improved in 80–90% of people by a single manoeuvre
    (e) Associated with neurological disease

4   Vertigo may be consequent upon:
    (a) Cardiovascular drugs
    (b) Hypoglycaemia
    (c) Myxoedema
    (d) Cerebellar haemorrhage
    (e) Bifocal glasses

Gastroenterology

Coeliac disease

Paul J Ciclitira

☐ INTRODUCTION

Coeliac disease is an acquired permanent enteropathy that is induced by the gluten contained within wheat, rye, barley and possibly oats. The pathological abnormalities are characterised by a flattened small intestinal mucosa with a lymphocytic infiltrate and by increased epithelial cell proliferation. This results in impaired absorptive function. Dermatitis herpetiformis is a related skin condition, in which there is an itchy, blistering skin eruption, which frequently affects the knees, elbows, buttocks and back, with deposition of granular immunoglobulin A (IgA) at the dermoepidermal junction. The latter also affects areas not involved with the rash. Most patients with dermatitis herpetiformis have a small intestinal enteropathy that improves on gluten withdrawal.

Areataeus the Cappadocian described coeliac disease in the second century AD: 'If the diarrhoea does not proceed from a slight cause of only one or two days' duration and if, in addition, the patient's general symptoms be debilitated by atrophy of the body the coeliac disease of a chronic nature is formed'. Aretaeus thought that the illness affected only adults. In 1887, Samuel Gee described the condition as we know it, when he noted that the disease affected people of all ages. He thought that 'to regulate the food was the main part of the treatment'. He reported on one child who was fed daily on a quart of the best Dutch mussels and 'throve wonderfully' but relapsed when the season for mussels was over.

In 1924, Haas described a treatment for coeliac disease. After the successful treatment of anorexia nervosa with a banana diet, he thought it logical to try this diet in children with coeliac disease and anorexia. This dietary treatment of coeliac disease continued well into the 1950s. Dicke – a Dutch paediatrician – observed that coeliac sprue diminished remarkably during the period of scarcity during the Second World War. After Swedish planes dropped bread into the Netherlands, however, children with coeliac disease relapsed rapidly.[1]

In 1954, Paulley *et al* reported the histology of coeliac jejunal mucosa obtained operatively at the time of partial gastrectomy. Shiner and Royer independently developed methods for biopsying the duodenum; Crosby then recognised the need for a more flexible instrument.[2]

☐ EPIDEMIOLOGY

Coeliac disease is thought to be a disorder of northern Europe and those countries to which Europeans have emigrated. Although the condition previously was thought to affect only one in 2,000 people of these populations, it now is known to affect about one in 100 people. Several studies suggest that the female to male ratio is 2:1, but the sexes are affected more equally in other series.

Patients with coeliac disease have increased mortality compared with the general population. Before the introduction of a gluten-free diet, mortality was reported to be 10–30%, but recent data show a mortality of 0.4%, with these deaths predominantly resulting from increased prevalence of lymphoma in the small intestine.[3]

☐ PATHOLOGY

The disease affects the mucosa of the proximal small intestine, with damage gradually decreasing in severity towards the distal small intestine. In severe cases, however, the lesions extend to the ileum. Abnormalities of the rectal mucosa also may be seen in severe cases.

Examination of the jejunal mucosa with a dissecting microscope shows abnormalities. In patients with untreated coeliac disease, the duodenal and jejunal mucosa may be flat, often with a mosaic pattern caused by intersection of deep depressions and elevated mounds, between which are crypts. The characteristic histological appearance is a loss of the normal villous architecture at a ratio of between 5:1 and 3:1. General flattening of the mucosa occurs, which can vary from mild to partial villous atrophy with a total absence of villi. The thickness of the mucosa may be increased because of the increased depth of the crypts and because of infiltration of plasma cells and lymphocytes to the lamina propria. Crypt cells normally migrate to the tip of the villi in 3–5 days, but in untreated coeliac disease, this is reduced to 1–2 days.

Some degree of patchiness can be seen in the abnormalities of the small intestine; this is more often the case in patients with dermatitis herpetiformis. The epithelium is infiltrated with lymphocytes, 70% of which are CD8-positive suppressor/cytotoxic cells, 5% CD4-positive helper/inducer cells and 20% CD3-positive, CD4 negative and CD8 negative. The number of intraepithelial lymphocytes that express the more primitive gamma/delta receptors is also increased; the role of these remains unclear. Abnormalities in histology are classified as type 0 (with pre-infiltrative lesions), type 1 (infiltrative lesions), type 2 (hyperplastic lesions), type 3 (destructive lesions, in which partial to severe villus atrophy is present) and type 4 (hypoplasic lesions, which is considered to be the end-stage of gluten sensitive enteropathy, with deposition of collagen between the mucosa and submucosa (collagenous sprue)). The latter condition frequently is unresponsive to treatment with steroids and immunosuppressive agents.[4]

☐ CLASSIFICATION OF COELIAC DISEASE

Coeliac disease can be classified as follows:

- ☐ undiagnosed coeliac disease
- ☐ silent coeliac disease: a group of patients without symptoms

☐   latent coeliac disease: patients who have genetic susceptibility, sometimes with positive serology but normal small intestinal histology

☐   normal individuals.

☐ COELIAC MUCOSA AND AUTOIMMUNE RESPONSE

In patients with active coeliac disease, the lamina propria is expanded in volume because of the recruitment of T lymphocytes, plasma cells and dendritic macrophages, which express human leucocyte antigen (HLA) molecules, intercellular adhesion molecule 1 (ICAM-1) and CD25 (interleukin 2), and an infiltrate indicative of a T cell-mediated immune response. Gluten-sensitive T cells, which are DQ2-restricted, can be obtained from the small intestinal mucosa. When activated, these cells secrete γ interferon, with an increase in matrix metalloproteinases that activate degradation of extracellular matrix proteins.

A group of intraepithelial lymphocytes that express γ/δ T-cell receptors are thought to form part of an innate rather than acquired immunity. Intraepithelial lymphocytes with identified monoclonal T-cell receptor gene rearrangements are associated with refractory coeliac disease and the development of enteropathy-associated T-cell lymphoma.[3]

☐ GENETIC SUSCEPTIBILITY TO COELIAC DISEASE

Coeliac disease is a strongly inherited condition. Segregation studies have shown the prevalence of affected first-degree relatives to be 10–15% and concordance in HLA identical siblings to be 30–50%. The prevalence of concordance in monozygotic twins ranges from 70% to 100%, which suggests that environmental factors also may be important. Some studies may have underestimated concordance, however, because of unproven monozygosity and durations of follow-up insufficient to exclude the future development of coeliac disease. On the basis of a sibling recurrence risk of 10% and a population prevalence of 0.0033, the sibling relative risk (λs) in patients with coeliac disease is 30.

Coeliac disease has the strongest HLA association of any complex disease, with more than 60% of cases in Caucasian populations being associated with the HLA DQ2 haplotype. Human leucocyte antigen clearly is one important locus that affects disease susceptibility; however, most people with a DQ2 haplotype do not develop coeliac disease. Haplotype sharing probabilities across the HLA region in affected sibling pairs suggest that genes within the major histocompatibility complex (MHC) contribute no more than 40% of the sibling familial risk of coeliac disease, making non-HLA link genes the stronger determinant. Although these data must be interpreted with caution, the non-HLA genetic risk in coeliac disease probably is oligogenic rather than polygenic.

HLA association

The association between major histocompatibility complex and coeliac disease first was recognised with HLA-A1 and HLA-B8, but closer associations subsequently have been found with HLA-DR3 and HLA-DQ2. Current evidence suggests that the primary HLA susceptibility lies in the DQ alleles HLA-DQA1*0501 and HLA-DQB1*0201, which encode DQ2 and are associated with HLA-A1-B8-DR3 as part of an extended haplotype.[5] Here the DQ2 is encoded in *cis*; however, DQ2 also may be encoded in *trans* in DR5/DR7 heterozygotes. HLA-DQA1 β0105 and DQB1*0201 alleles are present in more than 90% of Caucasian parents. In southern European populations, where the overall prevalence of the DQ2 haplotype is low, an additional association is seen with the HLA DR4-DQ8 haplotype.

The hypothesis is that a unique DQ2 molecule confers susceptibility to coeliac disease. This was tested in a study that used microsatellite markers that flank the HLA class II region to establish the parental origin of the DQ alleles. The results did not support the presence of a rare mutation within the DQ alleles or the presence of an HLA-linked gene nearly in linkage disequilibrium with the DQ locus.[6] Development of coeliac disease thus seems to depend on the presence of common non-mutated HLA haplotypes. Peptide binding studies suggest that the DQ2 and DQ8 molecules play a key role in disease pathogenesis: by presenting gliadin to T cells, they trigger the inflammatory response.[7]

Non-HLA susceptibility gene

Attempts to find non-HLA disease susceptibility genes in patients with coeliac disease have involved genome-wide linkage studies as well as a targeted candidate gene approach. A number of groups have studied the cytotoxic T lymphocyte-associated gene (CTLA-4) on chromosome 2q33.[8]

Two genome-wide linkage studies have been published to date. Zhong *et al* performed an autosomal screen with 328 microsatellite markers in 45 affected sibling pairs from the west coast of southern Ireland.[9] They found evidence of linkage, with logarithm of the odds scores >2.0 in five areas. A number of other genome screens are under way in other countries. A number of other loci are likely to be proposed, and, although some agreement may be seen between the studies, many of these loci may fail to be reproduced in follow-up studies.

□ ROLE OF GLUTEN AS AN ANTIGEN

The precise structure of the part of gluten that causes damage in patients with coeliac disease remains unclear. Wheat grains have three major constituents that are separated by milling: the outer husk or bran, the germ and the endosperm of white flour. The endosperm constitutes 70–72% of the whole grain by weight and contains the toxic components.

Proteins in cereals are stored in one of two forms: the prolamins (ethanol-soluble fraction) and the glutenins. Prolamins from different cereals have different terms: gliadins are from wheat, secalins from rye, hordeins from barley, avenins from oats and zeins from coeliac non-toxic maize.

Wheat proteins are divided into classes according to their solubility characteristics: gliadins are soluble in 40–90% ethanol. Glutenins are insoluble in neutral aqueous solution, saline or ethanol. The gliadins may be further subdivided into α, β, γ and Ω subfractions according to their relative electrophoretic mobility or α, β and Ω according to their N-terminal amino acid sequences. Molecular masses of the gliadins range from 32 kD to 58 kD.

A growing number of DQ2-restricted gluten epitopes have been shown to stimulate T-cell clones derived from the intestinal mucosa of patients with coeliac disease.[10] The optimal requirement for MHC binding and T-cell stimulation is 10–15 residues, and a peptic–tryptic or chymotryptic digest of gluten contains many suitable peptides. These peptides can be cultured with gluten-specific T-cell clones, which can be tested for stimulation and cytokine production. Arentz-Hantzen *et al* described a sequence within α-gliadin that contains two overlapping immuno-dominant epitopes to which the vast majority of adult coeliac T-cell clones respond.[11,12] These peptides are resistant to normal luminal digestion and, *in vivo*, are toxic to the intestine of patients with coeliac disease.

Role of tissue transglutaminase

Anti-tissue transglutaminase (tTG) antibody titres fall and can become undetectable during a gluten-free diet, which suggests that B-cell activity depends on persistent antigen presentation. tTG-gliadin complexes have been proposed to stimulate gluten-specific T cells to induce anti tTG antibody production. T and B cells are likely to recognise different parts of this antigen complex, with T cells reacting to the smaller gliadin peptides and B cells responding to the larger 76 kD tTG enzyme, which is analogous to a hapten carrier. The unanswered question is whether these antibodies play a role in pathogenesis or represent a bystander phenomenon.

In patients with coeliac disease, tTG seems to have an important role in modifying gluten epitopes before they are recognised by T-cells; in fact, responses depend crucially on deamidation of key glutamine residues.[11] *In vitro*, tTG permits or enhances T-cell responses to the identified gliadin epitopes. Prolamins have a high proportion of glutamine residues and are excellent substrates for tTG, although only selective residues seem to be targeted.

□ CAN WE IMPROVE ON THE CURRENT GLUTEN-FREE DIET?

Refinements in the techniques for measuring gluten in food, which use monoclonal antibodies to the toxic epitopes, will help ensure appropriate labelling of foodstuffs and help patients with coeliac disease avoid inadvertent ingestion of gluten proteins. Advances have been made in our understanding of the pathogenesis of coeliac disease and the potential development of novel therapies. It should not be forgotten that a strict gluten-free diet is a safe and effective treatment.

REFERENCES

1   Dicke WK, Weijers HA, van der Kamer JH. Coeliac disease. II. The presence in wheat of a factor having a deleterious effect in cases of coeliac disease. *Acta Paediatrica* 1953;42:34–42.

2   American Gastroenterological Association medical position statement: celiac sprue. *Gastroenterology* 2001;**120**;1522–5.

3   Cellier C, Delabesse E, Helmer C, Patey N *et al.* Refractory sprue, coeliac disease, and enteropathy-associated T-cell lymphoma. French Coeliac Disease Study Group. *Lancet* 2000;**356**:203–8.

4   Marsh MN. Gluten, major histocompatibility complex, and the small intestine. A molecular and immunobiologic approach to the spectrum of gluten sensitivity ('celiac sprue'). *Gastroenterology* 1992;**102**:330–54.

5   Sollid LM, Markussen G, Ek J, Gjerde H *et al.* Evidence for a primary association of celiac disease to a particular HLA-DQ alpha/beta heterodimer. *J Exp Med* 1989;**169**:345–50.

6   Brett PM, Yiannakou JY, Morris MA, Vaughan R *et al.* Common HLA alleles, rather than rare mutants, confer susceptibility to coeliac disease. *Ann Human Genetics* 1999;**63**:217–25.

7   Shidrawi RG, Parnell ND, Ciclitira PJ, Travers P *et al.* Binding of gluten-derived peptides to the HLA-DQ2 (alpha1*0501, beta1*0201) molecule, assessed in a cellular assay. *Clin Exp Immunol* 1998;**111**:158–65.

8   Djilali-Saiah I, Schmitz J, Harfouch-Hammond, Mougenot JF *et al.* CTLA-4 gene polymorphism is associated with predisposition to coeliac disease. *Gut* 1998;**43**:187–9.

9   Zhong F, McCombs CC, Olson JM, Elston RC *et al.* An autosomal screen for genes that predispose to celiac disease in the western counties of Ireland. *Nat Genet* 1996;**14**:329–33.

10 Lundin KEA, Scott H, Hansen T, Paulsen G *et al.* Gliadin-specific, HLA-DQ (α1*0501, β1*0201) restricted T-cells isolated from the small intestinal mucosa of coeliac disease patients. *J Exp Med* 1993;**178**:187–96.

11 Arentz-Hansen H, McAdam SN, Molberg O *et al.* Coeliac lesion T-cells recognise epitopes that cluster in regions of gliadins rich in proline residues. *Gastroenterology* 2002;**123**:803–9.

12 Arentz-Hansen H, Korner R, Molberg O, Quarsten H *et al.* The intestinal T cell response to alpha-gliadin in adult celiac disease is focused on a single deamidated glutamine targeted by tissue transglutaminase. *J Exp Med* 2000;**191**:603–12.

☐ GASTROENTEROLOGY SELF ASSESSMENT QUESTIONS

Coeliac disease

1   Coeliac disease – general:
   (a) Coeliac disease is a temporary condition
   (b) Coeliac disease is a strongly inherited condition
   (c) Coeliac disease can be treated with a banana diet
   (d) Coeliac disease affects one in 100 people in Europe

2   Coeliac disease – pathology
   (a) Coeliac disease only affects the colon
   (b) Coeliac disease is associated with lymphocytic infiltration of the small intestinal mucosa
   (c) Coeliac disease exhibits crypt hyperplasia in the small intestine
   (d) In coeliac disease, villus atrophy is seen in the small intestine
   (e) The time taken for the crypt cells to reach the villus tips in untreated coeliac disease is reduced

3   Coeliac disease – genetics:
   (a) Coeliac disease is associated with human leucocyte antigen (HLA)-DQ2
   (b) Coeliac disease is associated with HLA-DQ8
   (c) Coeliac disease is associated with HLA-B2
   (d) Coeliac disease is associated with HLA DR3
   (e) Coeliac disease is associated with HLA DR5/7

4   Coeliac disease – immunology
   (a) Coeliac disease is associated with an increased prevalence of immunoglobulin A deficiency
   (b) Tissue transglutaminase antibodies invariably are raised in the untreated condition
   (c) Patients can continue to ingest barley
   (d) If untreated, coeliac disease is associated with an increased prevalence of gastrointestinal malignancy
   (e) Coeliac disease has an association with inflammatory bowel disease

Dermatology

Psoriasis: advances in management

Christopher EM Griffiths

☐ INTRODUCTION

Psoriasis is a chronic inflammatory skin disease that affects about 2% of the population of the United Kingdom. The disease manifests most commonly as red, heavily scaled plaques on the extensor aspects of the elbows, knees, lower back and scalp, although any skin surface may be affected (Fig 1). The nails are involved in 50% of people with psoriasis, and an inflammatory seronegative arthritis occurs in 15%.[1] The most common form of psoriasis, which accounts for 85% of cases, is chronic plaque psoriasis. Rarer forms include guttate psoriasis, erythroderma, flexural psoriasis and generalised pustular psoriasis. Psoriasis is recognised to produce a very significant downturn in quality of life for those it affects; indeed, impairment of quality of life in patients with psoriasis is equivalent to or worse than the impairment for other medical conditions such as cardiac insufficiency, asthma and diabetes.[2] The 'leper complex' still abounds for people with skin disease, which results in a lack of sympathy from the general public.

The age of onset for psoriasis has two peak incidences. In most cases (75%), psoriasis occurs for the first time before the age of 40 years, with a second peak

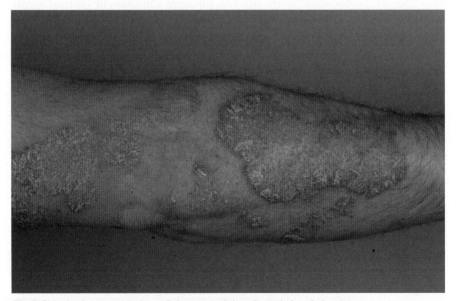

Fig 1 Chronic plaque psoriasis: well demarcated, heavily scaled, red plaques.

between the ages of 55 and 60 years. A strong family history usually is present in patients with early onset disease (<40 years of age). Considerable research efforts have focused on elucidating the immunogenetics of psoriasis. To date, eight distinct chromosomal loci (although no genes or gene products) have been identified, with the strongest link to chromosome 6 at or close to the locus for major histocompatibility complex (MHC)-1; indeed, 65% of patients with early onset psoriasis are positive for human leucocyte antigen (HLA)-Cw6. Monozygotic twin concordancy is 72% for psoriasis, which implies that development of the characteristic skin lesions is dependent on a confluence of genetic predisposition and environmental trigger factors. Such triggers include streptococcal pharyngitis or laryngitis; skin trauma (Koebner phenomenon); drugs such as β-blockers, non-steroidal anti-inflammatory drugs and anti-malarials; and stress.

The classic histological features of psoriasis include epidermal keratinocyte proliferation and loss of differentiation, angiogenesis and an inflammatory infiltrate. This infiltrate contains memory effector (CD45RO+) T cells that secrete Th1 cytokines such as interferon γ and interleukin 2. As in most inflammatory diseases, significant activity of the proinflammatory cytokine tumour necrosis factor-α (TNF-α), is seen in psoriatic plaques.[3]

Most cases of psoriasis (75%) are classified as 'mild', with less than 5% of the body's surface area being affected. Patients with mild disease usually can be managed in primary care with the use of topical preparations such as vitamin D_3 analogues, coal tar, topical corticosteroids and emollients. Patients with moderate or severe disease, however, need referral to secondary care for treatments such as phototherapy, photochemotherapy (PUVA), inpatient admission or systemic agents including methotrexate, ciclosporin and acitretin (a retinoid). Despite the current availability of treatments for severe disease, a considerable unmet need for the treatment of psoriasis, particularly the severe form, is well recognised. A survey of members of the National Psoriasis Foundation – a support group for patients with psoriasis in North America – showed that only 22% of patients were satisfied with current treatments.[4] Second-line therapies for psoriasis are not without risk, and, in fact, psoriasis cannot be cleared without some element of toxicity, such as skin cancer with photochemotherapy, hypertension and nephrotoxicity with ciclosporin, or bone marrow suppression and hepatotoxicity with methotrexate. Furthermore, current systemic therapies are more likely to produce cumulative organ toxicity if they are used in the long term. Relatively safe and effective systemic therapies that can be used over the long term for continuous control of this currently incurable disease thus are needed.

Knowledge of the immunopathogenesis of psoriasis coupled with the advent of recombinant DNA technology in the form of biological therapies (biologics) has facilitated new treatment paradigms for the management of severe psoriasis. Biologics are defined by the American Food and Drug Administration as 'derived from living material – human, plant, animal or micro-organism and used for the treatment, prevention or cure of disease in humans.' The introduction of biologics for the management of severe psoriasis follows their important addition to the armamentarium for inflammatory diseases such as rheumatoid arthritis and Crohn's disease. Psoriasis has two key biologic approaches: T-cell targeting and cytokine modulation, particularly inhibition of TNF-α.

This paper will discuss two T cell-targeted approaches for psoriasis – alefacept and efalizumab. Both are approved in the United States for the treatment of psoriasis, and efalizumab is approved in the United Kingdom. The TNF-α inhibitors are better known in general medicine, as they have been used for several years for the management of inflammatory arthritis. Two will be discussed: etanercept, which is licensed in the United States and United Kingdom for the treatment of psoriasis and psoriatic arthritis, and infliximab, which as yet is unlicensed for psoriatic arthritis or psoriasis.

☐ T CELL-TARGETED BIOLOGICS

Alefacept

Alefacept is a fusion protein of lymphocyte function-associated antigen-3 (LFA-3) and immunoglobulin G1 (IgG1).[5] Alefacept binds to the T-cell receptor CD2 and inhibits secondary T-cell activation that occurs after binding of CD2 to LFA-3 on antigen-presenting cells. A secondary mechanism of action seems to be via apoptosis of circulating CD45RO+ T cells that are dependent on granzyme release from natural killer cells: CD45RO+ T cells are apoptosed preferentially because they express high levels of CD2.

Alefacept is administered on a weekly basis by intravenous or intramuscular fixed-dose injection (7.5 or 15 mg) for a 12-week cycle. Up to nine cycles have been used safely. Clinical response is relatively modest: reductions in psoriasis area severity index (PASI: a measure of clinical severity of psoriasis) of 75% (PASI 75) are achieved in only 20% of patients by 12 weeks of treatment. Furthermore, onset of improvement is slow: on average, eight weeks pass before significant clinical improvement is apparent in patients who are going to respond. Improvement in psoriasis correlates with a reduction in the numbers of peripheral T cells. Patients thus need regular monitoring of peripheral CD4 T-cell counts, but safety in the short term seems to be good. Some patients who respond achieve long-term remission, which obviates the need for further treatment. Only a modest improvement is seen in patients with psoriatic arthritis.

Efalizumab

Efalizumab is a humanised monoclonal antibody to CD11a (LFA-1).[6] This biologic has a dual mechanism of action predicated on blocking LFA-1-mediated adhesion to intercellular adhesion molecule–1 (ICAM-1). This inhibits T-cell activation and adhesion of circulating T cells to endothelial cells that express ICAM-1, thus preventing cutaneous trafficking of T cells.

Efalizumab is self-administered once a week by 1 mg/kg subcutaneous injection. Onset of action is relatively quick: the first significant clinical improvement is seen within two weeks of starting treatment and, overall, 25% of patients achieve PASI 75 by 12 weeks of treatment (Fig 2). Patients who respond by 12 weeks can be treated continuously, as data is available for up to three years of continuous safe control. Safety seems to be good in the short term, and monitoring beyond three months is limited to regular full blood counts because of sporadic reports of thrombocytopaenia. As with other T cell-targeted biologics, efficacy for psoriatic arthritis is only modest.

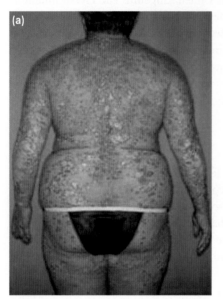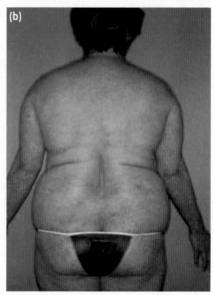

Fig 2 Woman aged 45 years with extensive psoriasis before (a) and after (b) successful treatment with efalizumab over 12 weeks. (Courtesy of Serono.)

☐ TNF-α INHIBITION

Etanercept

Etanercept is a recombinant fusion protein that consists of the two extracellular ligand-binding portions of the p75 TNF receptor linked to the F_c portion of human immunoglobulin G.[7] This biologic has been used for several years for the treatment of inflammatory arthritis.

Etanercept is self-administered by twice weekly subcutaneous injections of 25 or 50 mg. Response is good, with 34% of patients on 25 mg and 49% of patients on 50 mg achieving PASI 75 by week 12. Extension of treatment duration to 24 weeks increases the number of responders to 44% and 59% for patients taking 25 and 50 mg twice weekly, respectively. Etanercept is approved for up to 24 weeks of continuous therapy in the management of psoriasis and also is highly effective for the treatment of psoriatic arthritis. The drug is well tolerated, although about one third of patients develop injection site reactions consisting of transient, urticated plaques. The side effects of TNF-α inhibitors as a group are discussed below.

Infliximab

Infliximab is a chimeric monoclonal antibody to TNF-α.[8] Infliximab is delivered by intravenous infusion, and the standard regimen comprises 5 mg/kg at the start of treatment and two and six weeks later, followed by repeat infusions every eight weeks irrespective of the clinical activity of the psoriasis. This regimen was developed for the treatment of rheumatoid arthritis in combination with methotrexate, but to date only case reports have shown efficacy of the combination of methotrexate and infliximab in patients with psoriasis. Infliximab is approved for the treatment of rheumatoid arthritis, fistulating Crohn's disease and ankylosing spondylitis. Compared with alefacept, efalizumab and etanercept, infliximab is significantly more effective in the short term and is faster acting. More than 80% of patients with psoriasis treated with infliximab achieve PASI 75 by 10 weeks of treatment and 60% within six weeks. Psoriatic arthritis also improves significantly with infliximab treatment. At present, no studies of the efficacy of long-term treatment (more than six months) with infliximab for psoriasis have been published.

Side effects

Side effects of TNF-α inhibitors are well known because of their extensive use in the management of rheumatoid arthritis. Before etanercept or infliximab are started, patients should be screened for active tuberculosis, because of reports of reactivation of tuberculosis (more so with infliximab than etanercept). Demyelination, cardiac failure and lymphoma have been reported, and antinuclear antibodies and anti-DNA antibodies are frequent but rarely proceed to lupus erythermatosus (particularly with infliximab). Patients who receive infusions of infliximab are at risk of infusion or anaphylactic reactions, although no good evidence shows that these are related to the development of antibodies to infliximab.

Interestingly, some patients who receive TNF-α inhibitors for psoriasis, rheumatoid arthritis or Crohn's disease have developed an atopic dermatitis-like skin eruption. This is probably the result of a shift in the cutaneous cytokine profile towards Th2 cytokines, which is more characteristic of atopic dermatitis.

☐ FUTURE BIOLOGICS

A number of other biologics are in development for the management of psoriasis.[9]

Adalimumab is a human, monoclonal antibody to TNF-α that is approved in the United Kingdom for the treatment of rheumatoid arthritis. It is delivered by subcutaneous injection at a dose of 40 mg on alternate weeks. Initial evidence from clinical trials indicates that this is a highly effective treatment for psoriasis, with 53% of patients achieving PASI 75 over 12 weeks.

Another development is the targeting of interleukin 12 – a key proinflammatory cytokine produced by cutaneous Langerhans cells. Preliminary evidence indicates that a single intravenous infusion of interleukin-12 p40 antibody significantly improves psoriasis, with 100% of patients in the highest dose group achieving PASI 75 within 16 weeks of infusion.[10]

National Institute for Health and Clinical Excellence guidelines for the clinical use of biologics for psoriasis are awaited, but the challenge for dermatologists is how to use these as part of the current armamentarium of systemic therapies for severe disease. Efalizumab and etanercept are likely to be used only in patients with psoriasis who are unsuitable for and/or unresponsive to additional systemic therapies. As yet, no head-to-head randomised controlled trials of one biologic against another or of a biologic against a traditional systemic therapy, such as methotrexate, have been undertaken.

The use of biologics for psoriasis is an important example of translational medicine: we now have therapies targeted to key immune pathways in this disease and advancement of therapy is much less a case of serendipity and more of a concerted reductionist approach. Furthermore, the observation that only a subset of patients treated with alefacept or efalizumab achieved significant clinical improvement begs the question as to whether pharmacogenomics predicated on identification of single nucleotide polymorphisms of the CD2 receptor or CD11a could dictate or predict outcomes with alefacept and efalizumab, respectively. The other conclusion is that chronic plaque psoriasis may be a spectrum of skin disorders that are genotypically different, phenotypically similar but not identical and that could be 'identified' by individual response to biologic therapies.

The advent of biologics in the management of severe psoriasis is salient and may provide a glimpse of the long-awaited goal of treatment – long-term, safe, continuous therapy.

REFERENCES

1   Griffiths CEM, Camp RDR, Barker JNWN. Psoriasis. In: Burns DA, Breathnach SM, Cox NH, Griffiths CEM (eds), *Rook's textbook of dermatology*. Oxford: Blackwell Sciences, 2004.

2   Finlay AY, Coles EC. The effect of severe psoriasis on the quality of life of 369 patients. *Br J Dermatol* 1995;**132**:236–44.

3   Griffiths CEM. The immunological basis of psoriasis. *J Eur Acad Dermatol Venereol* 2003; **17**:1–5.

4   Kruger G, Koo J, Lebwohl M *et al.* The impact of psoriasis on quality of life: results of a 1998 National Psoriasis Foundation patient-membership survey. *Arch Dermatol* 2001;**137**:280–4.

5   Ellis CN, Kruerger GG. Treatment of chronic plaque psoriasis by selective targeting of memory effector T lymphocytes. *N Engl J Med* 2001;**345**:248–55.

6   Gordon KB, Papp KA, Hamilton TK *et al.* Efalizumab for patients with moderate to severe plaque psoriasis: a randomised controlled trial. *JAMA* 2003;**290**:3073–80.

7   Leonardi CL, Powers JL, Matheson RT *et al.* Etanercept as monotherapy in patients with psoriasis. *N Engl J Med* 2003;**349**:2014–22.

8   Gottlieb AB, Evans R, Li S *et al.* Infliximab induction therapy for patients with severe plaque-type psoriasis: a randomised, double-blind, placebo-controlled trial. *J Am Acad Dermatol* 2004;**51**:534–42.

9   Gottlieb AB. Psoriasis: emerging therapeutic strategies. *Nat Rev Drug Discov* 2005;**4**:19–24.

10 Kauffman CL, Aria N, Toichi E *et al.* A phase I study evaluating the safety, pharmacokinetics, and clinical response of a human IL-12 p40 antibody in subject with plaque psoriasis. *J Invest Dermatol* 2004;**123**:1037–44.

Photosensitivity disorders

John Hawk

□ INTRODUCTION

The photosensitivity disorders, or photodermatoses, are distinct from the normal ultraviolet radiation (UVR)-induced effects of sunburn, tanning, ageing and cancer. They potentially occur in all people and may affect around 10–15% of the population in the United Kingdom. They are categorised as:

- □ probably immunologically mediated disorders – polymorphic light eruption (the most common of all photodermatoses), actinic prurigo, hydroa vacciniforme, chronic actinic dermatitis and solar urticaria

- □ DNA repair-defective disorders – predominantly the cancer-prone xeroderma pigmentosum

- □ chemical and drug photosensitivity caused by exogenous drugs or endogenous chemicals in the porphyrias

- □ light-exacerbated dermatoses – disorders worsened or precipitated by, but not caused by, light.

Pathogenic mechanisms in many of these disorders have been understood poorly until recently, but they are being clarified steadily.

□ PROBABLY IMMUNOLOGICALLY MEDIATED DISORDERS

Polymorphic light eruption

Polymorphic light eruption (PLE) is the most common of the probably immunologically mediated disorders (Fig 1).[1] Colloquially, but incorrectly, PLE is known as prickly heat, which is, in fact, an entirely separate disorder of excessive sweating. In fact, PLE is an intermittent sunlight or artificial UVR-induced eruption of particularly temperate climatic regions. It more commonly affects women of any race within hours to rarely days of exposure, usually in summer or on sunny vacations and occasionally in winter if snow is on the ground. The resultant rash is non-scarring, itchy, erythematous, usually papular, sometimes plaque-like, vesicular, bullous or often mixed. It usually affects only some exposed, rarely covered skin. Regularly exposed areas such as the face and backs of hands often may be spared. The disorder persists for days to a week or so after exposure ceases until total clearance, and is often worse in spring, becoming gradually less severe as summer progresses.

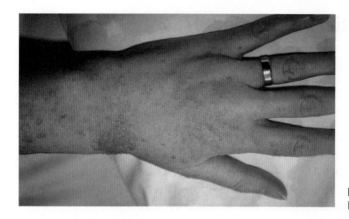

Fig 1 Polymorphic light eruption.

The UVR wavelengths that induce PLE have not been established precisely, but they seem to vary widely between patients, which suggests that many cutaneous molecular absorbers may initiate the disorder. Serial skin biopsies from patients after low-dose, solar-simulated irradiation have shown increased numbers of dermal and epidermal antigen-presenting cells within hours, along with an early, predominantly CD4+, perivascular T-lymphocytic cellular infiltrate that becomes mostly CD8+ within days. This differs from the immunosuppressive response seen in normal people, as does the pattern of expression of E-selectin, vascular cell adhesion molecule-1 and intercellular adhesion molecule-1 in the skin of irradiated patients. Furthermore, autologous peripheral blood lymphocytes, but not normal keratinocytes, are stimulated *in vitro* by UVR-irradiated PLE through presumed UVR-induced antigen production in the former. All these facts together strongly suggest that PLE is a delayed type hypersensitivity immunological reaction – arguably to UVR-induced endogenous cutaneous antigen. The reasons for this apparent abnormality of response largely seem to have a genetic basis:[2] families of patients with PLE are affected some three times more often than the general population, and both of some 70% of identical twins but only 30% of non-identical twins are affected. As only up to about 20% of the population expresses the disorder, however, environmental factors and disease penetrance also seem to be important. The nature of this genetic abnormality seems likely to be a reduced capacity of the patient for normal UVR-induced cutaneous immunosuppression during the induction phase of antigen recognition: patient susceptibility to dinitrochlorobenzene skin sensitisation after solar-simulated irradiation is higher than in normal controls,[3] although no difference is seen in the elicitation response after sensitisation has been achieved.[4] In addition, recent work suggests that specific features of patients with PLE that allow this abnormality may well include an increased number of antigen-presenting Langerhans cells in the skin of patients with PLE compared with normal people, as well as a conceivably reduced capacity to handle free radical insult through a genetically determined depletion of glutathione.[5] Cutaneous molecular absorbers of UVR that initiate the rash of PLE have not been identified as yet, and a variety of these are likely to be responsible, presumably becoming antigenic themselves or leading to putative antigen production through secondary free radical activity.

Treatment of mild PLE is by the restriction of exposure to UVR, covering up with appropriately protective clothing and the application of high-protection, broad-spectrum sunscreens. In patients affected more severely and frequently, regular prophylactic phototherapy is helpful for months – almost certainly through immunosuppressive activity – with follow-up courses needed annually. For occasional attacks of PLE or if the rash develops in spite of the above measures, however, brief courses of oral steroids, perhaps prednisolone 25–30 mg at earliest disease onset and then each morning until clear for a maximum of about 10 days every 2–3 months, almost always are rapidly effective. Oral azathioprine or ciclosporin also may be required rarely for unremitting disease.

Actinic prurigo

Actinic prurigo (AP) is a rare, sunlight-induced, papular or nodular, extremely itchy, usually excoriated eruption of light-exposed (and to a lesser extent covered) skin, sometimes associated also with acute PLE-like attacks (Fig 2).[1] Actinic prurigo most commonly has onset in childhood, is usually worse in summer and may slowly remit or, more rarely, persist indefinitely. As in PLE, widely varying wavelengths of UVR seem able to induce the rash. A relation between the two conditions and thus an immunological basis also for AP is suggested by the regular association of the condition with PLE in the same patient or their family, that some patients with actinic prurigo later develop PLE (or the reverse), that the perivascular mononuclear cell infiltrate of early AP resembles that of PLE and that some patients with genetic AP have clinical PLE but atypical lesional persistence. Actinic prurigo thus may be a persistent variant of PLE. The fact that more than 80% of British Caucasian patients have human leucocyte antigen type DRB1*04 (DR4), which is present in only 30% of normal people and patients with PLE, and that 60% compared with 6% have its subtype DRB1*0407,[6] suggests this feature very likely may be the determinant that transforms PLE into AP.

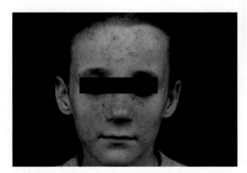

Fig 2 Actinic prurigo.

Mild AP rarely may be managed by the restriction of sun exposure, use of appropriately protective clothing, regular application of high-protection broad-spectrum sunscreens and, if rash is present, topical steroids and emollients. Patients who respond poorly sometimes may do well with occasional courses of oral steroids for flares, but for more persistent disease, prophylactic low-dose phototherapy, as in PLE, sometimes may be helpful. Much more reliable in suitable patients, however, is oral thalidomide (50–100 mg nightly until clearance over weeks and adjusted thereafter to as low a dose as possible), although a high risk of teratogenicity and a moderate risk of gradual development of unpleasant peripheral neuropathy necessitate extreme care in its use. Failing this, oral ciclosporin also may help.

Hydroa vacciniforme

Hydroa vacciniforme closely resembles PLE in its clinical behaviour (Fig 3),[1] except that it mostly affects children and always leaves disfiguring pock scars, perhaps because the reaction takes place at a vulnerable skin site or leads to a toxic photoproduct. In addition, hydroa vacciniforme seems unresponsive to almost all therapy, apart perhaps from strong sunscreens and prophylactic phototherapy (although the latter may sometimes induce the rash instead). Fortunately, however, the condition frequently resolves in adolescence.

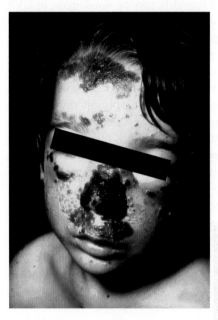

Fig 3 Hydroa vacciniforme.

Chronic actinic dermatitis

Chronic actinic dermatitis (CAD) is a not uncommon UVR-induced (and, rarely, short-wavelength visible light-induced) eczema of the exposed sites (Fig 4).[6] It is persistent but often slowly remitting, often incapacitating and very rarely suicide-inducing. The affected sites are patchily or confluently covered with an extremely itchy eruption. In severe cases, this is markedly thickened and florid and sometimes spreads to covered sites, although the depths of skin creases, finger webs and upper

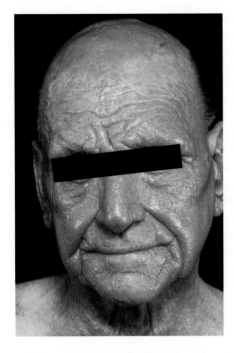

Fig 4 Chronic actinic dermatitis.

eyelids sometimes may be spared. In severe cases, the eruption and its histology may have the features of cutaneous T-cell lymphoma, and abnormal lymphocytes also may circulate in the peripheral blood, but progression to malignancy in ordinary CAD seems not to occur. The disorder most commonly affects older men and, more rarely, younger patients with atopic eczema and occasionally patients infected with human immunodeficiency virus. It also is associated often with contact dermatitis to a variety of allergens (frequently airborne allergens), such as the sesquiterpene lactone from *Compositae* plants, colophony from pine trees and perfumes from flowers, as well as topical medicaments. The condition usually is worse in summer or after sun exposure – a fact often not noted by the patient.

Chronic actinic dermatitis is reproducible at all skin sites in the absence of exogenous photosensitiser with the use of ultraviolet and, very rarely visible, irradiation – frequently at considerably lower than the smallest doses that cause sunburn. Furthermore, the clinical and histological appearances, the dermal infiltrate, which contains a predominance of CD8+ T-cells, and the expression of adhesion molecules all resemble those of the known delayed type hypersensitivity response, allergic contact dermatitis. This suggests, therefore, that CAD may be a similar reaction, but, by inference, against cutaneous photoinduced endogenous antigen. This reaction may be facilitated by the fact that CAD often occurs in association with pre-existing, widespread, often airborne contact dermatitis to exogenous sensitisers, which arguably may enhance cutaneous immune function enough to enable putative recognition of endogenous photoantigen. Alternatively, or as well, chronic photodamage may impair UVR-induced cutaneous immuno-suppression, such that endogenous UVR-induced skin photoantigen is recognised more easily, as apparently also occurs genetically in PLE, particularly because elderly outdoor workers or leisure enthusiasts are affected most often. In addition, the photoaged skin of such people may lead to slower putative antigen removal, as well as easier penetration of associated contact allergens. Molecular absorbers of UVR that initiate the CAD rash have not been identified definitively, but DNA, RNA or a similar or associated molecule seems likely to be involved in at least some instances.[7]

Careful avoidance of exposure to UVR and, if necessary, visible light (even from fluorescent room lighting) and relevant contact allergens, is essential. Computer and television screens are safe. Appropriate cover with clothing and the use of non-irritating, broad-spectrum, high-protection sunscreens of low allergenic potential often also are helpful. Although rarely effective alone, topical steroids or intermittent therapy with oral steroids also usually are necessary. For resistant disease, prolonged phototherapy with low-dose psoralen plus exposure to ultraviolet light A or perhaps narrowband ultraviolet light B also may be helpful, although often they are tolerated poorly initially, except under high-dose systemic and topical steroid cover or oral immunosuppressive therapy, such as ciclosporin, azathioprine or mycophenolate mofetil. In addition, topical tacrolimus occasionally is helpful.

Solar urticaria

Solar urticaria (SU) is an uncommon wealing disorder of both sexes at any age, but with slight female predominance and peak onset in the second and third decades (Fig 5).[8] Itching, burning and hive formation (rarely redness alone), just of exposed sites occur within minutes of sun exposure and fade in an hour or so. Confluent rash with a sharp cut-off at lines of clothing or multiple individual lesions may occur, while generalised wealing on occasion may lead to anaphylactic-type responses.

All UVR and short visible-light wavelengths may induce SU, but the exact spectrum is essentially constant for any given patient. Mast cell degranulation with histamine release plays a major role in causation, presumably because of an immediate type hypersensitivity response against endogenous photoinduced antigen.

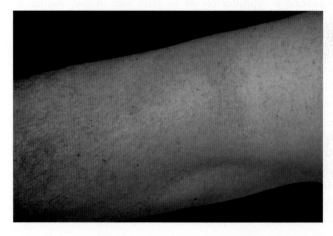

Fig 5 Solar urticaria.

Patients with mild SU occasionally respond just to care in sunlight, the use of appropriate clothing and sunscreens (particularly if the patient is sensitive only to short wavelength UVR) or, more reliably, to non-sedating antihistamines an hour or so before exposure – often in highish doses. In many patients, however, this is insufficient, and UVR phototherapy, given carefully to avoid evoking the rash, is helpful on occasion. In patients whose disease is more resistant, plasma exchange sometimes may be very effective for months to years. Beyond that, ciclosporin and intravenous immunoglobulin very occasionally seem to be helpful, but a group of patients do not respond to any therapy and remain extraordinarily inconvenienced.

☐ DNA REPAIR-DEFECTIVE DISORDERS

Xeroderma pigmentosum

Xeroderma pigmentosum (XP) is an autosomal recessive condition with an estimated incidence of one in 250,000 in the United Kingdom (Fig 6).[9] Patients have marked photosensitivity (the inducing radiation being short wavelength UVR) and show premature, severe onset of skin ageing and all types of skin cancer. Many patients also show easy skin sunburning, with blistering after even minimal sun exposure starting from an early age. Within a few years, practically all unprotected patients then develop at least some skin dryness, pigmentation and freckling. Actinic keratoses, basal cell carcinomas, squamous carcinomas and melanomas then tend to have onset on exposed areas within a few more years. Severe photophobia, keratitis, and corneal opacification and neovascularisation, also are common. About 30% of

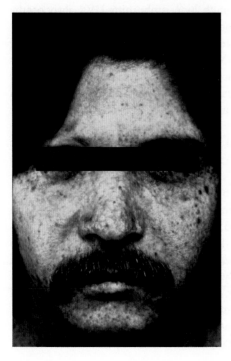

Fig 6 Xeroderma pigmentosum.

patients also present in late childhood, with impaired mental, physical, neurological or sexual function, while the incidence of internal cancer is also increased moderately. Eight different genetic groups represent various different faults in UVR-induced DNA repair.

Treatment requires lifelong rigorous photoprotection, including maximal sunlight avoidance; the use of broad-spectrum sunscreen preparations; and the wearing of wide-brimmed hats, sunglasses, UVR-absorbing contact lenses and tightly woven clothing. Oral retinoids have been used successfully as chemopreventive agents, however, although rebound tumour growth on drug cessation is a major disadvantage. Cryotherapy and other surgical techniques are used to manage premalignant and malignant lesions. Recently, a bacteriophage-derived DNA repair enzyme, T4 endonuclease V (T4N5), incorporated into a liposomal delivery vehicle applied to the skin also has been introduced as a potentially effective prophylactic therapy. A study of 20 patients who received the active preparation developed markedly fewer actinic keratoses and basal cell carcinomas than controls over a year, with persistence of the effect for months after treatment cessation.[10] The study was too small to show any changes in the incidence of squamous cell carcinoma or melanoma. This treatment is awaiting administrative approval for distribution as a drug.

☐ DRUG- AND CHEMICAL-INDUCED PHOTOSENSITIVITY

Exogenous drug- and chemical-induced photosensitivity

Exogenous drug- and chemical-induced photosensitivity comprises inflammatory reactions induced by usually long-wavelength, non-sunburning UVR absorbed by molecules in the skin derived from an oral drug or topically applied chemical.[11] Absorption and transfer of the radiation to nearby vulnerable tissues occur directly or after secondary free radical formation. Many drugs are potential photosensitisers (Table 1), but individual susceptibility is so variable that often no reaction at all may occur except with a few drugs – such as, for example, amiodarone, with which reactions are usual. Patients on all such drugs should initially expose their skin to the sun more cautiously than usual until they learn the nature of their reaction rather than not have the drugs prescribed at all if needed. Several distinct reaction patterns occur, which apparently are dependent on the drug's exact location in the skin. Oral drug-induced photosensitivity leads most commonly to sunburn-like reactions after a few hours, rarely to skin fragility with blistering and broken skin of the exposed areas, very rarely to a burning sensation (occasionally also with redness and sometimes wealing) and very rarely indeed to separation of the tips of the fingernails from the nail plate. Topical chemical-induced photosensitivity also leads to sunburn-like reactions – but usually in bizarre skin patterns from the skin's random contact with sensitising plants (commonly known as phytophotodermatitis (Fig 7)) – or, not uncommonly, to itchy, irregular, poorly localised reactions of eczema not seen with oral drugs, particularly after continuing topical medicine or cosmetic use. Treatment comprises avoidance of excessive exposure to sunlight or, if possible, the product, or rarely evening dosing of drug if pharmacokinetics permit.

Table 1 Selection of past and present oral drugs incriminated as possible photosensitisers.

Class	Drug
Analgesics	Azapropazone
	Naproxen
	Piroxicam
	Benoxaprofen (in past)
Antibiotics	Nalidixic acid
	Sulphonamides
	Tetracyclines
Antidepressants	Protryptiline
Antiepileptics	Carbamazepine (relatively common)
Cardiac drugs	Amiodarone (very common)
Diuretics	Thiazides
Psoralens (universal)	
Tranquillisers	Chlorpromazine (relatively common, particularly in past)
	Diazepam

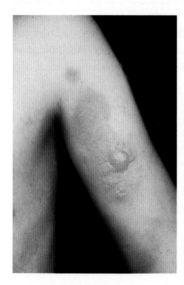

Fig 7 Phytophotodermatitis.

Endogenous drug- and chemical-induced photosensitivity

Endogenous drug- and chemical-induced photosensitivity comprises just the cutaneous porphyrias – either hepatic, in which the long-wavelength UVR-absorbing chemical, porphyrin, accumulates markedly in the liver and skin, or erythropoietic, in which porphyrin accumulates in red blood cells, which regularly traverse the skin.[12] These diseases are all defects of haem biosynthetic enzyme function, in which the disease-inducing porphyrins are present excessively as a by-product, and all produce reactions that mimic drug- and chemical-induced photosensitivity, apparently again dependent on the location of porphyrins in the skin.

Erythropoietic protoporphyria (EPP) is the most typically photosensitive condition. It leads from usually early childhood to a severe burning pain without skin change within about 20 minutes of sun exposure; this then lasts for hours to days. Liver disease is a rare accompaniment in severe cases. Porphyria cutanea tarda (PCT) and variegate porphyria (VP) instead lead in adults to fragility, blistering and broken skin of exposed areas, especially the backs of the hands, in summer, with moderate liver changes not uncommon. Potentially disabling acute systemic attacks also are possible in VP. Treatment other than sun avoidance is difficult except in PCT, in which alcohol restriction and regular venesection or low-dose chloroquine are effective over 6–12 months. Erythropoietic protoporphyria may respond moderately to administration of high-dose beta-carotene in summer, or perhaps sometimes phototherapy. Variegate porphyria requires the strict prophylactic avoidance of alcohol, oestrogens and liver enzyme-inducing drugs, along with haem derivative infusions and symptomatic therapy if acute attacks occur.

Dermatoses exacerbated by UVR

Certain dermatoses not initiated by UVR exposure, particularly seborrhoeic eczema, (Fig 8) lupus and much more rarely psoriasis may be exacerbated by exposure.[13] In some cases, immunological events associated with their underlying pathogenesis presumably are modified, while pre-existing inflammation may be exacerbated in others. On occasion, particularly in seborrhoeic eczema, the underlying disease may

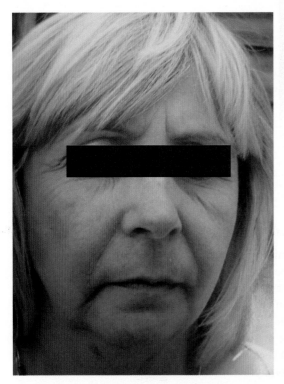

Fig 8 Light-exacerbated seborrhoeic eczema.

be worsened significantly, even if it is only mild – sometimes subclinical – to begin with.[14] Often, however, the disorder may be unaffected or more likely improved by irradiation. If sunlight does cause exacerbations, the eruption may develop or worsen at all exposed sites or, more usually, just at those typical of the disorder. Treatment is by the restriction of UVR exposure, use of cover with appropriate clothing, application of high-protection sunscreens and, most particularly, assiduous therapy of the underlying disorder (even if minimal), the last of which alone frequently may clear the light sensitivity completely.[13] Failing this, courses of low-dose UVB or PUVA therapy, as for PLE, may be carefully tried in conditions that usually respond to such treatment, including seborrhoeic eczema, but not in disorders such as cutaneous lupus, in which the aggravation of systemic features is a potential severe hazard.

REFERENCES

1   Norris PG, Hawk JLM. The idiopathic photodermatoses: polymorphic light eruption, actinic prurigo and hydroa vacciniforme. In: Hawk JLM (ed), *Photodermatology*. London: Arnold, 1999: 178–90.

2   McGregor JM, Grabczynska S, Vaughan R, Hawk JL *et al*. Genetic modeling of abnormal photosensitivity in families with polymorphic light eruption and actinic prurigo. *J Invest Dermatol* 2000;**115**:471–6.

3   van de Pas CB, Kelly DA, Seed PT, Young AR *et al*. Ultraviolet-radiation-induced erythema and suppression of contact hypersensitivity responses in patients with polymorphic light eruption. *J Invest Dermatol* 2004;**122**:295–9.

4   Palmer RA, Hawk JLM, Young AR, Walker SL. The effect of solar-simulated radiation on the elicitation phase of contact hypersensitivity does not differ between controls and patients with polymorphic light eruption. *J Invest Dermatol* 2005;**124**:1308–12.

5   Millard TP, Hawk JLM, Fryer AA, McGregor JM. Protective effect of glutathione S-transferase *GSTP1* Val[105] against polymorphic light eruption. *Br J Dermatol* 2003;**149**(Suppl 64):88–9.

6   Menagé H du P, Hawk JLM. The idiopathic photodermatoses: chronic actinic dermatitis. In: Hawk JLM (ed), *Photodermatology*. London: Arnold, 1999: 190–202.

7   Menagé H du P, Harrison GI, Potten CS, Young AR *et al*. The action spectrum for induction of chronic actinic dermatitis is similar to that for sunburn inflammation. *Photochem Photobiol* 1995;**62**:976–9.

8   Hölzle E. The idiopathic photodermatoses: solar urticaria. In: Hawk JLM (ed), *Photodermatology*. London: Arnold, 1999: 203–10.

9   Norris PG, Lehmann AR. The DNA repair defective photodermatoses. In: Hawk JLM (ed), *Photodermatology*. London: Arnold, 1999: 211–21.

10 Yarosh D, Klein J, O'Connor A, Hawk J *et al*. Effect of topically applied T4 endonuclease V in liposomes on skin cancer in xeroderma pigmentosum: a randomised study. *Lancet* 2001;**357**:926–9.

11 Ferguson J. Chemical- and drug-induced photosensitivity. In: Hawk JLM (ed), *Photodermatology*. London: Arnold, 1999: 222–33.

12 Elder GH. The porphyrias. In: Hawk JLM (ed), *Photodermatology*. London: Arnold, 1999: 233–44.

13 Morison WL, Towne LE, Hönig B. The photoaggravated dermatoses. In: Hawk JLM (ed), *Photodermatology*. London: Arnold, 1999: 199–212.

14 Palmer RA, Hawk JL. Light-induced seborrhoeic eczema: severe photoprovocation from subclinical disease. *Photodermatol Photoimmunol Photomed* 2004:**20**:62–3.

☐ DERMATOLOGY SELF ASSESSMENT QUESTIONS

Psoriasis

1   Chronic plaque psoriasis:
    (a) Affects 0.2% of the population of the United Kingdom
    (b) Affects 2% of the population of the United Kingdom
    (c) Has 100% concordance in monozygotic twins
    (d) Is strongly associated with human leucocyte antigen-Cw6
    (e) Affects the nails in 50% of cases

2   Efalizumab:
    (a) Is a monoclonal antibody to CD11a
    (b) Blocks T-cell binding to vascular endothelium
    (c) Is an effective treatment for psoriatic arthritis
    (d) Belongs to the group of biological therapies known as tumour necrosis factor-α inhibitors
    (e) Produces significant clinical improvement in more than 75% of patients

3   Infliximab:
    (a) Is a chimeric monoclonal antibody to tumour necrosis factor-α
    (b) Is a T cell-targeted biologic
    (c) In most patients produces significant (>75%) improvements in psoriasis within 10 weeks of starting treatment
    (d) May reactivate tuberculosis
    (e) Has been associated with cardiac failure

4   Etanercept:
    (a) Is a monoclonal antibody to tumour necrosis factor-α
    (b) Is delivered by intravenous infusion
    (c) Is an effective treatment for psoriatic arthritis
    (d) Is delivered by subcutaneous injection
    (e) After 12 weeks of treatment produces 75% improvements in the clinical severity of psoriasis in about one-third of patients

Photosensitivity disorders

1   Polymorphic light eruption:
    (a) Seems to be a delayed type hypersensitivity immunological reaction against endogenous, ultraviolet radiation-induced skin antigen
    (b) Is the most common photosensitivity disorder
    (c) Is colloquially but incorrectly known as prickly heat
    (d) Seems to be a sporadically occurring disorder with no genetic basis
    (e) Responds rarely to oral steroids or prophylactic phototherapy

2   Chronic actinic dermatitis:
  (a) Typically affects young, female, gardening enthusiasts
  (b) Seems to be a contact dermatitis-like reaction against endogenous,
       ultraviolet radiation-induced skin antigen
  (c) Almost always persists indefinitely
  (d) Often is extraordinarily distressing and has on occasion led to suicide
  (e) Is reasonably responsive to therapy once a correct diagnosis is made

3   In drug- and chemical-induced photosensitivity:
  (a) Potentially photosensitising drugs should not be prescribed to anybody
       who will be in the sun in summer or on sunny holidays
  (b) Many potentially photosensitising drugs are idiosyncratic in their degree
       of photosensitising effect and often may produce no noticeable effect at all
  (c) Patients on a potentially photosensitising drug should be very careful in
       the sun to begin with until they discover if they have been photosensitised
       significantly
  (d) The porphyrias are a form of chemical photosensitivity and may present
       with similar clinical features to drug photosensitivity
  (e) Photosensitisers exert their effect by not absorbing sunlight and so
       directing more of this light into the vulnerable adjacent skin

4   Xeroderma pigmentosum:
  (a) Is a common cause of skin cancer in the general population
  (b) Is a disease of impaired repair of ultraviolet radiation-induced DNA
       damage
  (c) Is inherited as an autosomal recessive disorder
  (d) Improves spontaneously in adulthood
  (e) Responds somewhat to oral retinoids and a topical preparation of
       liposome-delivered DNA repair enzyme

5   Light-exacerbated dermatoses:
  (a) Are in fact all dermatoses if the sunlight is strong enough
  (b) Can be expressed severely in sunlight even if otherwise subclinical
  (c) Usually respond even in severe instances to assiduous therapy of the
       underlying disorder, even if subclinical
  (d) Generally do well with low-dose phototherapy if not responsive to other
       measures
  (e) Are readily distinguishable clinically from true photodermatoses

Obesity

Psychosocial burden of obesity in children

Jane Wardle

☐ INTRODUCTION

Social and psychological research has documented powerful negative stereotyping of obese people, with many studies showing that they are seen as unattractive, unsuitable dating and sexual partners, discontent with themselves, weak willed and emotionally impaired.[1] Children as young as five years make similar judgements about obesity. In one study, children aged 5–7 years were shown a series of sets of three pictures of a fat, normal-weight and thin child and asked to choose the one who was 'cleverest', 'kindest', 'laziest', and so on.[2] The fat image was chosen least for the positive adjectives (clever: 13%; kind: 21%; happy: 13%; pretty: 5%; like to play with: 8%) and most for the negative adjectives (selfish: 57%; stupid: 61%; lazy: 72%; tells lies: 55%; few friends: 58%).[2] Negative stereotyping of obesity is not restricted to the general public; even health professionals who would never consciously endorse negative attitudes, nonetheless reveal their prejudices on word association tasks.[3]

Stigmatisation of obesity is likely to lead to discrimination and social exclusion. In a seven-year follow-up of more than 10,000 adolescents, Gortmaker and colleagues showed that the obese adolescents had poorer educational, occupational and social trajectories than the normal weight adolescents, even after adolescent school performance and parental socio-economic status were controlled for.[4] Many studies, both quantitative and qualitative, have documented social exclusion, bullying and teasing of obese children and adolescents. Puhl and Brownell described the daily ritual of taunts and humiliation that obese children and adolescents experience in American high schools, not only from peers but also from teachers.[1]

Teasing is also common for overweight and obese British adolescents. In a longitudinal cohort study of almost 6,000 adolescents from 36 schools in South London,[5] 54% of obese children reported being teased at school at age 11 years compared with 30% of overweight and 5% of normal-weight children. Teasing at home showed the same pattern, ranging from 6% in normal-weight children through 17% and 24% in overweight and obese children. Teasing was reported equally often by boys and girls, and rates did not differ by ethnicity or socio-economic background.

Given that obesity carries a significant social burden in the form of stigmatisation, social rejection and public humiliation, it would be expected to have negative consequences for body image, self-esteem and mood. This could be especially important in adolescence, when appearance is particularly salient to self-image. Adolescence is a stage of life at which identities are being formed, so the effects may be life long. In 1985, the National Institutes of Health highlighted the devastating psychosocial consequences of obesity when they said, 'Obesity creates an enormous psychological burden...in terms of suffering, the burden may be the greatest adverse effect of obesity'.[6] Similar statements have appeared in recent guidelines for the treatment of obesity in the United Kingdom.

The aim of this paper is to review the evidence for adverse psychological consequences of obesity in childhood and adolescence and to consider the implications for healthcare professionals.

☐ OBESITY AND BODY IMAGE

Extensive literature is available on body image in children and young adults, largely stimulated by concerns raised in the 1970s about excessive weight preoccupation and dieting in young women. In the adolescent sample described above, a small sex difference was seen in perceived weight at baseline, with more girls than boys feeling overweight. The most surprising observation, however, was that even among the obese adolescents, the proportion who selected 'I am very overweight' was only 25%.

More significant for understanding the psychological costs of obesity are measures of hedonic rather than perceptual appraisal – how people feel about their appearance rather than the size they believe themselves to be. This can be a simple rating of body dissatisfaction or a more complex psychometric measure looking at 'body esteem'. In a review of the literature, Ricciardelli and McCabe concluded that consistent findings show an inverse relation between body mass index and body dissatisfaction, with the strongest effects seen in girls.[7] Since that review was published, about a dozen large studies have supported this conclusion.[8] Body dissatisfaction may be slightly lower in black than white American adolescents, and similar ethnic differences are seen in British adolescents.

Teasing seems to be one of the strongest determinants of dissatisfaction, suggesting that family and school tolerance for teasing and bullying might contribute to a milieu in which overweight and obese children develop a negative self-image. Most importantly, body dissatisfaction is associated with higher levels of binge eating,[9] which indicates that its effects go beyond the impact on self-image.

☐ SELF-ESTEEM

The 'looking glass' or 'self-reflected appraisal' model proposes that self-esteem is a reflection of how we think others see us. This implies that self-esteem should be dramatically lower in obese people because of teasing and social exclusion. However, two reviews of the literature have indicated surprisingly weak associations between obesity and self-esteem,[10,11] with many studies finding no association with body size. Effects are larger when the measure of self-esteem includes 'body esteem', reflecting the established association with body image. There is also a suggestion that effects were stronger in adolescents than children of younger ages, and slightly more consistent in girls than boys. The picture has not changed greatly since these reviews: some studies find modest associations between obesity, self-esteem and weight, and some find no effects.[8] The conclusion of the community studies has to be that obese children and adolescents are able to feel pride in their abilities outside of the domain of body shape, just like normal-weight children, and although there might be a small effect on average, most overweight and obese children have self-esteem scores within the normal range.

Several studies have shown that body dissatisfaction is associated with lower self-esteem. Our studies have shown the same: obese adolescents who are not dissatisfied with their appearance do not have lower self-esteem. This suggests that introjection of the social view of a larger body size as unacceptable is a necessary step before adverse effects on self-esteem.[12]

In general, findings from clinical samples show lower levels of self-esteem in obese children than in obese or normal-weight community controls.[13] People who seek treatment for obesity have been found to be more distressed than those who do not,[14] which may account for these findings. Alternatively, when a person is singled out for treatment, this could induce feelings of lower self-esteem by implying personal responsibility for the obesity and personal failure in not controlling it. Nevertheless, even among clinical samples, the mean self-esteem of obese children is not always lower than that of controls,[15] although mean scores may mask significant problems in some people.[16]

☐ DEPRESSION

Depression is the most serious of the potential psychological consequences of childhood obesity. As with the self-esteem connection, the idea that obese children have high rates of depression seems to be well entrenched – at least in the media – but the epidemiological evidence again gives little support. Studies of community samples of adolescents and young adults generally failed to find an association between depression and obesity.[17] One exception was a longitudinal study, in which the results were negative for cross-sectional analyses, but boys who were obese at all four time points between childhood and late adolescence had a very slightly higher prevalence of depression.[18] Another community study found a small correlation between body mass index and depressive symptoms in girls but not boys, but no data were presented on the obese subgroup *per se*.[19]

Friedman and Brownell found a very small association between obesity and depression, but they hypothesised that sex, socio-economic status or ethnicity could be moderating variables.[11] We tested this hypothesis in two community studies of adolescents. We found a small association between obesity and depression in both samples, but the effect sizes did not differ by sex, ethnicity or socio-economic status. Analysis of the results in terms of the odds ratio for having a depression score in the clinical range showed that, as expected, being female or coming from a lower socio-economic background raised the risk of depression, but no effect at all was seen for obese adolescents compared with those with a normal-weight status.[20]

Rates of psychological disorders are considerably higher in clinical samples of obese children and adolescents.[21] In one of the few studies to have included both clinical and population samples of obese young people, the clinical group were significantly more depressed than non-obese controls, but no difference was seen between obese and non-obese community controls.[22] Another similar study also found increased rates of depression in clinical groups, while the non-clinical obese group did not differ from normal-weight controls in diagnoses of depression according to the *Diagnostic and statistical manual of mental disorders*, although they had very slightly higher scores on the Children's Depression Inventory.[13] It is worth noting, however, that obese control groups often have significantly lower body mass indexes than clinical groups.[13,23]

The most likely explanation for the differences in results between clinical and community samples is that obese children and adolescents who are depressed are more likely to present for treatment. This is not surprising, because depression could motivate the child or parents to seek help. Depressed people also evaluate many aspects of themselves and their circumstances negatively, as part of the depressive cognitive style, so this could extend to any weight problem. What needs to be considered is whether the obesity–depression association seen in clinical settings should be interpreted as a coincidental comorbidity or different facets of one problem. In light of the consistently negative findings in the community studies, we have to conclude that obesity *per se* does not significantly raise the risk of depression. The number of extremely obese children in most community samples will always be low, however, and where concurrent disease and severe physical limitations exist, more powerful effects on psychological well-being could be present.

☐ CLINICAL IMPLICATIONS

The results discussed in this review confirm the significant social costs of obesity. On average, obese children are less popular at school; are more likely to be bullied (or to bully), teased and humiliated over their weight; are discriminated against in their educational or occupational options; and have more difficulty dating and eventually marrying. Most obese children and adolescents are aware of the fact that they are fat and know that they fall short of prevailing standards of beauty. Notwithstanding this appalling array of social handicaps, the evidence is that obese children express pride in other aspects of their appearance and abilities and the impact on global self-esteem is comparatively small. In addition, although obese children in community samples might score very slightly higher on measures of depressed mood than normal-weight children, the proportion that meets any clinical criterion is not increased.

These findings raise several important questions:

☐ How is it possible that the severe social burden of obesity does not translate into serious psychological consequences?

☐ Why is belief that obesity is linked with lower self-esteem and depression so widespread given the paucity of scientific support for this association?

☐ What are the implications for treatment?

The apparent resilience of obese children is reminiscent of findings from children with other disfiguring conditions. Studies of young people with visible disorders, such as port-wine stains, jug ears or cleft palates, generally concur that although their opinion of their body image is more negative, the disfigurement does not inevitably create the deeper sense of low self-worth that could be expected to lead to depression.[22] Members of stigmatised groups have been shown to have ways of protecting their view of themselves, and this might also apply in the case of obesity. One method is for the person to regard the impact of obesity on their appearance as less severe than others' perceptions. This may come from reassurance that they receive from family and friends that they have, for example, other compensatory attractive characteristics. The issue has never been investigated systematically in obese children or adolescents, but it may prove a useful avenue of research.

The survival of the 'myth' of the psychological burden of obesity is a striking phenomenon. One possible explanation is that clinicians help to perpetuate this myth as a consequence of seeing obese children who are disproportionately likely to be depressed, which understandably creates the impression that the two conditions are related closely. In addition, we all share the negative stereotyping of obese people[3] – one facet of which is to attribute them with emotional difficulties. We might therefore 'see' emotional problems that are not there, as a consequence of the biasing effect of the social stereotype.

What are the implications for treatment and prevention? First, it is critical to assess self-esteem or depression objectively before drawing any conclusion about individual patients. Obese patients who are depressed should be treated appropriately, with behavioural or pharmacological treatments, rather than being assumed to be depressed as an inevitable consequence of obesity. Second, health professionals should avoid comments or judgements that imply that obesity is unattractive or unacceptable; obese patients are vulnerable to comments from significant others, and the doctor's appraisal can affect both their self-image and their attitude to treatment. With children, it may be possible to build elements designed to enhance physical confidence and self-esteem into a treatment programme. For example, many severely obese children will have been excluded from sports at school or have avoided sports lessons, which can mean their athletic competencies are even more limited than necessary. Additional skill training or encouragement to take up sports where a large body mass is helpful (such as shot-putting) can provide a boost to self-confidence.

Part of the negative stereotyping of obesity comes from the notion that obese people are lazy, greedy or generally lacking in self-control. Medical science has shown beyond any doubt that obesity is a strikingly genetically determined condition. The 'explanation' for why one person is obese while another living in an equally 'obeseogenic' environment is lean is largely that the two are different genetically. Our data on childhood obesity from a large twin study show that differences in body mass index at age five years are accounted for 60% by genetics and 40% by environment.[24] By adulthood, the genetic component is higher, while the shared environment effect is lower.[25] The fact that genes contribute so significantly to adiposity does not mean that weight cannot be modified – after all, most of the children who are obese now would not have been obese if they had been raised in the 1950s – but it does mean that obese children have to work exceptionally hard to stay out of positive energy balance. Our clinical experience is that children and parents welcome information on the genetic contribution to obesity. Attribution of some of the problem to genes can take away some of the 'blame' and promote wellbeing in the child and family.

Finally, the larger issue of social attitudes to obesity and tolerance of the discrimination, social exclusion and cruelty that can damage the lives of obese children needs to be considered. Neither families nor schools should permit teasing about weight. Teasing a child in a wheelchair would not be tolerated and the same attitude should be taken to other disabilities, including obesity.

REFERENCES

1   Puhl R, Brownell KD. Bias, discrimination, and obesity. *Obes Res* 2001;**9**:788–805.

2   Wardle J, Volz C, Golding C. Social variation in attitudes to obesity in children. *Int J Obes Relat Metab Disord* 1995;**19**:562–9.

3   Teachman BA, Brownell KD. Implicit anti-fat bias among health professionals: is anyone immune? *Int J Obes Relat Metab Disord* 2001;**25**:1525–31.

4   Gortmaker SL, Must A, Perrin JM, Sobol AM *et al.* Social and economic consequences of overweight in adolescence and young adulthood. *N Engl J Med* 1993;**329**:1008–12.

5   Wardle J, Jarvis MJ, Steggles N, Sutton S *et al.* Socioeconomic disparities in cancer-risk behaviors in adolescence: baseline results from the Health and Behaviour in Teenagers Study (HABITS). *Prev Med* 2003;**36**:721–30.

6   Ricciardelli LA, McCabe MP. Children's body image concerns and eating disturbance: a review of the literature. *Clin Psychol Rev* 2001;**21**:325–44.

7   National Institutes of Health. What is the evidence that obesity has adverse effects on health? In: *Health implications of obesity. NIH consensus statement online 1985 Feb 11–13*. Bethesda: National Institutes of Health, 1985. www.ncbi.nlm.nih.gov/books/bv.fcgi?rid=hstat4.section.1103 (last accessed 7 February 2005)

8   Wardle J, Cooke L. The impact of obesity on psychological well-being. In: Sabin M, Hamilton-Shield J (eds), *Childhood obesity*. Oxford: Elsevier, 2005.

9   Wardle J, Waller J, Rapoport L. Body dissatisfaction and binge eating in obese women: the role of restraint and depression. *Obes Res* 2001;**9**:778–87.

10 French SA, Story M, Perry CL. Self-esteem and obesity in children and adolescents: a literature review. *Obes Res* 1995;**3**:479–90.

11 Friedman MA, Brownell KD. Psychological correlates of obesity: moving to the next research generation. *Psychol Bull* 1995;**117**:3–20.

12 Sands ER, Wardle J. Internalization of ideal body shapes in 9–12-year-old girls. *Int J Eat Disord* 2003;**33**:193–204.

13 Erermis S, Cetin N, Tamar M, Bukusoglu N *et al.* Is obesity a risk factor for psychopathology among adolescents? *Pediatr Int* 2004;**46**:296–301.

14 Fitzgibbon ML, Stolley MR, Kirschenbaum DS. Obese people who seek treatment have different characteristics than those who do not seek treatment. *Health Psychol* 1993;**12**:342–5.

15 Israel AC, Ivanova MY. Global and dimensional self-esteem in preadolescent and early adolescent children who are overweight: age and gender differences. *Int J Eat Disord* 2002;**31**:424–9.

16 Zeller MH, Saelens BE, Roehrig H, Kirk S *et al.* Psychological adjustment of obese youth presenting for weight management treatment. *Obes Res* 2004;**12**:1576–86.

17 Eisenberg ME, Neumark-Sztainer D, Story M. Associations of weight-based teasing and emotional well-being among adolescents. *Arch Pediatr Adolesc Med* 2003;**157**:733–8.

18 Mustillo S, Worthman C, Erkanli A, Keeler G *et al.* Obesity and psychiatric disorder: developmental trajectories. *Pediatrics* 2003;**111**:851–9.

19 Erickson SJ, Robinson TN, Haydel KF, Killen JD. Are overweight children unhappy?: body

mass index, depressive symptoms, and overweight concerns in elementary school children. *Arch Pediatr Adolesc Med* 2000;**154**:931–5.

20   Wardle J, Williamson S, Johnson F, Edwards C. The psychological consequences of obesity in adolescence: cultural moderators of the obesity-depression association. *Int J Obes* (submitted).

21   Vila G, Zipper E, Dabbas M, Bertrand C *et al.* Mental disorders in obese children and adolescents. *Psychosom Med* 2004;**66**:387–94.

22   Britz B, Siegfried W, Ziegler A, Lamertz C *et al.* Rates of psychiatric disorders in a clinical study group of adolescents with extreme obesity and in obese adolescents ascertained via a population based study. *Int J Obes Relat Metab Disord* 2000;**24**:1707–14.

23   Crocker J, Cornwell B, Major B. The stigma of overweight: affective consequences of attributional ambiguity. *J Pers Soc Psychol* 1993;**64**:60–70.

24   Koeppen-Schomerus G, Wardle J, Plomin R. A genetic analysis of weight and overweight in 4-year-old twin pairs. *Int J Obes Relat Metab Disord* 2001;**25**:838–44.

25   Maes HH, Neale MC, Eaves LJ. Genetic and environmental factors in relative body weight and human adiposity. *Behav Genet* 1997;**27**:325–51.

☐ OBESITY SELF ASSESSMENT QUESTIONS

Psychosocial burden of obesity in children

1   The following factors have been proposed as moderating variables of the relation between depression and obesity:
  (a) Sex
  (b) Ethnicity
  (c) Socioeconomic status
  (d) Marital status
  (e) Duration of obesity

2   Obese people are often stereotyped as:
  (a) Weak-willed
  (b) Stupid
  (c) Happy
  (d) Selfish
  (e) Kind

3   Most obese children and adolescents:
  (a) Are depressed
  (b) Are dissatisfied with their body shape
  (c) Are teased at school
  (d) Have low self esteem
  (e) Know that they are obese

Immunosuppression

Immunosuppressive drugs in renal transplantation

Anthony Warrens

☐ INTRODUCTION

Immunosuppression in renal transplantation used to be relatively simple! When renal transplantation first became routine in the 1960s, the only effective available therapy was the combination of corticosteroids and azathioprine. By the early 1980s, a third new agent, ciclosporin, had been introduced and showed a marked reduction in rejection. This then became the standard therapy for the next 10 years or more. The principal variation around this time was whether this triple therapy was supplemented with an antibody; polyclonal antilymphocyte preparations (such as antilymphocyte globulin) and the monoclonal antibody OKT3, which is specific for the ε chain of CD3, were introduced variably, depending on an individual's perceived immunological risk. The threshold for their use was set rather higher in Europe than in North America, where antibody induction often was regarded as 'standard' therapy. These antibody preparations also were used to treat intractable rejection, and still are, when pulsed intravenous steroids proved ineffective.

All this changed, however, in the latter half of the last decade, when an amazing burgeoning of new therapeutic options occurred. Some of these represented only minor variations in what then was available, but others genuinely represented novel therapeutic strategies:

☐ Calcineurin inhibitors (CNIs):
  • A new microemulsion formulation of ciclosporin (Neoral™) superseded Sandimmune™ and offered more reliable pharmacokinetics for this drug which has a notoriously narrow therapeutic window.
  • Tacrolimus was introduced – this is a different molecule with a similar mechanism of action.

☐ Antimetabolites:
  • The mycophenolic acid (MPA) prodrug, mycophenolate mofetil (MMF), was introduced as an alternative to the purine antagonist azathioprine. A second MPA prodrug, mycophenolate sodium, has now also been developed.

☐ Interleukin 2 (IL-2) receptor blockers:
  • Two monoclonal antibodies specific for the α chain (CD25) of the IL-2 receptor were introduced – basiliximab and daclizumab. Both had been produced as a result of recombinant DNA technology.

☐ Mammalian target of rapamycin (mTOR) inhibitors:
  • Sirolimus (originally known as rapamycin) and the more recently introduced everolimus inhibit this molecule, which helps the T lymphocyte to enter the cell cycle on receipt of the signal generated when IL-2 reacts with its surface receptor.

Fig 1 summarises the timescale of these developments:

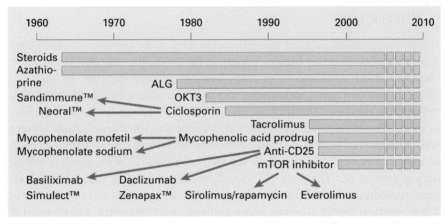

Fig 1 Development of immunosuppression in renal transplantation. Timeline of the introduction of immunosuppressive drugs currently used in renal transplantation. A line begins at the introduction of the first agent of a given class, and currently available agents are shown adjacent to the label.

This considerable increase in the number of therapeutic options clearly provides management opportunities that previously were not available. The rapidity with which these drugs were introduced, however, means that it has not been possible to conduct the rational sequential comparisons that ideally would have been performed. Rather, the drive to introduce them often has been commercial or anecdotal. This issue was underscored by the survey of immunosuppressive practice undertaken in 2002 by the British Transplantation Society in preparation for its submission to the National Institute for Clinical Excellence. This showed that the 20 units surveyed in the United Kingdom were using 10 different immunosuppressive regimens (www.bts.org). Clearly, no 'standard therapy' for recipients of renal transplants exists in 2005. Almost all agents currently in use, however, act, at least in part, by inhibiting part of the sequence of T-cell activation (Fig 2). This allows for an immunologically rational approach to the development of regimens.

☐ DEVELOPMENTS IN EXISTING CLASSES OF IMMUNOSUPPRESSIVE DRUGS

Calcineurin inhibitors (CNIs)

Rather to the surprise of the transplantation community, the microemulsion preparation of Ciclosporin (Neoral™) in some studies was associated with

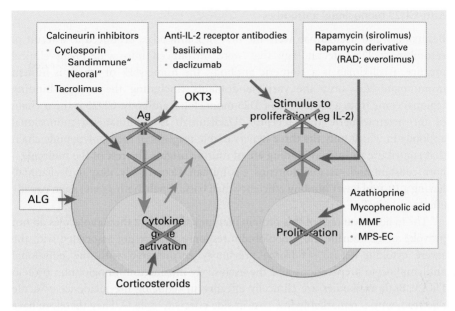

Fig 2 Sites of action of currently used immunosuppressive drugs on the activation cascade of the helper T lymphocyte. Two helper T cells are depicted for ease of illustration. The cascade of activation is illustrated in red arrows: antigen (Ag) is recognised and a signal is transduced to the nucleus, where a range of cytokine genes are activated. One such cytokine, interleukin 2 (IL-2), is secreted and binds to its receptor on the surfaces of secreting and other cells. This generates another signal that causes cell proliferation and, as a result, activation. The points at which each class of drug acts is shown with a red cross. ALG = antilymphocyte globulin (representing all polyclonal sera in use); MMF = mycophenolate mofetil; MPS-EC = enteric coated mycophenolate sodium.

improved graft outcome not merely easier pharmacokinetics.[1] Initially, however, it proved somewhat harder to show a significant difference between tacrolimus and ciclosporin. The early hope that tacrolimus would display less nephrotoxicity was not borne out, although the pattern of side effects of the two agents is different. For a while, choice of side-effect profile became the principal clinical driving force for some units when determining which of the two agents to prescribe. For example, if the hirsutism or gingival overgrowth common with ciclosporin proved intolerable, the patient might be switched to tacrolimus. Conversely, patients with tacrolimus-associated alopecia might be converted to ciclosporin. Increasing evidence also shows that ciclosporin is associated with more hypertension and hyperlipidaemia than tacrolimus,[2] an issue potentially of great importance given the dominance of vascular disease in the long-term outcome after transplantation. It now is becoming clear, however, that tacrolimus is a more potent immunosuppressive drug with a lower incidence of acute rejection generally and of refractory, steroid-resistant acute rejection in particular.[3] Increasingly, therefore, tacrolimus is the CNI of choice in patients at significant immunological risk, whereas ciclosporin is sometimes seen as the CNI of choice in patients perceived at risk of overzealous immunosuppression.

Anti-CD25 monoclonal antibodies

Basiliximab and daclizumab were the first two antibodies produced as a result of recombinant DNA technology that were introduced into widespread clinical practice. Basiliximab is a chimeric antibody, the framework of which is human immunoglobulin; only the variable domains (including the antigen-binding regions) come from a mouse anti-CD25 monoclonal antibody. CD25 is the α chain of the heterotrimeric IL-2 receptor. Daclizumab is a humanised monoclonal antibody in which only the three hypervariable reagents of each polypeptide chain that contribute to antigen binding are of murine origin. The rest of the molecule – both constant and variable domains – is human. Remarkably, despite daclizumab having a 10-fold lower binding efficiency than basiliximab, both agents seem equally effective clinically.

The major advantage of this protein manipulation is that these molecules do not provoke an antimurine immunoglobulin response and are not associated with the severe cytokine-release syndrome previously encountered with the polyclonal antilymphocyte preparations and the exclusively murine immunoglobulin protein OKT3. Both antibodies are clinically effective in reducing the incidence of acute rejection, with a remarkably low cost in side effects to date.[4,5] They therefore have very rapidly found a place as induction agents in patients perceived to require rather more immunosuppression. The use of these agents is still increasing.

Antimetabolites

The introduction of MMF as an alternative to azathioprine clearly presented a significant improvement in terms of decreased acute rejection. This was shown in three very large multicentre trials that involved almost 1500 patients.[6] Mycophenolate mofetil represents a significant theoretical advantage over azathioprine. The latter is a competitive antagonist of purine synthesis, while MMF is a prodrug of mycophenolic acid (MPA), which is a non-competitive inhibitor of one enzyme in the guanylate monophosphate (GMP) synthetic pathway. This enzyme, inosine monophosphate dehydrogenase (IMPDH), is part of the 'de novo' pathway of GMP synthesis that focuses the antimetabolite activity on lymphocytes rather than other purine synthetic cells. In addition, MPA has greater activity against the type II isoform of IMPDH, which is the dominant form in activated lymphocytes. In other words, this agent's action is more focused on the cell in which immunosuppression is particularly needed in the transplant scenario – the activated lymphocyte. Most experience with this agent has been with MMF, although a second MPA prodrug, mycophenolate sodium, recently became available.

mTOR inhibitors

Sirolimus, originally know as rapamycin, is the prototype drug in this group. It has a different mechanism of action to any of the other classes of immunosuppressive drugs previously mentioned. It inhibits the so-called 'third signal' of T-cell activation generated by the engagement of IL-2 with its receptor. This inhibition prevents the cell entering the cell cycle and proliferating. As it was not an obvious replacement for any single pre-existing drug or class of drug, it has taken some time to work out the role of this agent. Initial studies envisaged it as a replacement for azathioprine or MMF or as adjunct to CNI and steroid therapy. Certainly, in this context, it was found to contribute additional immunosuppression – for example, by decreasing acute rejection.[7]

More recent studies, however, have shown that it can replace CNIs when used with MMF and steroids.[8] This offers the major advantage of allowing the circumvention of CNI-related nephrotoxicity; however, its role remains unclear. An alternative mTOR inhibitor, everolimus (previously known as rapamycin-derivative (RAD)) also became available recently.

☐ DEVELOPMENTS IN NEW CLASSES OF IMMUNOSUPPRESSIVE DRUGS

As if the above list was not enough, several additional immunosuppressive drugs are at a fairly mature stage in preclinical and clinical development. Alemtuzumab (Campath-IH) is another monoclonal antibody and is specific for the small molecule CD52 (whose function is unknown). It has been shown to generate profound immunosuppression in the transplant context.[9] Consequently, this is hoped to allow avoidance of some of the other drugs and their adverse effects.

FTY720 is particularly interesting, as it does not focus on inhibiting the activation process of T cells. Rather, it modulates lymphocyte migratory patterns. It has been shown to be effective in reducing rejection in clinical renal transplantation.[10]

Finally, a group of agents are being developed to inhibit pyrimidine synthesis. One of these is based on leflunomide – a drug well known to rheumatologists – and it too has been shown to be efficacious in renal transplantation.[11]

This list of new drugs could go on for page after page and no doubt will do so in future articles such as this.

☐ REFOCUSING THE APPROACH TO IMMUNOSUPPRESSION

Over the last 20 years, we have become extremely good at decreasing acute rejection. Indeed, it is now very unusual to lose a graft to acute rejection. Some evidence, however, suggests that we have allowed the balance between adequate immunosuppression and avoidance of the adverse effects of these drugs to swing too far towards minimising rejection. The most common cause of graft loss is now death of recipients with functioning transplants. The most common cause of this premature death is cardiovascular disease. The second most common cause of graft loss is chronic allograft nephropathy. This term has rather superseded 'chronic rejection', as this process is now recognised not necessarily to be predominantly immunological. Indeed, many of the problems are vascular and are, at least in part, contributed by the immunosuppressive drugs used.

Accordingly, the focus in managing these patients is now on decreasing the level of immunosuppression, but no unanimity exists about the priorities in this process. Many people favour the withdrawal of corticosteroids as early as possible – indeed, some people are now transplanting people with no or minimal steroids. On the other hand, some people believe that the principal villain in this piece is the CNI, because of its associated chronic nephrotoxicity. That is why many people are focusing on the use of more potent immunosuppressive agents, such as MMF or sirolimus, as adjunctive therapy to minimise or eliminate the need for CNIs. Where consensus will fall in this debate remains unclear, but the battle of immunosuppression of the renal transplant recipient certainly will continue over the next few years.

One final point that relates to the phenomenon of chronic allograft nephropathy derives from the prominence of fibrosis in this pathological process. Mycophenolate mofetil and sirolimus are known to have antifibrotic effects, and tacrolimus may be less profibrotic than ciclosporin. Indeed, coronary artery stents impregnated with sirolimus have been shown to decrease the rate of restenosis after percutaneous transluminal angioplasty.[12] This contributes an additional fillip to altering the profile of immunosuppression.

□ CONCLUSION

This is an exciting time in the immunotherapy of patients who undergo renal transplants. More opportunities are available in 2005 than ever before in the history of renal transplantation. We have the opportunity of offering our patients the customised immunotherapeutic regimen that best meets the changing needs of their transplant. This hopefully will lead to a prolongation of the life of these transplants and, therefore, of their recipients.

REFERENCES

1   Shah MB, Martin JE, Schroeder TJ, First MR. The evaluation of the safety and tolerability of two formulations of cyclosporine: neoral and sandimmune. A meta-analysis. *Transplantation* 1999;**67**:1411–7.

2   Baid-Agrawal S, Delmonico FL, Tolkoff-Rubin NE, Farrell M *et al.* Cardiovascular risk profile after conversion from cyclosporine A to tacrolimus in stable renal transplant recipients. *Transplantation* 2004;**77**:1199–202.

3   Margreiter R. Efficacy and safety of tacrolimus compared with ciclosporin microemulsion in renal transplantation: a randomised multicentre study. *Lancet* 2002;**359**:741–6.

4   Nashan B, Moore R, Amlot P, Schmidt AG *et al.* Randomised trial of basiliximab versus placebo for control of acute cellular rejection in renal allograft recipients. *Lancet* 1997; **350**:1193–8.

5   Vincenti F, Kirkman R, Light S, Bumgardner G *et al.* Interleukin-2-receptor blockade with daclizumab to prevent acute rejection in renal transplantation. *N Engl J Med* 1998;**338**:161–5.

6   Halloran P, Mathew T, Tomlanovich S, Groth C *et al.* Mycophenolate mofetil in renal allograft recipients: a pooled efficacy analysis of three randomized, double-blind, clinical studies in prevention of rejection. *Transplantation* 1997;**63**:39–47.

7   Kahan BD. Efficacy of sirolimus compared with azathioprine for reduction of acute renal allograft rejection: a randomised multicentre study. *Lancet* 2000;**356**:194–202.

8   Groth CG, Backman L, Morales JM, Calne R *et al.* Sirolimus (rapamycin)-based therapy in human renal transplantation: similar efficacy and different toxicity compared with cyclosporine. *Transplantation* 1999;**67**:1036–42.

9   Knechtle SJ, Fernandez LA, Pirsch JD, Becker BN *et al.* Campath-1H in renal transplantation: the University of Wisconsin experience. *Surgery* 2004;**136**:754–60.

10   Tedesco-Silva H, Mourad G, Kahan BD, Boira JG *et al.* FTY720, a novel immunomodulator: efficacy and safety results from the first phase 2A study in de novo renal transplantation. *Transplantation* 2004;77:1826–33.

11   Williams JW, Mital D, Chong A, Kottayil A *et al.* Experiences with leflunomide in solid organ transplantation. *Transplantation* 2002;73:358–66.

12   Fajadet J, Morice MC, Bode C, Barragan P *et al.* Maintenance of long-term clinical benefit with sirolimus-eluting coronary stents: three-year results of the RAVEL trial. *Circulation* 2005;111:1040–4.

Biological agents

David Isenberg

□ INTRODUCTION

Nearly fifty years have passed since 6-mercaptopurine was shown to inhibit antibody synthesis and allograft rejection[1] in laboratory animals.[2] This drug – an inhibitor of purine metabolism – and its analogue azathioprine, subsequently were used to prevent rejection of organ grafts. The use of these drugs heralded the era of immunological intervention as a means of treating, not just failure of organ transplantation, but a wide range of autoimmune diseases from organ-specific conditions such as polymyositis to non-organ-specific disorders such as systemic lupus erythematosus. Although successful in many conditions, and on occasion life saving, the problem with these drugs (and corticosteroids, which had been introduced a little earlier by Hench and colleagues[3]) is their non-specific 'nature', which leads to a high frequency of side effects. These side effects include an increased predisposition to infection; bone-marrow toxicity; potential harm to the fetus (limiting their use in pregnant patients); and, in the case of steroids, an increased risk of hypertension, diabetes and osteoporosis.

Not surprisingly, therefore, in the past two decades the search has been on for the kind of 'magic bullet' first envisaged by Ehrlich when he developed the notion of antibodies as a chemical that might bind to and specifically kill microbes or tumour cells. Like many truly original ideas, his thoughts about the nature of antibodies were virtually ignored for half a century. A reappraisal of his work and advances in technology combined to confirm the broad truth of his assertion.

□ RECENT DEVELOPMENTS

The past decade has seen the remarkable development of a new generation of biological disease-modifying agents that increasingly consist of humanised monoclonal antibodies or receptor antagonists targeted against specific cytokines or cell-surface molecules. The hope, not entirely borne out in practice, has been that more specific targeting would provide more effective and safer treatments than the traditional immunosuppressive drugs.

Among the successful examples of this sort of targeting, Miller et al showed that the number of new cerebral lesions in patients with multiple sclerosis was statistically significantly reduced when a monoclonal antibody (natalizumab) that binds to α_4 intergrin was used.[4] Likewise, Lebwohl and colleagues showed that efalizumab – an antibody that binds to LFA1 (CD11A) – could be strikingly effective in patients with psoriasis.[5] It is in the subspecialty of rheumatology, however, that biological agents have had the biggest impact. Since the earliest demonstrations, in the mid-Nineties, that blocking TNF-α was highly effective in reducing inflammation and synovitis,[6,7] three TNF-α blockers (infliximab, etanercept and adalimumab) have become widely available and are used routinely in the treatment of rheumatoid arthritis. For financial reasons (these drugs cost around £10,000 per patient per year), the drugs are restricted to patients who have failed two conventional 'so-called' disease-modifying drugs [reviewed in 'Rheumatoid arthritis – management'[8]]. They seem to work best in conjunction with methotrexate, and increasing evidence shows that this combination of drugs genuinely reduces the previously inexorable passage of patients with rheumatoid arthritis from inflammatory synovitis to multiple bone erosion with frequent requirements for surgery, including joint replacement. Increasing pressure to use these drugs much earlier in the course of rheumatoid arthritis seems highly likely. Increasing evidence also shows that they are effective in patients with psoriatic arthritis and ankylosing spondylitis. Intriguingly, blockade of TNF-α, notably using infliximab, also has been shown to be of benefit in patients with Crohn's disease.[9]

The blocking of other targets including interleukin 1 (using anakinra) and a recombinant interleukin (IL) 1 receptor antagonist has been shown to be effective clinically and to reduce the rate of joint erosion.[8] This approach has not proved to be as effective as TNF-α blockade, however, and is more troublesome for the patient, as it has to be given daily. Blockade of IL-6 also may turn out to be more effective in patients with rheumatoid arthritis.

In November 1997, a genetically engineered chimeric monoclonal antibody that blocks the CD20 antigen (a pan B-cell surface glycoprotein that appears at the pre-B stage and disappears during differentiation into plasma cells) was approved by the American Food and Drug Administration for the treatment of non-Hodgkin's lymphoma. More than 300,000 patients around the world have been treated with this drug, which has been used as a single agent and in combination with chemo-therapeutics and immunoadjuvants such as interferon alpha 2a, IL-2 and granulocyte–macrophage colony-stimulating factor. When combined with chemo-therapeutics, the anti-CD20 antibody rituximab has response rates in 81–97% of patients with non-Hodgkin's lymphoma and induces complete remission in 34–74% [reviewed in 'Rituximab therapy for follicular lymphoma: a comprehensive review of its efficacy as primary treatment, treatment for relapsed disease, re-treatment and maintenance'[10]]. Going against the 'T-cell grail', Edwards and colleagues have encouraged the belief that B cells play a critical role in the development of rheumatoid arthritis. It was logical therefore for them to use rituximab as a therapy for this condition. In a recently published double-blind controlled trial, more than 40% of patients with rheumatoid arthritis treated with rituximab in combination with methotrexate or cyclophosphamide achieved a notable response rate designated ACR 50.[11] As reported in cancer trials, adverse events with rituximab were of only mild or moderate intensity and often resolved without complications. As this approach requires just two infusions of rituximab, which may last for periods of around a year, this treatment is potentially advantageous for patients with rheumatoid arthritis compared with the TNF-α blockers: etanercept, for example, involves twice-weekly self-administered injections, while infliximab is given as an infusion once every four to eight weeks.

Given the success of rituximab in the treatment of rheumatoid arthritis, it was logical to extend this approach to patients with systemic lupus erythematosus (SLE), which is acknowledged widely to be strongly mediated by antibodies. Indeed, a number of small open-label trials [reviewed in 'Anti B cell therapy (rituximab) in the treatment of autoimmune diseases'[12]] have indicated the likely benefit of this approach. The capacity of B-cell depletion (induced by a combination of rituximab, cyclophosphamide and steroids) to improve a wide range of the clinical features of SLE and to lower DNA antibody and urine protein:creatinine ratios in patients with SLE who fail conventional immunosuppressive therapy has been impressive. A double-blind controlled trial of this therapy is being planned.

□ SUMMARY

Biological therapy offers the major potential advance of highly targeted intervention that cannot be achieved with more 'classic' immunosuppression. We are in the relative early days of this type of treatment, however, and the long-term side effects of, for example, TNF-α blockade, still need to be established. Nevertheless, to date, biological therapies do seem to offer a very useful advance in a wide variety of autoimmune diseases, notably in patients for whom conventional immunosuppression clearly is inadequate.

REFERENCES

1 Schwartz R, Stack J, Dameshak W. Effect of 6-mercaptopurine on antibody production. *Proc Soc Exp Biol Med* 1958;**99**:164–7.

2 Schwartz R, Dameshak W. The effects of 6-mercaptopurine on homograft reactions. *J Clin Invest* 1960;**39**:952–8.

3 Hench PS, Kendall EC, Slocumb CH, Polley HF. Effects of a hormone on the adrenal cortex (17 hydroxy-II dehydrocorticosterone compound E) and of pituitary adrenocorticotrophic hormone on rheumatoid arthritis. *Ann Rheum Dis* 1949;**8**:97–104.

4 Miller DH, Khan OA, Sheremata WA *et al.* A controlled trial of natalizumab for relapsing multiple sclerosis. *N Engl J Med* 2003;**348**:15–23.

5 Lebwohl M, Tyring SK, Hamilton TK *et al.* A novel targeted T-cell modulator, efalizumab, for plaque psoriasis. *N Engl J Med* 2003;**349**:2004–13.

6 Elliott MJ, Maini RN, Feldmann M *et al.* Randomised double-blind comparison of chimeric monoclonal antibody to tumour necrosis factor alpha (cA2) versus placebo in rheumatoid arthritis. *Lancet* 1994;**344**:1105–10.

7 Rankin EC, Choy EH, Kassimos D *et al.* The therapeutic effects of an engineered human anti-tumour necrosis factor alpha antibody (CDP571) in rheumatoid arthritis. *Br J Rheum* 1995;**34**:334–42.

8 Bingham SJ, Quinn MA, Emery P. Rheumatoid arthritis – management. In: Maddison PJ, Isenberg DA, Woo P *et al*, *Oxford textbook of rheumatology*. Oxford: Oxford University Press, 2004:719–32.

9 Dhillon S, Loftus EV. Medical therapy of Crohn's disease. *Curr Treat Options Gastroenterol* 2005;**8**:19–30.

10   Cohen Y, Solal-Celigny P, Polliack A. Rituximab therapy for follicular lymphoma: a comprehensive review of its efficacy as primary treatment, treatment for relapsed disease, re-treatment and maintenance. *Haematologica* 2003:**88**;811–23.

11   Edwards JC, Szczepanski L, Szehinski J *et al.* Efficacy of B-cell-targeted therapy with rituximab in patients with rheumatoid arthritis. *N Engl J Med* 2004;**350**:2572–81.

12   Kazkaz H, Isenberg D. Anti B cell therapy (rituximab) in the treatment of autoimmune diseases. *Curr Opin Pharmacol* 2004;**4**:398–402.

Unwanted sequelae of immunosuppression

Gavin Spickett

☐ INTRODUCTION

Most of the adverse sequelae of immunosuppressive drugs relate to the immunosuppression itself. All of the drugs used also have other side effects, some of which can lead to severe organ toxicity. An awareness of the mode of action of the drugs is of material assistance in predicting adverse events and planning appropriate monitoring. Table 1 identifies the major problems that can arise.

☐ PRE-TREATMENT PLANNING

Before immunosuppressive drugs are used, pretreatment testing is desirable, as it may predict future problems and certainly gives a baseline against which subsequent changes can be evaluated. Appropriate testing is determined by the drug or drugs selected. Testing will include liver and renal function, blood cell counts and differential white cell counts: it is important that the differential white cell count – not just the total white cell count – is measured. Interpretation of baseline tests may be influenced by the disease being treated: for example, lymphopaenia and neutropaenia may be found commonly in active systemic lupus erythematosus as part of the autoimmune process and may be indicators for more rather than less immunosuppression.

Table 1 Types of adverse events during immunosuppression.

Idiosyncratic	Rashes, nausea, vomiting, etc.
Allergic	Anaphylaxis (biologics)
Secondary to mode of action	Infection: bacterial, mycobacterial, viral, fungal, parasitic
Autoimmune	Anti-TNF agents: generation of antinuclear and anti-ds-DNA antibodies; arthritis?
Bone-marrow suppression	Anaemia, thrombocytopenia, neutropenia
Neoplasia	Secondary to infection: lymphoma (Epstein-Barr virus) or cutaneous/cervical (human papillomavirus)
Organ-specific toxicity	Neuropathy (vincristine) Liver and kidney damage (ciclosporin, tacrolimus, methotrexate) Cardiac damage (tacrolimus) Haemorrhagic cystitis (cyclophosphamide) Lung damage (methotrexate)
Miscellaneous	Hypersensitivity/pyrexia of unknown origin (azathioprine)

TNF = tumour necrosis factor

Specific drugs may require specific testing. For example, measurement of thiopurine methyltransferase is valuable in predicting the side effects of azathioprine. Patients who are homozygously deficient for the enzyme will be at high risk of severe bone marrow toxicity from azathioprine, while heterozygous deficiency requires the standard dose to be halved. Because of the known toxicity of methotrexate, pretreatment chest radiograph and liver function tests are essential. Biologic agents, such as high-dose intravenous immunoglobulin, need special precautions in view of the side effects, and patients with impaired renal function, deficiency of immunoglobulin A and high levels of rheumatoid factors and cryoglobulins are at significantly increased risk of severe side effects. Highly lymphocytotoxic drugs such as rituximab and fludaribine merit baseline assessment of immunoglobulins and lymphocyte subsets (not just a total lymphocyte count). The risk of autoantibody generation by anti-tumour necrosis factor (TNF) agents means that baseline autoantibody screening is essential.

Knowledge of the patient's previous infection and immunisation status is critical. Pre-existent infection must be controlled before immunosuppression is started. Previous tuberculous infection, especially if treated inadequately, may merit regular prophylaxis. Likewise, the use of vaccination against varicella zoster virus may be appropriate. Any immunisation programme clearly must be carried out before the immunosuppression starts, but this may not be possible. It is critical that live vaccines are not used during immunosuppression because of the risks of dissemination and severe vaccine-induced disease. Close family contacts should also avoid live vaccines to avoid person-to-person transmission. Even after a course of immunosuppression has been completed, immune function may remain impaired significantly for years afterwards, so vaccination should be approached with caution. Although toxoid and subunit vaccines may be safe, they also may be useless. Annual vaccination against influenza is recommended for immunosuppressed people, but this is a group that it is hardly likely to benefit. More logical is to vaccinate all close contacts and give the patient a standby supply of an anti-influenza drug.

Patients, carers and the primary healthcare team must be aware of the risks of infection and the action to be taken if a patient on immunosuppressive drugs develops shingles, for example. Informed consent is essential, and patients must understand the risks and benefits. Evidence of the discussion must be recorded in the case notes. Other actions may be required: for example, sperm banking in men or consideration of ovarian conservation when drugs with a high incidence of infertility are used (such as cyclophosphamide).

□ MONITORING OF THERAPY

For each drug, a clear plan should be established to monitor side effects and efficacy. At the outset, clarity is needed about who will be responsible for prescribing and monitoring. General practitioners will not have expert knowledge of immunosuppressive drugs and therefore may refuse to prescribe these medications. Shared care guidelines may help, but these need to have clarity about monitoring and actions to be taken when results are obtained.

The reasons for monitoring need to be established: is it for toxicity, prediction of treatment failure or compliance? How will the results be acted upon and by whom? For example, will the results of monitoring CD4-positive T-cell counts influence the use of prophylaxis? Table 2 identifies the established risk thresholds in patients with human immunodeficiency virus (HIV) but which will apply to other immunosuppressed states.

Table 2 Risks of infection in relation to CD4+ T cell counts.

CD4+ T cell count (cells/mm³)	Infection
<400	Candida
<200	Pneumocystis carinii pneumonia
<100	Toxoplasmosis
<75	Atypical mycobacteria (mycobacteria avium intracellulare)
<50	Cytomegalovirus

When a programme for monitoring is selected, the correct parameters must be chosen. Use of total white count rarely is valuable, so a full differential count is needed. For example, a therapeutic effect is unlikely to be obtained with cyclophosphamide unless lymphopaenia is generated. The degree of lymphopaenia therefore must be monitored and set off against other bone marrow toxicity through observation of platelet and neutrophil counts. Monitoring of lymphocyte subsets certainly will be essential during the use of high-intensity immunosuppression with anti-OKT3, antilymphocyte globulin, alemtuzumab and rituximab, because it is essential to know that the target population has been removed by the dose administered and because considerable batch-to-batch variability exists. For agents predominantly active against B cells, monitoring of total immunoglobulins may be helpful but does not give any indication of actual antibody function. A detailed knowledge of the mode of actions of the drugs used therefore is critical to the planning of appropriate monitoring schedules. This also includes knowledge of the duration of action of the immunosuppressive drugs and, in particular, which axis of the immune system will be affected. The effects of tacrolimus and ciclosporin are rapidly reversible when the drugs are withdrawn, whereas the effects of cytotoxic drugs such as azathioprine and cyclophosphamide may persist for years after their withdrawal.

Other testing that may be relevant in the context of biologic agents will be for the development of the host's immune response against the agent. This may include antimouse antibodies when murine anti-OKT3 is used and anti-chimera antibodies when fusion molecules, such as etanercept, are used.

☐ DRUG MONITORING

Monitoring of drug levels is well established in the context of the use of ciclosporin and tacrolimus to prevent graft rejection. The value of drug monitoring when these drugs are used for the management of autoimmune disease is not well established, and many specialists do not bother because lower doses deemed not to present a significant risk of toxicity are used. Measurement of drug levels does have value, however, as it allows individualisation of the dosing and also enables compliance to be monitored. Personal experience has shown how widely trough levels vary in patients who receive similar weight-related doses. Trough levels are essential, and random levels have little value except to determine compliance. For immuno-suppression in autoimmune disease, trough levels of 100–200 ng/ml ciclosporin and 5–10 ng/ml tacrolimus usually are adequate; much higher levels are used for prevention of graft rejection.

☐ USE OF PROPHYLACTIC DRUGS TO MITIGATE SIDE EFFECTS

No agreed consensus exists on the use of prophylaxis against infection in the context of immunosuppressive therapy. The experience in HIV makes it clear, however, that reproducible thresholds for infections can be mapped to the CD4+ lymphocyte count (see Table 2). Thus where T-cell lymphopaenia is an expected effect of the drug regimen, prophylaxis may be desirable; however, how far the prophylaxis should be taken is unresolved. Prophylaxis against *Pneumocystis carinii* pneumonia (PCP) is accepted as sensible for cyclophosphamide, but whether antiviral prophy-laxis should be started immediately is unresolved. The more prophylactic drugs that are used, the more compliance will be reduced and the greater the risk of drug interactions and toxicity from the prophylactic agents. Prophylaxis against PCP usually is obtained with cotrimoxazole, and, again, no consensus exists on the optimum regimen; this drug would be undesirable in the context of drugs such as azathioprine and methotrexate because of the potential for additive bone marrow toxicity. Corticosteroids in doses higher than an equivalent of 20 mg/day prednisolone also increase the risk of PCP (although this risk usually is not recognised): high-dose steroids are significantly lymphocytotoxic, whereas low doses are anti-inflammatory.

Where B cells particularly are targeted, a different antibiotic regimen, such as low-dose penicillin, macrolide or tetracycline, may be appropriate. No optimum regimen has been determined yet. Persistent B-cell lymphopaenia and reduced levels of serum immunoglobulins may warrant prophylactic immunoglobulin replacement.

Another unresolved issue is whether to use folic acid or folinic acid to mitigate the side effects of methotrexate. One of the modes of action of methotrexate is the inhibition of dihydrofolate reductase, which converts folic acid to folinic acid – the active agent in the bone marrow. Haematologists have always used folinic acid rescue to preserve bone marrow function after chemotherapy with methotrexate, as this bypasses the block induced by the methotrexate. Methotrexate, however, also inhibits 5-amino-imidazole-4-carboxamide ribonucleotide transformylase, increases adenosine levels (which is lymphocytotoxic) and inhibits production of TNF, interleukin (IL)-6 and IL-8, thus suppressing inflammation. How these different actions combine to produce a clinical effect is unclear. Rheumatological practice usually is to use folic acid. Studies with folic and folinic acid have shown benefit in reducing adverse effects, but no critical evaluation of which agent should be used, or whether they are interchangeable, has been made. Folinic acid seems the more logical agent to use from a theoretical standpoint.

Where immunosuppressive regimens include medium-term to long-term use of corticosteroids, baseline bone mineral density values and the desirability of bone protection must be considered. Most of the bone loss in patients who take steroids comes within the first few months of therapy, when the doses are highest, and it is sensible therefore to institute prophylaxis early, with a bisphosphonate, calcium and vitamin D.

☐ MALIGNANCY

Malignancy is a major long-term complication of immunosuppression, particularly viral-induced malignancy such as Epstein-Barr virus-induced lymphoma, infections with human papillomavirus and Kaposi's sarcoma. Cyclophosphamide also increases the risk of myeloid leukaemia and bladder tumours. Doctors should be aware of the risks and ensure appropriate surveillance. Suspicious cutaneous lesions should be referred immediately. Lymphomas may be identified by the appearance of monoclonal proteins on serum electrophoresis and changes in immunoglobulin profiles.

☐ MONITORING OF IMMUNE FUNCTION

Traps exist for the unwary when monitoring immune parameters. Lymphocyte subsets show a distinct circadian rhythm and are affected directly by intercurrent infection, as well as the disease process. Monitoring therefore can be interpreted only in the light of a clear understanding of the patient's status. Samples must be taken at a consistent time. Peripheral blood lymphocyte counts give only a snapshot of circulating levels and no information at all about immunological reactions in a target tissue, such as a graft undergoing rejection. Indeed, the fall in peripheral count may be the result of transit of cells out of the circulation into the graft. Lymphocytes are recirculating constantly through tissues, with an average circulation time of 48–72 hours. Trends over time are more valuable than single snapshots.

Measurement of lymphocyte function in vitro is possible but time consuming, difficult to standardise, very expensive and, in practice, of little value in clinical management during immunosuppression. It may have a role after immuno-suppression has been completed, however, to monitor the recovery of function. When cytotoxic agents have been used, recovery of immune function may take up to two years, requiring reconstitution of the immune system by new emigrants from bone marrow and thymus. Contrary to published wisdom, the thymus is active, although less efficient, well into old age. The appearance of naïve recent emigrants and their conversion into T and B memory cells is possible. After such immunological reconstitution, the immune system will require re-education, which may mean reimmunisation against common pathogens. The humoral immune response can be monitored and will give a good idea of the adequacy of immune function. Persistent B lymphocyte deficiency may occur, with failure of recovery of antibody production. For those with poor or absent recovery of B-cell function after high-intensity immunosuppression, regular prophylactic intravenous immuno-globulin in replacement doses may be needed (0.2–0.6 g/kg every 2–3 weeks, determined by trough immunoglobulin G levels).

☐ CONCLUSION

To identify adequate clinical studies, or even reviews, that evaluate the optimum monitoring regimens for immunosuppressive drugs is almost impossible, and monitoring tends to be mentioned only as a couple of lines in papers about drug actions, with little practical guidance and often little thought about the appropriateness. Much that is written is superficial and not based on understanding of the drugs or the tests themselves. Despite this, the risks of getting it wrong are high, with resultant morbidity and mortality. Many current guidelines and recommendations are illogical. To summarise the four 'P's, sequelae may be:

- ☐ predictable from knowledge of drug actions

- ☐ preventable by monitoring

- ☐ precluded by prophylactic measures

- ☐ post-mortem-inducing when ignored!

FURTHER READING

Bhat G, Schroeder TJ. Clinical role of immunologic monitoring during OKT3 treatment. *Transplant Proc* 1997;**29**(Suppl. 8A):21S–6S.

Hale DA. Biological effects of induction immunosuppression. *Curr Opin Immunol* 2004;**16**:565–70.

Halloran PF. Immunosuppressive drugs for kidney transplantation. *N Engl J Med* 2004;**351**:2 715–29.

Helbert M, Breuer J. Monitoring patients with HIV disease. *J Clin Pathol* 2000;**53**:266–72.

Hickman PE, Potter JM, Pesce AJ. Clinical chemistry and post-liver-transplant monitoring. *Clin Chem* 1997;**43**:1546–54.

Hutchinson P, Chadban SJ, Atkins RC, Holdsworth SR. Laboratory assessment of immune function in renal transplant patients. *Nephrol Dial Transplant* 2003;**18**:983–9.

Masri MA, Stephan A, Barbari S, Rizk A *et al.* Pre- and posttransplant immunologic monitoring: why, when, and how? *Transplant Proc* 2002;**34**:2482–4.

Ortiz Z, Shea B, Suarez Almazor M, Moher D *et al.* Folic acid and folinic acid for reducing side effects in patients receiving methotrexate for rheumatoid arthritis. *Cochrane Database Syst Rev* 2000;**2**:CD000951.

☐ IMMUNOSUPPRESSION SELF ASSESSMENT QUESTIONS

Immunosuppressive drugs in renal transplantation

1   The following drugs are calcineurin inhibitors:
    (a) Ciclosporin
    (b) Tacrolimus
    (c) Sirolimus
    (d) Mycophenolate mofetil
    (e) Leflunomide

2   Tacrolimus:
    (a) Is a more potent immunosuppressive drug than ciclosporin
    (b) More commonly causes gingival hyperplasia than ciclosporin
    (c) Has comparable nephrotoxicity to ciclosporin
    (d) May be favoured in chronic allograft nephropathy for its less profibrotic effect
    (e) May be associated with a worse cardiovascular risk profile than ciclosporin

3   Clinically available anti-interleukin 2 receptor antibodies:
    (a) Are specific for CD25
    (b) Act by binding CD4+ CD25+ regulatory cells
    (c) Are derived, in part, from mouse monoclonal antibodies
    (d) Inhibit mammalian target of rapamycin (mTOR)
    (e) Have significant anti-fibrotic effect

Biological agents

1   Historical aspects:
    (a) Philip Hench was responsible for the introduction of corticosteroids in the late 1940s
    (b) The side-effects of corticosteroids were appreciated as soon as the drugs became available
    (c) Robert Schwartz showed that methotrexate could alter the synthesis of antibodies
    (d) The first renal transplant was performed in 1976
    (e) The first heart transplant was performed in 1989

2   Immunological connections:
    (a) Antigen-presenting cells present antigen to B cells
    (b) B cells may act as antigen-presenting cells
    (c) Accessory molecules are required for efficient interaction between antigen-presenting cells and T cells
    (d) T-helper cells help B cells produce antigen
    (e) Antibodies are produced by plasma cells

3   Current biological therapies:
   (a) Tumour necrosis factor-α is thought to be a key molecule in the immunopathogenesis of rheumatoid arthritis
   (b) Etanercept is an antibody that blocks production of tumour necrosis factor
   (c) Infliximab is a fully humanised, human monoclonal, anti-tumour necrosis factor-α antibody
   (d) Antibodies to interleukin 1 have yet to be made available in the treatment of rheumatoid arthritis
   (e) Anti-tumour necrosis factor-α antibodies have shown benefit in the treatment of psoriatic arthritis and ankylosing spondylitis

4   Biological therapies in other conditions:
   (a) Rituximab (anti-CD20) is a fully humanised monoclonal antibody
   (b) Rituximab was introduced for the treatment of lymphoma
   (c) Evidence from double-blind, controlled trials shows that rituximab is of value in the treatment of rheumatoid arthritis
   (d) Evidence from trials shows that natalizumab is beneficial in patients with multiple sclerosis
   (e) Antibodies to LFA3 are of no value in the treatment of psoriasis

Unwanted sequelae of immunosuppression

1   Work-up before azathioprine therapy starts should include the following:
   (a) Measurement of dihydrofolate reductase
   (b) Liver function tests
   (c) Lung function tests
   (d) Rheumatoid factor
   (e) Differential white cell count

2   Side effects of cyclosphosphamide include:
   (a) *Pneumocystis carinii* pneumonia
   (b) Myeloid leukaemia
   (c) Severe depletion of B lymphocytes
   (d) Bladder neoplasia
   (e) Induction of autoimmunity

3   Return of immunological function after therapeutic immunosuppression with lymphotoxic drugs:
   (a) Is dependent on recent thymic emigrants
   (b) Is usually complete within 3–6 months
   (c) Is unlikely to occur in the elderly because of thymic atrophy
   (d) Leads to a naïve immune system that requires reimmunisation
   (e) May be incomplete, with poor B-cell function

Vascular risk factors

Prevention of atherosclerosis in diabetes

Paul Durrington

☐ INTRODUCTION

In both type 1 and type 2 diabetes, atherosclerosis is the largest cause of morbidity and premature mortality. The risk of cardiovascular disease (CVD) in patients with type 2 diabetes is increased two to fourfold,[1] and in patients with type 1 diabetes, risk is increased from early adulthood.[2] In addition, survival rates are lower in patients with diabetes after acute myocardial infarction and coronary intervention procedures.[3] The incidences of peripheral vascular disease and stroke also are increased greatly in patients with diabetes. An excellent case thus exists for trying to prevent the clinical consequences of atherosclerosis in patients with diabetes.

☐ REDUCING CVD RISK

Until recently, the case for the meticulous management of glycaemia and blood pressure in patients with diabetes was accepted by diabetologists, but the value of using specific lipid-lowering drugs in the management of diabetic dyslipidaemia (raised serum triglycerides and low high-density lipoprotein (HDL) cholesterol) and CVD risk was contentious. Nonetheless, it clearly was evident that some more effective means of decreasing CVD risk than glycaemic control and treatment of high blood pressure was required.

Glycaemic control and CVD risk

In neither type 1 nor type 2 diabetes does evidence show that glycaemic control actually does significantly decrease CVD risk.[4,5] In the case of type 2 diabetes, this is probably because a state of high CVD risk often exists for many years before the onset of hyperglycaemia severe enough for the diagnosis of diabetes. During this pre-diabetic phase, obesity and insulin resistance typically are present and are associated with dyslipidaemia and hypertension.[6,7] Unsurprisingly, these risk factors often lead to the development of coronary heart disease during the chronic state of high CVD risk that exists before hyperglycaemia is of diabetic proportions. This also accounts for the progressive increase in the prevalence of diabetes in the years after myocardial infarction and unstable angina.[8] Treatment of glycaemia at this stage can have no discernible impact in reversing CVD risk. In type 1 diabetes, many young adults will have had years of diabetes poorly controlled in childhood. This, together with the development of nephropathy (which even at the stage of microalbuminuria can cause marked deteriorations in lipid profiles and blood pressure[9]), accounts for the high CVD risk in these patients, which glycaemic control cannot be expected to reduce.

Blood pressure and CVD risk

Meticulous control of blood pressure can be expected to decrease CVD risk and is of utmost importance. In meta-analyses of randomised clinical trials of antihypertensive drugs, however, the reduction in coronary risk was only about half that reported with the statin drugs,[10,11] and coronary risk accounts for most CVD risk. Randomised clinical trials of statins against placebo or usual care show an approximately linear relation between the extent of reductions in low-density lipoprotein (LDL) cholesterol and the decrease in coronary heart disease risk (Fig 1). For each 1% reduction in LDL cholesterol, patients randomised to receive statin as opposed to placebo or usual care have 1.25% decreases in coronary risk.[13–22] In practical terms, where glycaemic and blood pressure targets often are difficult to achieve in practice, cholesterol targets often are relatively easy to reach.[23]

☐ LIPID LOWERING IN PATIENTS WITH DIABETES

The reluctance of doctors to treat patients with diabetes with statins resulted from the lack of specific trials in this patient group. In secondary prevention trials (those

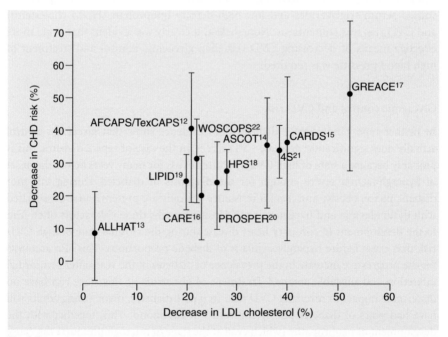

Fig 1 Percentage reduction in relative risk of coronary heart disease (CHD) in randomised clinical trials of statins as a function of the decrease in LDL on active intervention rather than placebo or usual care. Vertical bars are 95% confidence intervals, and the result is statistically significant if these do not cross zero.

in which participants had pre-existing CVD), substantial numbers of patients had type 2 diabetes for the reasons described above. It was possible, therefore, to be reasonably certain that statins would decrease relative CHD risk in patients with type 2 diabetes at least as effectively as in non-diabetic patients (Table 1). Statins have thus come to be accepted as being indicated in the secondary prevention of CVD in patients with diabetes.

Table 1 Randomised clinical trials of statin treatment compared with placebo or usual care in patients with type 2 diabetes.

Study	Diabetes		All participants	
	No. of patients	Difference in CVD endpoint between active treatment and placebo or usual care (%)	No. of patients	Difference in CVD endpoint between active treatment and placebo or usual care (%)
Secondary prevention				
4S[27]	483	−42	4,444	−34
CARE[24]	586	−25	4,157	−24
LIPID[19]	782	−19	9,014	−24
GREACE[25]	313	−58	1,600	−51
Heart Protection Study[26]	1,981	−15	20,536	−24
Primary prevention				
Heart Protection Study[26]	2,912	−31	NA	NA
CARDS[15]	2,838	−37	NA	NA

NA = not applicable.

The one trial that seems to prove the exception is the secondary prevention arm of the Heart Protection Study.[26] In this study, CVD risk decreased by only 15% in patients with diabetes compared with patients without diabetes, whereas in those patients with diabetes who had no clinical evidence of atherosclerotic vascular disease at randomisation, active statin treatment was associated with a reduction in CVD risk of around one third.[26] This probably was because by the time this study was carried out, doctors increasingly believed that evidence for the use of statins in patients with diabetes who already had clinically overt CHD was sufficiently convincing. This meant there was considerable use of add-in statin therapy in the patients with diabetes and coronary disease who had been allocated to placebo, so the difference in LDL cholesterol between these patients and those allocated to active simvastatin was eroded.

A study that specifically looked at primary prevention with statin therapy in patients with diabetes thus was needed to confirm and extend the Heart Protection Study's findings to inform diabetic practice. Although the American Diabetes Association recommended after the Heart Protection Study was published that patients with diabetes should, in general, receive a statin,[28] most healthcare systems did not reimburse the cost of these drugs in diabetes for the primary prevention of CVD.

□ COLLABORATIVE ATORVASTATIN DIABETES STUDY

The Collaborative AtoRvastatin Diabetes Study (CARDS) was pivotal.[15] This study compared the effectiveness and safety of atorvastatin 10 mg/day and placebo in the primary prevention of cardiovascular disease in 2,838 patients with type 2 diabetes without raised cholesterol levels.

Study design

To enter the trial, patients' serum LDL cholesterol levels had to be ≤4.14 mmol/l. Fasting serum triglycerides, however, could be elevated to as high as 6.78 mmol/l. The patients had to have one of the following cardiovascular risk factors in addition to their diabetes: hypertension, microalbuminuria or macroalbuminuria (with serum creatinine <150 μmol/l), retinopathy or smoking despite advice to stop. The primary endpoint was combined acute death from coronary heart disease, non-fatal (including silent) myocardial infarction, unstable angina that required hospital admission, resuscitated cardiac arrest, coronary revascularisation and stroke.

The study researchers calculated that for a reduction in clinical endpoints of 30% with active statin therapy compared with placebo about 2,800 patients would be necessary to give around 300 primary endpoints and to produce a statistically significant outcome. The study was anticipated to finish in June 2005, by which time patients, on average, would have been in the trial for 5–6 years. Given the strength of the evidence of a benefit from statins in many non-diabetic patients at this stage, however, if there had been a clear benefit in those actively treated, to have allowed patients in the trial to continue to receive placebo clearly would have been as unethical as allowing patients to continue with active therapy that produced some unforeseen adverse effect. The safety committee thus were empowered to stop the trial if a highly significant difference in favour of active therapy emerged earlier than the anticipated date of completion of the trial. In the event, the trial was terminated on these grounds after an average duration of 3.9 years.

Setting and participants

The study was conducted in 132 sites in the United Kingdom and the Republic of Ireland, with about one-third of patients recruited from general practice and two-thirds from hospital centres. Importantly, CARDS, unlike some statin trials, such as the Heart Protection Study, had no active treatment run-in before randomisation, when patients who believe they have experienced an adverse event would leave before randomisation. The first exposure of patients in CARDS to active treatment thus was after randomisation, so the intention-to-treat analysis captured all adverse events.

On average, the patients were aged 62 years, and, as is the case with type 2 diabetes, by and large they were overweight. Some 16% were treated for their diabetes with diet alone, 70% were on oral hypoglycaemic agents and 20% were taking insulin alone or in combination with oral agents.

Most patients (63%) had only a single CVD risk factor in addition to diabetes and, in general, this was mild hypertension. Overall, therefore, the patients' CVD risk was reduced by not including patients with higher than average cholesterol levels and increased again by one or sometimes more additional CVD risk factors. The patients' CVD risk, on average, thus was no more than would be typical of a type 2 diabetic population without pre-existing CVD. Partly because of this and partly because of the design of the trial, which aimed to limit any adverse effects from not receiving statin treatment, the mortality in the placebo group was similar to the standardised mortality rate in the general population.

Findings

Serum cholesterol at entry was 5.4 mmol/l (LDL cholesterol 3.1 mmol/l), and serum triglycerides were 1.7 mmol/l. Reductions in serum cholesterol, LDL cholesterol and triglycerides on atorvastatin as opposed to active treatment were 26%, 40% and 21%, respectively. This resulted in a 37% reduction in the primary endpoint (Fig 2), which included a 48% decrease in stroke. Tests of heterogeneity showed that the relative decrease in CVD risk was not influenced significantly by pretreatment lipid levels, even though before randomisation one-quarter of patients already had LDL cholesterol levels <2.6 mmol/l – the target for statin treatment in the United States. Age, sex, smoking, blood pressure and complications, such as retinopathy and nephropathy, also did not influence the relative decrease in CVD risk achieved with statin treatment. Thirty-seven (2.6%) cardiovascular deaths and 45 (3.2%) non-cardiovascular deaths occurred in the placebo group. Corresponding figures in the active treatment group were 25 (1.8%) and 36 (2.5%). Adverse events, such as elevated creatine kinase, muscle symptoms and increased liver transaminases, were no more frequent on active treatment than on placebo.

Event	Placebo*	Atorva-statin*	Hazard ratio	Risk reduction (95% confidence interval)
Primary endpoint	127 (9.0)	83 (5.8)		37% (17% to 52% $p = 0.001$
Acute coronary	77 (5.5)	51 (3.6)		36% (9% to 55%)
Coronary revascularisation	34 (2.4)	24 (1.7)		31% (−16% to 59%)
Stroke	39 (2.8)	21 (1.5)		48% (11% to 69%)

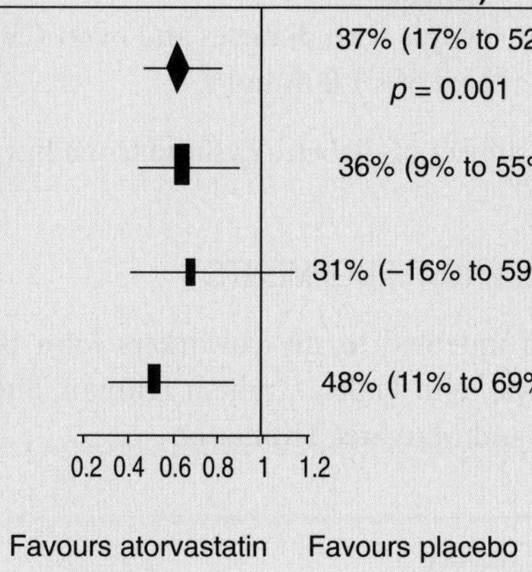

0.2 0.4 0.6 0.8 1 1.2

* No. of patients (% randomised)   Favours atorvastatin   Favours placebo

Fig 2. Results from CARDS.[15] Events in patients taking placebo and atorvastatin are shown as hazard ratios. The horizontal bars indicate 95% confidence intervals, and if these do not cross unity they are statistically significant. The hazard ratio also is presented as relative risk reduction (%) (95% CI).

☐ CONCLUSIONS

The results from CARDS provide direct evidence that a threshold level of LDL cholesterol for the introduction of statin treatment is no longer justified in patients with type 2 diabetes. The principal indication for statin treatment should be to reduce CVD risk. To identify reliably any patient with diabetes in the age range included in CARDS who safely could be deprived of statin therapy on the grounds of cost is probably impossible. Furthermore, the results from CARDS might reasonably be extrapolated to younger patients with type 2 diabetes, particularly in the presence of another risk factor; this is true even when the patient's current absolute CVD risk is not as high as the risk in CARDS, because their lifetime risk would be even greater. Many patients with type 1 diabetes also would be at higher absolute risk at a much younger age than many patients with type 2 diabetes included in CARDS (particularly if the onset of their disease was in childhood). Patients with type 1 diabetes who survive to the age of 50 years have the same level of CVD risk as non-diabetic people 20 years or more their senior.[2] Although no direct statin trial evidence is available in patients with type 1 diabetes, if these drugs are viewed as indicated for the reduction of CVD risk, they certainly are indicated in type 1 diabetes.

The latest recommendations from the American Diabetes Association since the publication of the Heart Protection Study and CARDS are that statin therapy should be used in:[29]

- ☐ people with diabetes aged >40 years with serum cholesterol ≥3.5 mmol/l (the lower limit for entry to HPS; CARDS had no lower limit) but without overt CVD to reduce LDL cholesterol by 30–40% regardless of baseline levels or to <2.6 mmol/l, whichever is lower

- ☐ adults with diabetes aged <40 years without overt CVD who are at increased CVD risk because of other risk factors or long duration of diabetes and who do not achieve LDL cholesterol <2.6 mmol/l with lifestyle modification

- ☐ people with diabetes and overt CVD, with the LDL cholesterol treatment goal of <1.8 mmol/l.

The subject of diabetic dyslipidaemia has recently been reviewed.[30]

☐ ACKNOWLEDGEMENTS

I am indebted to my coworkers John Betteridge, Helen Colhoun, Val Charlton-Menys, John Fuller, Graham Hitman, Shona Livingstone, Mike Mackness, Andrew Neil and Margaret Thomason.

REFERENCES

1 Stamler J, Vaccaro O, Neaton JD, Wentworth D. Diabetes, other risk factors, and 12-year cardiovascular mortality for men screened in the Multiple Risk Factor Intervention Trial. *Diabetes Care* 1993;16:434–44.

2 Laing SP, Swerdlow AJ, Slater SD, Burden AC *et al.* Mortality from heart disease in a cohort of 23,000 patients with insulin-treated diabetes. *Diabetologia* 2003;**46**:760–5.

3 Kirk A, Fisher M, MacIntyre P. Diabetes and survival after myocardial infarction: is cardiac rehabilitation an effective secondary prevention measure? *Pract Diab Int* 2004;**21**:267–75.

4 UK Prospective Diabetes Study Group. Intensive blood-glucose control with sulphonylureas or insulin compared with conventional treatment and risk of complications in patients with type 2 diabetes (UKPDS 33). *Lancet* 1998;**352**:837–53.

5 Diabetes Control and Complication Trial (DCCT) Research Group. Effect of intensive diabetes management on macrovascular events and risk factors in the diabetes control and complications trial. *Am J Cardiol* 1995;**75**:894–903.

6 Haffner SM, Stern MP, Hazuda HP, Mitchell BD *et al.* Cardiovascular risk factors in confirmed prediabetic individuals. Does the clock for coronary disease start ticking before the onset of clinical diabetes? *JAMA* 1990;**263**:2893–8.

7 Haffner SM, Mykkanen L, Festa A, Burke JP *et al.* Insulin-resistant prediabetic subjects have more atherogenic risk factors than insulin-sensitive prediabetic subjects: implications for preventing coronary heart disease during the prediabetic state. *Circulation* 2000;**101**: 975–80.

8 Farrer M, Fulcher G, Albers CJ, Neil HA *et al.* Patients undergoing coronary artery bypass surgery are at high risk of impaired glucose tolerance and diabetes mellitus during the first post-operative year. *Metabolism* 1995;**44**:1016–27.

9 Winocour PH, Durrington PN, Ishola M, Anderson DC *et al.* Influence of proteinuria on vascular disease, blood pressure, and lipoproteins in insulin-dependent diabetes mellitus. *BMJ (Clin Res Ed)* 1987;**294**:1648–51.

10 Collins R, MacMahon S. Blood pressure, antihypertensive drug treatment and the risks of stroke and of coronary heart disease. *Br Med Bull* 1994;**50**:272–98.

11 Law MR, Wald NJ, Rudnicka AR. Quantifying effect of statins on low density lipoprotein cholesterol, ischaemic heart disease, and stroke: systematic review and meta-analysis. *BMJ* 2003;**326**:1423.

12 Downs JR, Clearfield M, Weiss S, Whitney E *et al.* Primary prevention of acute coronary events with lovastatin in men and women with average cholesterol levels: results of the AFCAPS/TEXCAPS. Air Force/Texas Coronary Atherosclerosis Prevention Study. *JAMA* 1998;**279**:1615–22.

13 ALLHAT Officers and Coordinators for the ALLHAT Collaborative Research Group. Major outcomes in moderately hypercholesterolemic, hypertensive patients randomised to pravastatin vs usual care. The Antihypertensive and Lipid-Lowering Treatment to Prevent Heart Attack Trial (ALLHAT-LLT). *JAMA* 2002;**288**:2998–3007.

14 Sever PS, Dahlof B, Poulter NRM, Wedel H *et al.* Prevention of coronary and stroke events with atorvastatin in hypertensive patients who have average or lower-than-average cholesterol in the Anglo-Scandinavian Cardiac Outcomes Trial – Lipid lowering arm (ASCOT-LLA): a multicentre randomised controlled trial. *Lancet* 2003;**361**:1149–58.

15 Colhoun HM, Betteridge DJ, Durrington PN, Hitman GA *et al,* on behalf of the CARDS investigators. Primary prevention of cardiovascular disease with atorvastatin in type 2 diabetes in the Collaborative Atorvastatin Diabetes Study (CARDS): multicentre randomised placebo-controlled trial. *Lancet* 2004;**364**:685–96.

16 Sacks FM, Pfeffer MA, Moye LA, Rouleau JL *et al,* for the Cholesterol and Recurrent Events trial investigators. The effect of pravastatin on coronary events after myocardial infarction in patients with average cholesterol levels. *N Engl J Med* 1996;**335**:1001–9.

17 Athyros VG, Papageorgiou AA, Mercouris BR, Athyrou VV *et al.* Treatment with atorvastatin to the National Cholesterol Educational Program goal versus 'usual' care in secondary coronary heart disease prevention. The GREek Atorvastatin and Coronary heart-disease Evaluation (GREACE) Study. *Curr Med Res Opin* 2002;**18**:220–8.

18 Heart Protection Study Collaborative Group. MRC/BHF Heart Protection Study of cholesterol lowering with simvastatin in 20,536 high-risk individuals: a randomised placebo-controlled trial. *Lancet* 2002;**360**:7–22.

19 Long-Term Intervention with Pravastatin in Ischaemic Disease (LIPID) Study Group. Prevention of cardiovascular events and death with pravastatin in patients with coronary heart disease and a broad range of initial cholesterol levels. *N Engl J Med* 1998;**339**:1349–57.

20 Shepherd J, Blauw GJ, Murphy MB, Bollen EL *et al.* Pravastatin in elderly individuals at risk of vascular disease (PROSPER): a randomised controlled trial. *Lancet* 2002;**360**:1623–30.

21 Scandinavian Simvastatin Survival Study Group. Randomised trial of cholesterol lowering in 4444 patients with coronary heart disease: the Scandinavian Simvastatin Survival Study. *Lancet* 1994;**344**:1383–9.

22 Shepherd J, Cobbe SM, Ford I, Isles CG *et al*, for the West of Scotland Coronary Prevention Study Group. Prevention of coronary heart disease with pravastatin in men with hypercholesterolaemia. *N Engl J Med* 1995;**333**:1301–7.

23 Edwards R, Burns JA, McElduff P, Young RJ *et al.* Variations in process and outcomes of diabetes care by socio-economic status in Salford, UK. *Diabetologia* 2003;**46**:750–9.

24 Goldberg RB, Mellies MJ, Sacks FM, Moye LA *et al*, for the CARE investigators. Cardiovascular events and their reduction with pravastatin in diabetic and glucose-intolerant myocardial infarction survivors with average cholesterol levels: subgroup analyses in the Cholesterol and Recurrent Events (CARE) trial. *Circulation* 1998;**98**:2513–9.

25 Athyros VG, Papageorgiou AA, Symeonidis AN, Didangelos TP *et al.* Early benefit from structured care with atorvastatin in patients with coronary heart disease and diabetes. *Angiology* 2003;**54**:679–90.

26 Collins R, Armitage J, Parish S, Sleigh P *et al* for the Heart Protection Study Collaborative Group. MRC/BHF Heart Protection Study of cholesterol-lowering with simvastatin in 5963 people with diabetes: a randomised placebo-controlled trial. *Lancet* 2003;**361**:2005–16.

27 Haffner SM, Alexander CM, Cook TJ, Boccuzzi SJ *et al*, for the Scandinavian Simvastatin Survival Study Group. Reduced coronary events in simvastatin-treated patients with coronary heart disease and diabetes or impaired fasting glucose levels: subgroup analyses in the Scandinavian Simvastatin Survival Study. *Arch Intern Med* 1999;**159**:2661–7.

28 Haffner SM, for the American Diabetes Association. Dyslipidemia management in adults with diabetes. *Diabetes Care* 2004;**27**(Suppl):S68–71.

29 American Diabetes Association. Standards of medical care in diabetes. *Diabetes Care* 2005;**28** (Suppl 1):S4–36.

30 Durrington PN, Charlton-Menys V. Diabetic dyslipidaemia. In: Barnett AH (ed), *Best practice and research compendium: diabetes.* Amsterdam: Elsevier (in press).

Vascular dysfunction in atherosclerosis: importance of lifetime management

Marietta Charakida and John E Deanfield

☐ INTRODUCTION

Despite enormous improvements in the treatment of the clinical manifestations of atherosclerosis, this condition remains the leading cause of morbidity and mortality in Western society and is increasing dramatically in developing countries. This is largely the result of the limited resources that thus far have been directed at prevention compared with those spent on managing the late clinical phase of vascular disease.

Treatment of the cardiovascular consequences of atherosclerosis may prolong life, but often with disability. In contrast, preclinical management has the potential to delay cardiovascular events and thus prolong 'disability-free' life expectancy. A further important argument for prevention strategies is that treatments for clinical problems of necessity fail to help the substantial number of people in society whose first manifestation of vascular disease is sudden death, catastrophic stroke or myocardial infarction.[1]

That the atherosclerotic process begins decades before its clinical manifestations has long been recognised. Indeed, in 1953, in post-mortem studies, Enos *et al* showed the presence of coronary atherosclerotic plaques in 77% of young American soldiers who died in action in their teenage years and early twenties.[2] More recently, Stary observed macrovascular fatty streaks in 40% of young Americans who died of non-cardiac causes, as well as evidence of lipid-rich deposits in the coronary arteries of many children by the age of 13 years.[3] Findings of such pathological studies recently were confirmed by intravascular ultrasound. In a group of people dying of non-cardiac related causes who provided the donor hearts in a transplantation programme, atherosclerotic lesions were seen in 17% of those younger than 20 years of age, with a steep increase in the incidence over the next three decades.[4] This early atherosclerosis is linked to classic risk factors such as cholesterol, smoking and high blood pressure, and the levels in early life track future cardiovascular disease decades later.[5] These observations indicate the exciting potential for early treatment as an 'investment strategy' against future cardiovascular events.

☐ VASCULAR BIOLOGY OF ATHEROSCLEROSIS

In recent years, a considerable amount has been learnt about the vascular biology of atherosclerosis throughout its natural history. The importance of inflammation not only in determining the stability and risk of established lesions but also during the long evolution of plaques has been recognised. The vascular endothelium has been a major focus of research because of its key role as 'signal transducer' for genetic and environmental influences on this process.[6] Apart from being a physical barrier between the vessel wall and lumen, inflammation also has paracrine actions in response to mechanical and humoral signals. Endothelial cells secrete numerous mediators, such as nitric oxide, prostacyclin and endothelin, which modulate a range of functions, including vascular tone, leucocyte and platelet adhesion, coagulation and smooth muscle cell proliferation. In the presence of cardiovascular risk factors or increasing age, the endothelium becomes dysfunctional, adopting a phenotype that encourages recruitment and accumulation of inflammatory cells and low density lipoprotein (LDL) into the vessel wall. This initiates and progresses plaque development. Recently, it has been appreciated that endothelial function may be regulated not merely by the presence of damaging influences but also by the activity of endogenous repair systems, such as bone marrow-derived circulating endothelial progenitor cells.[7]

The bioavailability of nitric oxide (NO) is a key factor in determining endothelial function. Nitric oxide is formed from the N-guanino terminal of the amino acid L-arginine and from molecular oxygen by the constitutively expressed NO synthase (eNOS). Alterations in the activity of eNOS may affect NO synthesis.[8] Expression of this enzyme can be modulated by shear stress, atherogenic lipoproteins and cytokines. In addition, eNOS activity can be decreased by the presence of inhibitory substances, including asymmetric dimethyl arginine (ADMA) and caveolin-1. Deficiencies of cofactors such as tetrahydrobiopterin may also result in reduced production of NO.

Evidence suggests that increased degradation of NO by reactive oxygen species accounts for the large proportion of reduced NO bioavailability and impaired NO-mediated endothelium-dependent function. The increased oxidative stress can be the result of excess production of reactive oxygen species or reduced activity of antioxidant substances synthesised within the body or taken in the diet.[9]

□ CLINICAL TESTING OF ENDOTHELIAL FUNCTION

Over the last decade, a number of techniques have been developed to study NO-dependent regulation of vascular tone in different vascular beds. Evaluation of NO-mediated endothelial function in response to pharmacological or physical stimuli, such as acetycholine, bradykinin, serotonin, substance P and shear stress in the coronary and peripheral circulations, is possible. In particular, the non-invasive assessment of endothelial function using flow-mediated dilatation in the brachial artery has provided opportunities to assess endothelial-dependent conduit artery reactivity from as early as the first decade of life. Flow-mediated dilatation can be measured accurately and reproducibly, is largely dependent on local bioavailability of NO and correlates with endothelial function in the coronary arteries.[10] Furthermore, endothelial function studied in this way is related to the presence of classic cardiovascular risk factors and the number of endothelial progenitor cells in the circulation and predicts future cardiovascular events.[11,12] These ultrasound-based, non-invasive techniques can be performed from childhood and can be repeated, providing the opportunity to study the pathophysiology of the initiation and progression of early disease and to evaluate potential reversibility in response to lifestyle and pharmacological interventions.

The link between endothelial dysfunction, inflammation and structural changes in the arterial wall begins remarkably early. Javisalo and colleagues studied 79 apparently healthy Finnish children and showed that increased C-reactive protein was associated with reduced flow-mediated dilatation and increased thickness of the media of the carotid intima at an average age of just 10.5 years.[13]

□ RISK FACTORS FOR EARLY ENDOTHELIAL DYSFUNCTION

All the classic risk factors known to increase morbidity and mortality from vascular disease in later life cause endothelial dysfunction from the first decade and interact in a familiar detrimental manner – even during the earlier stages of atherosclerosis development. Endothelial dysfunction has been shown in children with familial hypercholesterolaemia, and the relation between LDL cholesterol and vascular function has been shown even within the 'normal range' present in children aged 9–11 years. Endothelial dysfunction also has been shown in people with hypertension and their relatives, implicating genetic factors. Furthermore, active and passive cigarette smoking cause endothelial dysfunction.

Early development of endothelial dysfunction has been shown in people with type 1 and type 2 diabetes, the latter of which is increasingly seen at a young age. The pathophysiology is multifactorial, but LDL cholesterol seems to be an important early factor.[14]

Age and sex are major influences on the clinical manifestations of atherosclerosis. Celemajer *et al* showed an age-related decline in endothelial function from the fourth decade in men – even in the absence of classic cardiovascular risk factors.[15] In women, the pattern of age-related decline was different, with a delayed but steeper deterioration from their mid-fifties. How much of the decline in vascular function is related to cumulative exposure to risk factors and how much is intrinsic to the processes of ageing remains unclear.

The observation that vascular function may be abnormal from the first decade of life emphasises the need for a better understanding of the genetic and environmental influences that may interact to initiate and progress early disease. In addition to clinical risk factors, a number of new adverse influences have been identified. For example, extrinsic inflammatory stimuli may induce endothelial dysfunction. These include minor viral upper respiratory tract infections in children, as well as chronic dental sepsis.[16] Obesity is a major proinflammatory influence that is likely to drive arterial disease in the next generation of patients. This is reaching epidemic proportions in many countries, particularly among the young. A graded relation between increased body mass index and endothelial function and arterial distensibility has been shown in teenagers.[17] The pathogenic mechanisms by which obesity induces vascular dysfunction are multifactorial and include the development of metabolic syndrome, enhanced production of proinflammatory cytokines, and adipose cell-derived factors, such as leptin and adiponectin.[18]

Over the last decade, interest has been increasing in the concept of 'vascular programming', with prenatal and early postnatal factors producing a permanent change in the risk profile for later arterial disease or in the arterial wall itself.[19] Birth weight and 'catch-up' growth in small infants have been linked to impairment of endothelial function by the second decade of life, as well as the subsequent development of hypertension, insulin resistance and increased cardiovascular events in adults.[20]

The genetic contribution to cardiovascular risk long has been recognised. Our group showed impaired endothelial function in the offspring of people with premature cardiovascular disease, even in the absence of classic cardiovascular risk factors. Polymorphisms in a variety of genes involved in regulation of endothelial biology influence vascular function, particularly in association with environmental risk factors. For example, we recently showed that a Glu[298]Asp substitution in the eNOS gene modifies flow-mediated dilatation during pregnancy and in cigarette smokers.[21,22] However, the interaction between the multiple genes involved in atherogenesis and the complex environmental influences cannot be studied in small selected cohorts. We therefore initiated a large, prospective, population-based study of vascular structure and function in 8,000 children followed from birth for risk factors, lifestyle and genetic characterisation (Avon longitudinal study of parents and children (ALSPAC)).[23] Vascular studies in children aged 10 years show that a broad range of endothelial-dependent and -independent function already is present, with values comparable in some children to those found in adults with risk factors. This very large study will facilitate the study of gene–environment interaction before the acquisition of major risk factors, as well as enabling prospective evaluation of the evolution of arterial structure and function into adulthood.

☐ TREATMENT APPROACHES

The presence of disturbed vascular biology and early atherosclerosis from childhood, together with the identification of factors that contribute to early disease, argues strongly in favour of a systematic approach to prevention initiated from a much earlier stage than in current clinical practice.

Lifestyle changes, including diet and exercise, are highly relevant in the young, and clear evidence shows that these can reverse rapidly the dysfunctional biology associated with atherogenesis, as well as improving later cardiovascular outcome. Woo *et al* showed that just six weeks of regular physical exercise in overweight teenagers improved endothelial function, with further benefit if exercise was maintained.[24] This improvement in vascular function as a result of exercise training is not restricted to the vessels in the exercising musculature and occurs independently from changes in lipids, blood pressure and glycaemic control. These findings are of real therapeutic interest, as evidence shows that lifestyle modifications in people with multiple risk factors can retard or prevent progression to clinical disease. For example, in a cohort with metabolic syndrome, an active interventional protocol reduced the risk of progression to diabetes by 58% within four years.[25] In a recent review, a combination of a range of healthy dietary factors – 'the Polymeal' – was estimated to produce a reduction in future cardiovascular risk equivalent to that achieved by a multiple medication ('the Polypill').[26]

Many people, however, are unable or unwilling to adopt a healthy lifestyle. The range of pharmacological agents now available has transformed the ability to improve cardiovascular risk profiles in such people. Statins produce major outcome benefits in primary and secondary prevention and can retard or reverse the atherosclerotic process. Vascular inflammation and endothelial function are improved rapidly both experimentally and in clinical studies. A number of key issues regarding statins will be resolved by ongoing clinical trials. For example, how much of the differential vascular outcome benefits of different statin regimens is attributable to the degree of LDL lowering and how much to 'non-LDL' effects, which may differ within the class, is unclear.[27] Furthermore, the relative benefit of low and high doses of individual agents is still not certain.

For the individual, evidence is accumulating that the optimal lifetime approach to risk reduction and event-free life prolongation requires treatment to lower levels of risk factors (for example, high blood pressure and cholesterol), earlier initiation of treatment and attention to multiple risk factors once global risk is elevated. This more aggressive approach has been supported by the heart protection study (HPS), as well as the Anglo-Scandinavian cardiac outcomes trial-lipid lowering arm (ASCOT-LLA) and collaborative atorvastatin diabetes study (CARDS), in which treatment with a statin produced major cardiovascular benefits in patients with hypertension and type 2 diabetics, respectively, despite modest dyslipidemia.[28,29] In high-risk young people, such as those with familial hypercholesterolaemia, smaller studies have indicated the safety and efficacy of statins, with restoration of endothelial function and regression of carotid atherosclerosis achieved, even in children.[30] These findings highlight the importance of early treatment for atherosclerosis and are likely, in the future, to be extended to other high-risk young people. Similar evidence for the benefit of more active and earlier treatment of high blood pressure has been obtained from a meta-analysis of the relation between blood pressure and vascular outcome, as well as in recent large prospective studies.[31] Blood-pressure lowering clearly is central to vascular benefit, but the relevant impact of different agents, such as angiotensin-converting enzyme inhibitors, angiotensin receptor blockers and calcium channel blockers, remains controversial.

As with lifestyle modifications, a multiple risk reduction strategy with different agents has been advocated to produce a reduction in global risk profile. Wald *et al* developed the concept of the 'polypill' for prevention of future cardiovascular events in high-risk people, and this approach is likely to be adopted in drug development.[32]

☐ CONCLUSION

A change in the approach to the management of atherosclerosis is required to reduce further its impact in society. Attention needs to be directed at modification of the adverse risk profile that drives the long preclinical phase of the disease, rather than merely developing better treatments for its clinical complications. Lifestyle modifications and pharmacological interventions are likely to be important for reducing the disease burden, and doctors, together with politicians and healthcare providers, need to be involved actively in developing population-based strategies and treatment approaches for individuals.

REFERENCES

1   Murabito JM, Evans JC, Larson MG, Levy D. Prognosis after the onset of coronary heart disease. An investigation of differences in outcome between the sexes according to initial coronary disease presentation. *Circulation* 1993;**88**:2548–55.

2   Enos WF, Holms RH, Beyer J. Coronary disease among United States soldiers killed in action in Korea; preliminary report. *JAMA* 1953;**152**:1090–3.

3   Stary HC. Evolution and progression of atherosclerotic lesions in coronary arteries of children and young adults. *Arteriosclerosis* 1989;**9** (1 Suppl):I19–32.

4   Tuzcu EM, Kapadia SR, Tutar E, Ziada KM *et al*. High prevalence of coronary atherosclerosis in asymptomatic teenagers and young adults: evidence from intravascular ultrasound. *Circulation* 2001;**103**:2705–10.

5   Stamler J, Daviglus ML, Garside DB, Dyer AR *et al*. Relationship of baseline serum cholesterol levels in 3 large cohorts of younger men to long-term coronary, cardiovascular, and all-cause mortality and to longevity. *JAMA* 2000;**284**:311–8.

6   Luscher TF, Noll G. The pathogenesis of cardiovascular disease: role of the endothelium as a target and mediator. *Atherosclerosis* 1995;**118** (Suppl):S81–90.

7   Hill JM, Zalos G, Halcox JP, Schenke WH *et al*. Circulating endothelial progenitor cells, vascular function, and cardiovascular risk. *N Engl J Med* 2003;**348**:593–600.

8   Moncada S, Higgs A. The L-arginine-nitric oxide pathway. *N Engl J Med* 1993;**329**:2002–12.

9   Hoeschen RJ. Oxidative stress and cardiovascular disease. *Can J Cardiol* 1997;**13**:1021–5.

10   Anderson TJ, Uehata A, Gerhard MD, Meredith IT *et al*. Close relation of endothelial function in the human coronary and peripheral circulations. *J Am Coll Cardiol* 1995;**26**:1235–41.

11   Gokce N, Keaney JF Jr, Hunter LM, Watkins MT *et al*. Risk stratification for postoperative cardiovascular events via noninvasive assessment of endothelial function: a prospective study. *Circulation* 2002;**105**:1567–72.

12   Neunteufl T, Heher S, Katzenschlager R, Wolfl G *et al*. Late prognostic value of flow-mediated dilation in the brachial artery of patients with chest pain. *Am J Cardiol* 2000;**86**:207–10.

13   Jarvisalo MJ, Harmoinen A, Hakanen M, Paakkunainen U *et al*. Elevated serum C-reactive protein levels and early arterial changes in healthy children. *Arterioscler Thromb Vasc Biol* 2002;**22**:1323–8.

14   Clarkson P, Celermajer DS, Donald AE, Sampson M *et al*. Impaired vascular reactivity in insulin-dependent diabetes mellitus is related to disease duration and low density lipoprotein cholesterol levels. *J Am Coll Cardiol* 1996;**28**:573–9.

15   Celermajer DS, Sorensen KE, Spiegelhalter DJ, Georgakopoulos D *et al*. Aging is associated with endothelial dysfunction in healthy men years before the age-related decline in women. *J Am Coll Cardiol* 1994;**24**:471–6.

16   Charakida M, Donald AE, Terese M, Leary S *et al*. Endothelial dysfunction in childhood infection. *Circulation* (in press).

17   Whincup PH, Gilg JA, Cook DG, Donald AE *et al*. Adiposity and higher blood cholesterol level are related to diminished arterial distensibility in adolescents. *Circulation* (in press).

18   Singhal A, Farooqi IS, Cole TJ, O'Rahilly S *et al*. Influence of leptin on arterial distensibility: a novel link between obesity and cardiovascular disease? *Circulation* 2002;**106**:1919–24.

19   Singhal A, Kattenhorn M, Cole TJ, Deanfield J *et al*. Preterm birth, vascular function, and risk factors for atherosclerosis. *Lancet* 2001;**358**:1159–60.

20 Singhal A, Fewtrell M, Cole TJ, Lucas A. Low nutrient intake and early growth for later insulin resistance in adolescents born preterm. *Lancet* 2003;**361**:1089–97.

21 Leeson CP, Hingorani AD, Mullen MJ, Jeerooburkhan N *et al.* Glu298Asp endothelial nitric oxide synthase gene polymorphism interacts with environmental and dietary factors to influence endothelial function. *Circ Res* 2002;**90**:1153–8.

22 Savvidou MD, Vallance PJ, Nicolaides KH, Hingorani AD. Endothelial nitric oxide synthase gene polymorphism and maternal vascular adaptation to pregnancy. *Hypertension* 2001;**38**:1289–93.

23 Golding J, Pembrey M, Jones R. ALSPAC – the Avon longitudinal study of parents and children. I. Study methodology. *Paediatr Perinat Epidemiol* 2001;**15**:74–87.

24 Woo KS, Chook P, Yu CW, Sung RY *et al.* Effects of diet and exercise on obesity-related vascular dysfunction in children. *Circulation* 2004;**109**:1981–6.

25 Tuomilehto J, Lindstrom J, Eriksson JG, Valle TT *et al.* Prevention of type 2 diabetes mellitus by changes in lifestyle among subjects with impaired glucose tolerance. *N Engl J Med* 2001;**344**:1343–50.

26 Franco OH, Bonneux L, de Laet C, Peeters A *et al.* The Polymeal: a more natural, safer, and probably tastier (than the Polypill) strategy to reduce cardiovascular disease by more than 75%. *BMJ* 2004;**329**:1447–50.

27 Halcox JP, Deanfield JE. Beyond the laboratory: clinical implications for statin pleiotropy. *Circulation* 2004;**109** (21 Suppl 1):II42–8.

28 Colhoun HM, Betteridge DJ, Durrington PN, Hitman GA *et al.* Primary prevention of cardiovascular disease with atorvastatin in type 2 diabetes in the collaborative atorvastatin diabetes study (CARDS): multicentre randomised placebo-controlled trial. *Lancet* 2004;**364**: 685–96.

29 Nambi V, Ballantyne CM. ASCOT-LLA and the primary prevention of coronary artery disease in hypertensive patients. *Curr Atheroscler Rep* 2004;**6**:353–8.

30 de Jongh S, Lilien MR, op't RJ, Stroes ES *et al.* Early statin therapy restores endothelial function in children with familial hypercholesterolemia. *J Am Coll Cardiol* 2002;**40**:2117–21.

31 Lewington S, Clarke R, Qizilbash N, Peto R *et al.* Age-specific relevance of usual blood pressure to vascular mortality: a meta-analysis of individual data for one million adults in 61 prospective studies. *Lancet* 2002;**360**:1903–13.

32 Wald NJ, Law MR. A strategy to reduce cardiovascular disease by more than 80%. *BMJ* 2003;**326**:1419.

☐ VASCULAR RISK FACTORS SELF ASSESSMENT QUESTIONS

Prevention of atherosclerosis in diabetes

1 Cardiovascular mortality in diabetes:
(a) Is increased in type 2 but not type 1 diabetes
(b) Is higher in diabetes partly because the case fatality associated with acute myocardial infarction is increased
(c) Is already increased by the time type 2 diabetes is diagnosed
(d) Is equivalent in type 1 diabetic patients aged 50 years to that in non-diabetics 20 years older
(e) Is greater at any given level of serum cholesterol than in otherwise similar non-diabetics

2 The treatment of diabetic dyslipidaemia with a statin:
(a) Is more risky than prescribing aspirin 75 mg daily
(b) Is likely to prevent more coronary events than the treatment of hypertension
(c) Reduces cardiovascular risk in proportion to the degree of low-density lipoprotein cholesterol lowering achieved
(d) Is indicated in both primary and secondary prevention of cardiovascular disease in patients with diabetes
(e) Is unnecessary if good glycaemic control is achieved

3 In clinical trials, the effectiveness of statins in decreasing cardiovascular events:
(a) Is directly related to the absolute risk
(b) Is similar regardless of whether cardiovascular risk is determined by high cholesterol levels, high blood pressure, age, smoking, sex or diabetes
(c) Is counterbalanced by an increase in non-cardiovascular complications
(d) Provides one of the few examples of pharmacotherapy that reduces all-cause mortality
(e) Has been specifically demonstrated in trials involving patients with type 1 diabetes

4 The Collaborative AtoRvastatin Diabetes Study (CARDS):
(a) Was stopped prematurely because the investigators became concerned about the high rate of unexplained side effects
(b) Was stopped prematurely because of a highly significant benefit in the actively treated patients notified to the investigators by the safety committee
(c) Did not include patients with raised fasting triglycerides (>2.3 mmol/l)
(d) Was conducted in patients whose levels of low-density lipoprotein cholesterol were <4.14 mmol/l with no lower limit
(e) Pre-treatment levels of low-density lipoprotein cholesterol were <2.6 mmol/l in one-quarter of randomised patients

5   The first guidelines for statin therapy issued since the publication of CARDS
     are those of the American Diabetes Association. These:
     (a) Recommend that all type 1 and 2 diabetic patients aged >40 years receive
         statin treatment if their serum cholesterol is 3.5 mmol/l or more
     (b) Are illogical because CARDS showed that there was no threshold of low-
         density lipoprotein cholesterol below which the statin was ineffective
     (c) Recommend that the overall aim of statin therapy should be a level of low-
         density lipoprotein cholesterol of <2.6 mmol/l
     (d) Recommend that type 1 and 2 diabetic patients aged <40 years can receive
         statin therapy if judged to be at high cardiovascular risk
     (e) Recommend that young patients at high cardiovascular risk are identified
         when they have overt cardiovascular disease, have had diabetes for several
         years or have other additional risk factors

Vascular dysfunction in atherosclerosis: importance of lifetime management

1   Endothelial dysfunction may reflect:
     (a) Decreased production of nitric oxide
     (b) Reduced numbers of endothelial progenitor cells
     (c) Increased production of endothelin-1
     (d) Increased degradation of nitric oxide
     (e) All of the above

2   Endothelial function testing:
     (a) Endothelial function testing in the peripheral arteries correlates with
         coronary tests
     (b) Endothelial function testing can be a good surrogate for future
         cardiovascular events
     (c) Endothelial function testing can be assessed non-invasively from the first
         decade of life
     (d) Non-invasive measures reflect local bioavailability of nitric oxide

3   Treatment approaches for vascular dysfunction:
     (a) Exercise and diet modification can restore endothelial function
     (b) Multiple risk factor intervention in metabolic syndrome can prevent
         progression to diabetes
     (c) Statins reduce clinical cardiovascular events in patients with type 2
         diabetes
     (d) Lowering levels of low-density lipoprotein cholesterol to <100 mg/dl with
         statins produces no cardiovascular benefit
     (e) Statins do not lower levels of C-reactive protein

Cardiology

Genetics of cardiomyopathy

Srijita Sen-Chowdhry and William McKenna

☐ INTRODUCTION

The cardiomyopathies were originally defined as heart muscle diseases of unknown cause and were classified into three main types: hypertrophic cardiomyopathy (HCM), dilated cardiomyopathy (DCM) and restrictive cardiomyopathy (RCM).[1] Clinical manifestations of the cardiomyopathies include systolic and diastolic impairment, arrhythmia and sudden death. One of the major advances of the past two decades has the been the recognition that the primary myocardial diseases have a genetic basis. The ramifications in the clinical arena have been manifold. First and foremost, awareness is growing of the need to evaluate the relatives of index cases to identify other individuals who may be at risk. Second, elucidation of the genetic aetiology of these diseases has provided insight into their pathogenesis, which has facilitated the development of specific therapies.

The central role of genetics in the cardiomyopathies has prompted calls for a revised system of classification that incorporates the molecular basis of these diseases and descriptive clinical features. The deficiencies in the current definitions are best illustrated by RCM. Characterised by impaired filling and reduced diastolic volume of either or both ventricles with normal or near-normal systolic function and wall thickness, this clinical entity occurs in association with a number of systemic disorders. In its primary form, however, RCM may be affiliated genetically with HCM, coexisting within the same family and resulting from an identical mutation.[2] Conversely, a distinct heart muscle disorder, arrhythmogenic right ventricular cardiomyopathy (ARVC), is little known among general physicians but has received increased attention of late as an important cause of arrhythmia and sudden death in young people.[3]

☐ PATTERNS OF INHERITANCE

Like many monogenic structural disorders, the cardiomyopathies typically are inherited as autosomal dominant traits with incomplete penetrance. This is true of the three main heart muscle diseases: HCM, DCM and ARVC. Penetrance may be age related; clinical manifestations often become apparent during the pubertal growth spurt but may arise at any age from infancy to later life. Both HCM and DCM are recognised in childhood; ARVC, in contrast, is rare before adolescence. Variable expressivity is characteristic. Phenocopies of HCM and certain kindreds with DCM may show X-linked, mitochondrial and autosomal recessive transmission; the latter also is seen in syndromic forms of ARVC.

In general, mutations are isolated readily when they exhibit high penetrance, low lethality and a clearly defined clinical phenotype. The familial basis of HCM was recognised long before that of the other cardiomyopathies, perhaps because of the relatively low penetrance of DCM and ARVC in many families. The difficulty in genotyping families affected by ARVC is compounded further by the breadth of phenotypic variation. In contrast, HCM has a penetrance of up to 70% in some kindreds and became the first cardiac disease to be genotyped successfully in 1990.[4]

☐ HYPERTROPHIC CARDIOMYOPATHY

A disease of the sarcomere

Cardiac β-myosin heavy chain was the first gene implicated in familial HCM and paved the way for a search for defects in other sarcomeric proteins. Over the last 10 years, causative mutations have been identified in α-tropomyosin, cardiac troponin T, troponin I and C, myosin binding protein-C, α-cardiac myosin heavy chain, regulatory and essential myosin light chain, cardiac actin and titin. This fostered the view that HCM was a disease of the sarcomere – the contractile apparatus of the cell. Analysis of genotype–phenotype associations overturned two of the fundamental tenets of HCM: the requirement of unexplained left ventricular hypertrophy for diagnosis and onset of disease expression by early adulthood. In many families, mutations in troponin T are characterised by subtle or absent hypertrophy but a high incidence of sudden death. Late-onset disease may occur in conjunction with mutations in myosin binding protein C.[4]

A more contemporary definition of HCM is that of an inherited heart muscle disorder caused by mutations in sarcomeric proteins, which results in myocyte disarray, with or without fibrosis, myocardial hypertrophy and small vessel disease (narrowing of intramural coronary arteries by medial thickening). Penetrance is incomplete and age related: 55% from the ages of 10–29 years, 75% from 30–49 and 95% in gene carriers over the age of 50.[5]

Phenocopies of HCM

The prevalence of HCM in the adult population is estimated at 1 in 500; however, only about 60% of adults with HCM have mutations in the sarcomeric genes known to cause disease. A small proportion of the remainder may have defects in components of the sarcomere that are yet to be identified, but this is unlikely to fully account for the discrepancy. An examination of the aetiology of HCM in early life suggests an alternative explanation. Most infants and young children (younger than three years) with left ventricular hypertrophy do not have sarcomeric disease; instead, metabolic disorders, mitochondrial cytopathies and syndromes with characteristic extracardiac features predominate. These disease states are termed phenocopies and may exist in some adults with apparent HCM, remaining unrecognised because of a lack of systematic screening. Routine measurement of levels of α-galactosidase A in plasma among adult male patients with HCM showed a 4% prevalence of previously undiagnosed Anderson-Fabry's disease.[6]

Timely detection of cardiac phenocopies of HCM is important for several reasons. First, the cardiac profile frequently is distinct from that of sarcomeric HCM, with an increased incidence of conduction disease and progression to cavity dilation and heart failure. Management of these disorders also requires vigilance for extracardiac complications, such as skeletal myopathy, renal impairment and neurological involvement. Furthermore, specific therapies, such as enzyme replacement in Anderson-Fabry's disease, may alter the natural history of the disease. Finally, recognition of recessive, X-linked and mitochondrial patterns of inheritance has major implications for familial assessment and genetic counselling.

A disease of energy deficit

The genetic, clinical and pathological heterogeneity of HCM has hitherto defied a unifying classification. Recent thinking suggests that deficient cellular energetics may be the missing link.[7] Most of the genetic defects previously identified in HCM lead to an aberration at some point along the pathway of synthesis, transfer, regulation and expenditure of adenosine triphosphate (ATP). The sarcomeric mutations have differing effects on contractility, but inefficient use of ATP is a shared consequence. The mitochondrial cytopathies and Friedreich's ataxia may interfere with synthesis of ATP, while lysosomal storage of glycosphingolipids in Fabry's disease may impair activity of respiratory chain enzymes. Mutations in adenosine 5'-phosphate (AMP)-activated protein kinase, the cellular fuel gauge, cause HCM with pre-excitation and conduction system disease.

The cellular deficit in ATP that results is thought to cause dysfunction of the sarcoplasmic reticulum's calcium reuptake pump. The prolonged cytosolic calcium transient may serve as the signal that ultimately triggers cellular hypertrophy, although the exact pathway remains to be elucidated.[7]

Energetic abnormalities also are seen in ischaemic heart disease and heart failure and, as such, have been considered a consequence of hypertrophy rather than the primary defect. Magnetic resonance spectroscopy, however, has shown the presence of the bioenergetic deficit in non-penetrant HCM gene carriers without hypertrophy, arguing against it being a secondary phenomenon.[8]

☐ DILATED CARDIOMYOPATHY

A familial disease

Once considered an idiopathic and sporadic disease, DCM is now recognised to be familial in at least 40–60% of cases. Many apparently secondary forms of DCM, notably alcoholic cardiomyopathy and peripartum cardiomyopathy, probably arise when incompletely penetrant genetic disease is unmasked by an additional insult to the myocardium (eg alcohol) or stress on the cardiovascular system (eg pregnancy or viral infection).

The prevalence of familial DCM has been underestimated for a number of reasons. First, disease expression frequently is incomplete in family members. Prospective evaluation of the asymptomatic relatives of patients with DCM showed isolated left ventricular enlargement in 20%, mild contractile impairment in 6% and frank DCM in an additional 3%.[9] Asymptomatic relatives with left ventricular enlargement showed histological and immunological changes similar to those with established disease.[10] A proportion of relatives with minor abnormalities progressed to overt DCM during follow up, underscoring the importance of detecting these changes as markers of early disease.[11] Variable and age-related penetrance is a second impediment to recognition of familial cases. In one Italian series, penetrance was 10% for those younger than 20 years, 34% between the ages of 20 and 30 years, 60% in those aged 30–40 years and 90% in those older than 40.[12] Estimation of the true prevalence of familial DCM therefore will need serial assessment of extended families over lengthy periods of follow up.

A disease of force deficit

Elucidation of the molecular aetiology of DCM has proved challenging because of its exceptional genetic heterogeneity. One of the first breakthroughs was the identification of dystrophin as the causative gene in X-linked familial DCM. Defects in dystrophin also are responsible for Duchenne and Becker muscular dystrophy. While patients with muscular dystrophy frequently develop DCM, involvement of the skeletal muscle is rare among patients with X-linked DCM, although serum creatine kinase muscle isoforms are increased in both. Dystrophin localises to the inner aspect of the myocyte cytoplasmic membrane (sarcolemma), binding to actin at its N-terminus and to the transmembrane dystrophin-glycoprotein complex at its C-terminus. Most of the mutations isolated in X-linked DCM affect the N-terminal domain.[13]

The first disease-causing gene to be isolated in autosomal dominant DCM was cardiac actin on chromosome 15q14. Actin is a sarcomeric thin filament with a dual function in cardiac myocytes. At one end, it interacts with other components of the sarcomere (β-myosin heavy chain, α-tropomyosin and the troponins) and has a key role in force generation within the contracting myocyte. At its other end, actin binds to the anchoring proteins dystrophin and α-actinin, thereby facilitating trans-mission of the contractile force to the sarcolemma and adjacent cardiac myocytes. Interestingly, mutations in the sarcomeric end of actin are associated with HCM, while defects in its anchoring end cause DCM, presumably via impaired transmission of force. A similar mechanism has been invoked for the DCM-related α-tropomyosin mutations, which are predicted to cause localised reversal of charge at the surface of the tropomyosin protein. This may disrupt the electrostatic interaction between tropomyosin and actin within the thin filament, thus compromising its function in transmitting force to adjacent sarcomeres.[13]

Mutations in a number of other sarcomeric genes, including β-myosin heavy chain, cardiac troponin T, troponin C and troponin I, also may result in DCM, often characterised by early onset disease expression and adverse prognosis.[13–16] A deficit in force generation by the sarcomere is thought to be the underlying mechanism. Conversely, the sarcomeric mutations that cause HCM may induce ventricular remodelling (ie, hypertrophy) through ineffective utilisation of ATP.

Impaired generation and transmission of force are therefore considered the key mechanisms that underlie disease expression in DCM. Both may be relevant in the case of titin[14] – a giant sarcomeric protein implicated in autosomal dominant DCM that binds to α-actinin, stabilises the myosin filament and confers elasticity to the sarcomere. Compromised linkage of the sarcomere, cytoskeleton and sarcolemma may serve as the 'final common pathway' of disease expression in DCM.[13,17] The finding of DCM mutations in the intermediate filament desmin, δ-sarcoglycan and β-sarcoglycan (both components of the dystrophin-glycoprotein complex), Cypher/Zasp (a Z-line protein that bridges the sarcomere to the cytoskeleton) and metavinculin (which connects actin filaments to the intercalated disc) lends support to this hypothesis.[17,18] Skeletal myopathy, which varies from subclinical to overt, may be an associated feature of some of these mutations.

Dilated cardiomyopathy with conduction defects

Dilated cardiomyopathy may occur in conjunction with conduction system disease, inherited as an autosomal dominant or X-linked trait. The dominant form has been linked to mutations in the LMNA gene on chromosome 1q21, which encodes two main isoforms (lamin A and C) by alternative splicing. The lamins are intermediate filament proteins of the inner nuclear membrane that confer mechanical strength to the nuclear envelope and may have a role in transcription regulation. The phenotypic spectrum associated with mutations in lamin A/C is broad, encompassing skeletal myopathies, progeria, Charcot-Marie-Tooth disease and familial partial lipodystrophy, as well as progressive atrioventricular block and DCM. Disruption of the integrity of the nuclear envelope, resulting in premature cell death, has been suggested as the molecular basis for these diseases. Emerin, another component of the nuclear membrane, has been implicated in the X-linked form of DCM with conduction system disease.[19]

A disease of cytoskeletal dysfunction

Despite the remarkable diversity of molecular mechanisms in DCM, the consequences at a cellular level are similar: neuroendocrine activation and local production of cytokines, maladaptive myocyte hypertrophy, apoptosis, fibrosis and progressive ventricular dilation and impairment. Recent studies show disruption of the N-terminus of dystrophin in both DCM and ischaemic heart failure. Dystrophin serves as the bridge between the cytoskeleton and the sarcolemma; its loss of integrity in the failing heart supports the premise of the final common pathway in DCM. Of note, dystrophin remodelling was reversible after support with a left ventricular assist device, which suggests that reduction of mechanical stress is critical to recovery of cellular and cardiac function.[20]

□ RESTRICTIVE CARDIOMYOPATHY

No longer idiopathic

Primary restrictive cardiomyopathy had long been considered idiopathic, although familial preponderance was described. More recently, a large family was reported in which several individuals had HCM, while others showed a classic RCM phenotype.[2] A novel missense mutation in Troponin I was isolated in all affected individuals. Nine unrelated patients with RCM subsequently were screened for mutations in Troponin I, and six were found to be positive. Restrictive cardiomyopathy therefore seems to be part of the spectrum of hereditary sarcomeric contractile protein disease.

A homozygous mutation in Troponin I also has been implicated in a family with recessive DCM,[16] underscoring the diverse clinical phenotypes that may be associated with mutations in the same gene.

☐ ARRHYTHMOGENIC RIGHT VENTRICULAR CARDIOMYOPATHY

A disease of cell adhesion

Arrhythmogenic right ventricular cardiomyopathy is a heart muscle disease that may result in ventricular arrhythmia and sudden death. The main pathological feature is progressive loss of myocardium, with fibrofatty replacement. Although a predilection for the right ventricle is traditionally one of the defining characteristics, left ventricular involvement is common and may predominate in some patients. The prevalence of familial disease usually is cited at around 30–50%, but this almost certainly is a conservative estimate. As in DCM, reduced penetrance and variable disease expression among relatives may give the false appearance of sporadic disease. An additional contributing factor in ARVC is the difficulty in establishing a clinical diagnosis; clinical findings in the early 'concealed' phase of the disease often are subtle and non-specific.

In most families, ARVC is inherited as an autosomal dominant trait. The molecular studies that led to identification of the first disease-causing gene, however, were conducted on a recessive variant known as Naxos syndrome: a triad of ARVC, palmoplantar keratoderma and woolly hair. The presence of easily discernible cutaneous features facilitated recognition of affected patients in this population. A two-base pair deletion in the plakoglobin gene was identified as the cause of Naxos disease in 2000. A homozygous deletion in the desmoplakin gene subsequently was isolated in an Ecuadorean family with a similar cardiocutaneous syndrome. Desmoplakin was also the first gene to be implicated in the more common dominant form of ARVC, followed by plakophilin-2; the latter may account for up to 25% of cases.[21]

Plakoglobin, desmoplakin and plakophilin are key components of desmosomes – the specialised adhesive junctions of cardiac and epithelial tissues that link the intermediate filaments and cytoplasmic membranes of adjacent cells. Tissue exposed to shear or frictional stress is dependent on the strength of this supporting network. Impaired desmosomal function consequent to a defect in one of the component proteins predisposes to myocyte detachment and death. Significant myocyte necrosis may be accompanied by an inflammatory response. The regenerative capacity of the myocardium is limited, necessitating repair by fibrofatty substitution. The relation between mechanical stress and loss of myocytes may explain why athletes often have structurally severe forms of the disease. The desmosomal proteins are newly recognised in ARVC but well known to dermatologists, with an established role in cutaneous disorders including epidermolysis bullosa, pemphigus vulgaris, palmoplantar keratoderma and familial hypotrichosis.

□ CONCLUSION

The cardiomyopathies, once defined as heart muscle diseases of unknown cause, now are known to be determined genetically. Sarcomeric defects predominate in HCM, while a wide range of metabolic defects may produce phenocopies; compromised cellular energetics may be the unifying mechanism. Loss of linkage between the sarcomere, cytoskeleton and sarcolemma may be the final common pathway in DCM. Primary restrictive cardiomyopathy seems to be part of the spectrum of sarcomeric contractile protein disease. The identification of mutations in plakoglobin, desmoplakin and plakophilin has led to the contemporary view of ARVC as a disease of cell adhesion.

Familial evaluation is mandatory once a diagnosis of cardiomyopathy has been established in an index case. Relatives often are asymptomatic and show incomplete disease expression but nonetheless may be at risk of complications. Reliance on a family history alone therefore is inadequate; first-degree relatives should be offered non-invasive cardiac evaluation, including 12-lead electrocardiogram (ECG) and transthoracic echocardiography, with exercise testing and ambulatory ECG monitoring as appropriate. As penetrance is variable and often age related, periodic rescreening may be needed, and second-degree relatives often require assessment. The identification of a disease-causing mutation within a family enables cascade screening, clarification of the diagnosis in borderline cases and reassurance of gene-negative people. Improved understanding of the pathogenesis of the heart muscle disorders ultimately may enhance the development of rational therapeutic strategies.

REFERENCES

1 Richardson P, McKenna W, Bristow M, Maisch B *et al.* Report of the 1995 World Health Organization/International Society and Federation of Cardiology Task Force on the definition and classification of cardiomyopathies. *Circulation* 1996;**93**:841–2.

2 Mogensen J, Kubo T, Duque M, Uribe W *et al.* Idiopathic restrictive cardiomyopathy is part of the clinical expression of cardiac troponin I mutations. *J Clin Invest* 2003;**111**:209–16.

3 Sen-Chowdhry S, Lowe MD, Sporton SC, McKenna WJ. Arrhythmogenic right ventricular cardiomyopathy: clinical presentation, diagnosis, and management. *Am J Med* 2004;**117**: 685–95.

4 Elliott P, McKenna WJ. Hypertrophic cardiomyopathy. *Lancet* 2004;**363**:1881–91.

5 Charron P, Carrier L, Dubourg O, Tesson F *et al.* Penetrance of familial hypertrophic cardiomyopathy. *Genet Couns* 1997;**8**:107–14.

6 Sachdev B, Takenaka T, Teraguchi H, Tei C *et al.* Prevalence of Anderson-Fabry disease in male patients with late onset hypertrophic cardiomyopathy. *Circulation* 2002;**105**:1407–11.

7 Ashrafian H, Redwood C, Blair E, Watkins H. Hypertrophic cardiomyopathy:a paradigm for myocardial energy depletion. *Trends Genet* 2003;**19**:263–8.

8 Crilley JG, Boehm EA, Blair E, Rajagopalan B *et al.* Hypertrophic cardiomyopathy due to sarcomeric gene mutations is characterized by impaired energy metabolism irrespective of the degree of hypertrophy. *J Am Coll Cardiol* 2003;**41**:1776–82.

9   Baig MK, Goldman JH, Caforio AL, Coonar AS *et al.* Familial dilated cardiomyopathy: cardiac abnormalities are common in asymptomatic relatives and may represent early disease. *J Am Coll Cardiol* 1998;**31**:195–201.

10   Mahon NG, Madden BP, Caforio AL, Elliott PM *et al.* Immunohistologic evidence of myocardial disease in apparently healthy relatives of patients with dilated cardiomyopathy. *J Am Coll Cardiol* 2002;**39**:455–62

11   Mahon NG, Murphy RT, MacRae CA, Caforio ALP *et al.* Echocardiographic evaluation in asymptomatic relatives of dilated cardiomyopathy patients reveals preclinical disease. *Ann Intern Med* 2005;**143**:108–15.

12   Mestroni L, Maisch B, McKenna WJ, Schwartz K *et al.* Guidelines for the study of familial dilated cardiomyopathies. Collaborative Research Group of the European Human and Capital Mobility Project on Familial Dilated Cardiomyopathy. *Eur Heart J* 1999;**20**:93–102.

13   Towbin JA, Bowles NE. The failing heart. *Nature* 2002;**415**:227–33.

14   Crispell KA, Hanson EL, Coates K, Toy W *et al.* Periodic rescreening is indicated for family members at risk of developing familial dilated cardiomyopathy. *J Am Coll Cardiol* 2002;**39**:1503–7.

15   Mogensen J, Murphy RT, Shaw T, Bahl A *et al.* Severe disease expression of cardiac troponin C and T mutations in patients with idiopathic dilated cardiomyopathy. *J Am Coll Cardiol* 2004;**44**:2033–40.

16   Murphy RT, Mogensen J, Shaw A, Kubo T *et al.* Novel mutation in cardiac troponin I in recessive idiopathic dilated cardiomyopathy. *Lancet* 2004;**363**:371–2.

17   Bowles NE, Bowles KR, Towbin JA. The 'final common pathway' hypothesis and inherited cardiovascular disease. The role of cytoskeletal proteins in dilated cardiomyopathy. *Herz* 2000;**25**:168–75.

18   Vatta M, Mohapatra B, Jimenez S, Sanchez X *et al.* Mutations in Cypher/ZASP in patients with dilated cardiomyopathy and left ventricular non-compaction. *J Am Coll Cardiol* 2003;**42**:2014–27.

19   Vohanka S, Vytopil M, Bednarik J, Lukas Z *et al.* A mutation in the X-linked Emery-Dreifuss muscular dystrophy gene in a patient affected with conduction cardiomyopathy. *Neuromuscul Disord* 2001;**11**:411–3.

20   Vatta M, Stetson SJ, Perez-Verdia A, Entman ML *et al.* Molecular remodelling of dystrophin in patients with end-stage cardiomyopathies and reversal in patients on assistance-device therapy. *Lancet* 2002;**359**:936–41.

21   Sen-Chowdhry S, Syrris P, McKenna WJ. Genetics of right ventricular cardiomyopathy. *J Cardio Electrophysiol* 2005;**16**:927–35.

Pulmonary hypertension

J Simon R Gibbs

☐ INTRODUCTION AND CLINICAL CLASSIFICATION

Pulmonary hypertension is elevation of pulmonary arterial pressure to a mean of 25 mmHg at rest or 30 mmHg on exercise. Pulmonary hypertension has a large number of causes, and these have been classified recently according to similarities in clinical presentation, where the pulmonary circulation is affected and response to treatment (Table 1, overleaf).[1]

Pulmonary arterial hypertension (PAH) includes a group of conditions associated with a progressive increase in resistance to blood flow in the lungs. This leads to right ventricular failure and premature death. Pulmonary arterial hypertension includes 'primary pulmonary hypertension', which is now classified as idiopathic and familial PAH, and other diseases that sometimes are associated with PAH. Idiopathic PAH may occur at any age and pursues a rapid downhill course: data from the National Institutes of Health showed a median survival of 2.8 years from diagnosis before the advent of recent disease-modifying therapies.[2] Certain clinical factors predict an adverse prognosis: extremes of age, fast rate of decline of symptoms and exercise capacity, syncope, haemoptysis and signs of right heart failure. In practice, the rate of deterioration is remarkably variable, and most patients currently only receive a diagnosis in an advanced state of the disease when their symptoms are equivalent to New York Heart Association (NYHA) functional class III or IV.

In the last 10 years, randomised clinical trials in patients mainly with the idiopathic, familial and connective tissue disease-associated forms of PAH have shown clear evidence of the benefit of new drug therapies. These important clinical breakthroughs not only have stimulated renewed clinical interest in what has been previously viewed as an untreatable group of diseases but have excited basic scientific interest in elucidating the mechanism of the disease, which as yet remains uncertain.

Left heart disease describes a group of conditions that give rise to pulmonary venous hypertension. Treatment with prostacyclin or endothelian antagonists is contraindicated, as these drugs increase morbidity and, in the case of prostacyclin, mortality in this situation.

The most common cause of pulmonary hypertension associated with lung diseases or hypoxaemia is chronic obstructive pulmonary disease. Some patients with interstitial lung disease may develop a pulmonary vasculopathy, with pulmonary hypertension out of proportion to the underlying lung disease. Sleep apnoea is an important diagnosis that should be considered in all patients, because treatment with non-invasive ventilation may improve symptoms significantly.

Table 1 Clinical classification of pulmonary hypertension. Reproduced from Ref 1 with permission from American College of Cardiology Foundation.

1	**Pulmonary arterial hypertension (PAH)**	
	1.1	Idiopathic (IPAH)
	1.2	Familial (FPAH)
	1.3	Associated with (APAH)
		1.3.1 Collagen vascular disease
		1.3.2 Congenital systemic-to-pulmonary shunts
		1.3.3 Portal hypertension
		1.3.4 HIV infection
		1.3.5 Drugs and toxins
		1.3.6 Other (thyroid disorders, glycogen storage disease, Gaucher disease, hereditary hemorrhagic telangiectasia, hemoglobinopathies, myeloproliferative disorders, splenectomy)
	1.4	Associated with significant venous or capillary involvement
		1.4.1 Pulmonary veno-occlusive disease (PVOD)
		1.4.2 Pulmonary capillary hemangiomatosis (PCH)
	1.5	Persistent pulmonary hypertension of the newborn
2	**Pulmonary hypertension with left heart disease**	
	2.1	Left-sided atrial or ventricular heart disease
	2.2	Left-sided valvular heart disease
3	**Pulmonary hypertension associated with lung diseases and/or hypoxemia**	
	3.1	Chronic obstructive pulmonary disease
	3.2	Interstitial lung disease
	3.3	Sleep-disordered breathing
	3.4	Alveolar hypoventilation disorders
	3.5	Chronic exposure to high altitude
	3.6	Developmental abnormalities
4	**Pulmonary hypertension due to chronic thrombotic and/or embolic disease**	
	4.1	Thromboembolic obstruction of proximal pulmonary arteries
	4.2	Thromboembolic obstruction of distal pulmonary arteries
	4.3	Non-thrombotic pulmonary embolism (tumour, parasites, foreign material)
5	**Miscellaneous**	
	Sarcoidosis, histiocytosis X, lymphangiomatosis, compression of pulmonary vessels (adenopathy, tumour, fibrosing mediastinitis)	

Chronic thrombotic or embolic disease includes patients who have incomplete resolution of pulmonary embolism or thrombosis. Such patients with proximal surgically accessible disease should be considered for pulmonary endarterectomy, whereas those with distal disease are deemed inoperable. This group also includes any other cause of embolism, such as pulmonary arterial sarcoma, which tends to present proximally in the pulmonary circulation.

☐ SCREENING

The main impediment to patients in the clinical course of their disease is getting a diagnosis of pulmonary hypertension. In the United Kingdom, the average delay between the onset of symptoms and diagnosis is 18–24 months. The most common misdiagnosis is bronchial asthma. Delays in diagnosis result in premature death, as well as delays in treatment until the illness is in a more advanced state.

The great majority of patients present with breathlessness, which may be associated with fatigue, syncope, angina, anorexia and weight loss, exercise-induced nausea and vomiting, ascites and dependent oedema.

A chest radiograph plus an electrocardiogram will suggest the diagnosis in about 80–90% of cases.[3] Abnormal spirometry will suggest an alternative diagnosis. Echocardiography can be used to confirm the suspicion of pulmonary hypertension.

Diagnosis of pulmonary hypertension with echocardiography focuses on the estimation of systolic pressure in the pulmonary artery with the peak tricuspid regurgitant velocity (V) and an estimate of right atrial pressure. The modified Bernoulli equation is used to calculate the pressure according to the formula:

☐   Estimated systolic pulmonary arterial pressure = $4V^2$ + right atrial pressure

Right atrial pressure can be estimated clinically or with echocardiographic measurement of the diameter of the inferior vena cava and the change in diameter with a sharp inspiration or sniff (Table 2). This method of estimating systolic pressure provides a different result from the definition of pulmonary hypertension, which is based on a mean pulmonary arterial pressure of 25 mmHg at rest or 30 mmHg on exercise. As the echocardiographic estimate depends on right atrial pressure, it is not possible to give a precise peak tricuspid velocity that corresponds to a mean pressure of 25 mmHg. In general, a resting velocity of 2.8–3.4 m/s will identify mild pulmonary hypertension in patients who have normal right atrial pressure.[4] False positive and false negative results may occur in this range, and cardiac catheterisation should be undertaken to reach a definitive diagnosis. It should be remembered that interpretation of an echocardiogram requires corroborating evidence from other measurements and observations.

Table 2 Semi-quantitative estimation of right atrial pressure by echocardiography.

Mean right atrial pressure (mmHg)	Diameter of inferior vena cava (mm)	Inspiratory collapse*
0–5	12–23	>50%
5–10	12–23	<50%
10–15	>23	>50%
15–20	>23	<50%

*Best tested by asking the patient to breathe in quickly or to sniff.

Echocardiography also may identify the cause of pulmonary hypertension – particularly left atrial or ventricular disease, aortic or mitral valve disease or congenital heart disease. Two important causes of pulmonary hypertension easily may be missed on a routine echocardiogram: diastolic dysfunction of the left ventricle and atrial septal defect. Left atrial enlargement in the presence of normal left ventricular systolic function should prompt a search for these diagnoses.

Screening with serum biomarkers is not standard practice. Brain natriuretic peptide may be raised in patients with pulmonary hypertension in the presence of right ventricular dysfunction and conversely may be normal in those with a normal-sized right ventricle despite pulmonary hypertension. Troponins may also be raised; in which case the differential diagnosis includes acute coronary syndromes, heart failure, myocarditis, cardiomyopathy, pulmonary embolism and chronic renal failure. Elevated troponins are associated with a worse prognosis.

☐ INVESTIGATION

To manage pulmonary hypertension, the clinician needs to know the aetiology and severity of the disease. The aetiology can be determined from cardiac and lung imaging, lung function tests, screening for sleep apnoea, cardiac catheterisation, arterial blood gases and blood tests to confirm or refute the aetiologies described in Table 1. The severity of pulmonary hypertension can be assessed by symptom severity according to a modified NYHA classification, distance on the six-minute walk test and severity of oxygen desaturation at peak exercise compared with baseline; haemodynamics measured by echocardiography; cardiac magnetic resonance imaging, cardiac catheterisation; and serum biomarkers, as mentioned above.

☐ PATHOPHYSIOLOGY OF PAH

The pathophysiological basis of PAH provides the rationale for current therapies. The major contributors to the disease and its progression seem to be proliferation of smooth muscle cells into the pulmonary arterial lumen, release of cytokines, thrombosis and vasoconstriction. More than half of familial cases have been found to have a mutation of BMPR2 – a member of the transforming growth factor beta superfamily of transmembrane proteins.[5] Some cases of idiopathic PAH also have been found to harbour such mutations. The effect of BMPR2 mutations on intracellular pathways is unclear as yet, but it likely influences proliferation of smooth muscle cells. The observation that only 10–20% of carriers of BMPR2 mutations will develop PAH suggests that environmental factors play a role in triggering its onset. In the next few years, whether additional gene mutations or polymorphisms contribute to the development of PAH will become clearer.

☐ TREATMENT OF PAH

Evidence from retrospective studies supports anticoagulation with warfarin for patients with idiopathic and anorexogen-induced PAH. Supportive therapy with oxygen, diuretics and digoxin may be needed.

Calcium channel blockers are reserved for the small number of patients who have a significant fall in pulmonary arterial pressure in response to a vasodilator challenge at cardiac catheterisation. Most evidence supports the use of nifedipine or diltiazem, which need to be used at high doses. Only about half of patients with idiopathic PAH will have a sustained response to this treatment, and those who do not should be considered for the other treatments described below. Calcium channel blockers should not be used in the absence of such a response, as they may cause deterioration.

At present, three classes of disease-modifying therapy are available: prostacyclins, endothelin antagonists and phosphodiesterase (PDE) type 5 inhibitors. Prostacyclin occurs naturally in the vascular endothelium and is antiproliferative, cytoprotective, an inhibitor of platelet aggregation and a vasodilator. Prostacyclin can be administered as epoprostenol, iloprost or treprostinil by continuous intravenous infusion; treprostinil by continuous subcutaneous infusion; or iloprost by electronic nebuliser. Endothelin receptor antagonists block either endothelin receptor A (ET_A) and ET_B receptors (bosentan) or ET_A only (sitaxsentan and ambrisentan). These receptor blockers antagonise the effect of the powerful vasoconstrictor and smooth muscle mitogen hormone endothelin-1 and can be taken orally. Sildenafil is a PDE type 5 inhibitor that increases intracellular cyclic guanosine monophosphate. This induces relaxation of, and has an antiproliferative effect on, vascular smooth muscle cells.

The development of these disease-modifying drug therapies initially was investigated in patients with the idiopathic and familial forms of PAH. Evidence from randomised trials of some of these agents now extends to PAH associated with anorexogens and connective tissue disease.[6–10] Some trials also have included patients with congenital heart disease, portal hypertension and human immunodeficiency virus. These trials mainly have targeted patients with functional NYHA class III disease, including small numbers of patients with class II and IV disease. The recent randomised trial of sildenafil included a significant proportion of patients with class II disease,[10] while the most evidence for benefit to patients with class IV disease comes from trials of epoprostenol. All of these agents have shown improvements in the distance on the six-minute walk test after 3–4 months of treatment, but very few patients become free of symptoms.

Registry data show a survival advantage for patients treated with disease-modifying therapies. For example, patients with idiopathic PAH treated with epoprostenol or conventional medical therapy had one-year survivals of 82% and 72%, two-year survivals of 74% and 53% and three-year survivals of 62% and 48%, respectively.[11] Follow-up of patients with idiopathic PAH in whom the first-line therapy was bosentan (to which other therapies could be added to or swapped with) showed survival of 96% at one year and 89% at two years. At these time points, 85% and 70% of patients, respectively, remained on bosentan monotherapy.[12]

The decision about which treatment to use is based on the severity and aetiology of PAH, as well as what is most suitable for the individual patient. Pulmonary hypertension may deteriorate despite treatment, and combination therapy with the disease-modifying drugs then may be the best course to take, although evidence for its efficacy in trials currently is limited. Lung transplantation and/or atrial septostomy may be considered for eligible patients with deterioration despite optimal drug therapy. All patients on treatment require vigilant follow-up, normally every three months, to include routine blood samples, six-minute walk test and echocardiography. Selected cases may need magnetic resonance imaging and cardiac catheterisation at less frequent intervals. Current evidence does not support the treatment of all forms of PAH with disease-modifying therapy. In Eisenmenger's syndrome and sickle cell disease, ongoing clinical trials will help determine the role of these therapies. They should be used in veno-occlusive disease with great caution, as they may cause pulmonary oedema.

Support for patients and carers is an essential part of clinical management. Women of child-bearing age require specialist contraceptive advice because of the high mortality associated with pregnancy.

☐ ORGANISATION OF CARE IN THE UNITED KINGDOM

Table 3 Pulmonary hypertension centres in the United Kingdom.

Location	Hospital
Cambridge	Papworth Hospital
Glasgow	Western Infirmary
London	Great Ormond Street Hospital*
	Hammersmith Hospital
	Royal Brompton Hospital
	Royal Free Hospital
Newcastle	Freeman Hospital
Sheffield	Royal Hallamshire Hospital

*Centre for children.

In 2001, the Department of Health designated seven hospital trusts in England to manage pulmonary hypertension through the National Specialist Commissioning Advisory Group. This followed the earlier designation of one centre in Scotland, based at Western Infirmary, Glasgow. These centres have specialist multidisciplinary teams able to offer diagnostic facilities, advanced access to care for patients, the full range of drug therapies and access to clinical trials. One centre is designated to manage children and has outreach clinics. All the centres have a substantial workload and clinical experience and participate in national audits. The need for access to 'expert' care has been emphasised in international guidelines.

The recommendation is that all patients with pulmonary arterial hypertension, chronic thrombotic and/or embolic disease or miscellaneous causes of pulmonary hypertension and those in whom the cause of pulmonary hypertension is not certain are referred to designated centres. Patients who are being referred should normally have undergone routine blood tests, electrocardiogram, chest X-ray, spirometry and echocardiography. As some patients with pulmonary hypertension may deteriorate rapidly, referral must not be delayed to complete more extensive investigations.

☐ CONCLUSIONS

Many forms of pulmonary hypertension are treatable. Major advances have been made in the treatment of some forms of pulmonary arterial hypertension. This has provided the imperative for well-coordinated clinical management and research, which is now available in the United Kingdom. Basic science research also is identifying new treatment targets as we come closer to understanding the mechanism of the disease.

REFERENCES

1 Simonneau G, Galie N, Rubin LJ, Langleben D *et al.* Clinical classification of pulmonary hypertension. *J Am Coll Cardiol* 2004;**43**:5S–12S.

2 D'Alonzo GE, Barst RJ, Ayres SM, Bergofsky EH *et al.* Survival in patients with primary pulmonary hypertension. Results from a national prospective registry. *Ann Intern Med* 1991; 115:343–9.

3 British Cardiac Society Guidelines and Medical Practice Committee, and approved by the British Thoracic Society and the British Society of Rheumatology. Recommendations on the management of pulmonary hypertension in clinical practice. *Heart* 2001;**86**(Suppl 1):I1–13.

4 Galie N, Torbicki A, Barst R, Dartevelle P *et al.* Guidelines on diagnosis and treatment of pulmonary arterial hypertension. The Task Force on Diagnosis and Treatment of Pulmonary Arterial Hypertension of the European Society of Cardiology. *Eur Heart J* 2004;**25**:2243–78.

5 Lane KB, Machado RD, Pauciulo MW, Thomson JR *et al.* Heterozygous germline mutations in BMPR2, encoding a TGF-beta receptor, cause familial primary pulmonary hypertension. The International PPH Consortium. *Nat Genet* 2000;**26**:81–4.

6 Barst RJ, Rubin LJ, Long WA, McGoon MD *et al.* A comparison of continuous intravenous epoprostenol (prostacyclin) with conventional therapy for primary pulmonary hypertension. The Primary Pulmonary Hypertension Study Group. *N Engl J Med* 1996;**334**:296–302.

7 Simmoneau G, Barst RJ, Galie N, Naeije R *et al.* Continuous subcutaneous infusion of treprostinil, a prostacyclin analogue, in patients with pulmonary arterial hypertension: a double-blind, randomized, placebo-controlled trial. *Am J Respir Crit Care Med* 2002;**165**: 800–4.

8 Olschewski H, Simmoneau G, Galie N, Higenbottam T *et al.* Inhaled iloprost for severe pulmonary hypertension. *N Engl J Med* 2002;**347**:322–9.

9 Rubin LJ, Badesch DB, Barst RJ, Galie N *et al.* Bosentan therapy for pulmonary arterial hypertension. *N Engl J Med* 2002;**346**:896–903.

10 Ghofrani HA *et al* for the Sildenafil 1140 Study Group. Efficacy and safety of sildenafil citrate in pulmonary arterial hypertension: results of a multinational, randomized, double-blind, placebo-controlled trial (Sildenafil Use in Pulmonary Arterial Hypertension Study). *Presented at the 70th Annual Meeting of the American College of Chest Physicians, Seattle, Washington, 23–28 October 2004* (Abstract).

11 McLaughlin VV, Presberg KW, Doyle RL, Abman SH *et al.* Prognosis of pulmonary arterial hypertension: ACCP evidence-based clinical practice guidelines. *Chest* 2004;**126**(Suppl 1): 78S–92S.

12 McLaughlin VV, Sitbon O, Badesch DB, Barst RJ *et al.* Survival with first-line bosentan in patients with primary pulmonary hypertension. *Eur Respir J* 2005;**25**:244–9.

Treatment of heart failure

John JV McMurray

□ INTRODUCTION

Heart failure remains one of the most common, costly, disabling and deadly medical conditions encountered by a wide range of doctors in primary and secondary care. The treatment of heart failure has advanced dramatically in the past 20 years and continues to develop apace. This review summarises current evidence-based treatment for heart failure and glimpses into the future treatment of this condition.

□ TREATMENT

Pharmacological treatment – reduced left ventricular systolic function

Diuretics

Diuretics are essential for relieving dyspnoea and signs of sodium and water retention and are needed in virtually all patients with symptomatic heart failure.[1] They are best used flexibly – that is, the dose can be adjusted according to the patient's social activities and clinical status. Diuretics need not be taken first thing every morning and may be postponed or even omitted if the patient has to travel or has another engagement that might be compromised by the effect of the treatment. Similarly, the daily dose may vary according to the patient's clinical condition. The dose may need to be increased – often only on a temporary basis – if evidence, such as increasing breathlessness, oedema or weight, suggests fluid retention. Conversely, the dose may need to be decreased if the patient has evidence of dehydration, such as unusually intense thirst, dizziness, low jugular venous pressure or increasing levels of urea. Diuretics should be used at the minimum dose needed to maintain 'dry weight' and to avoid electrolyte disorders (such as hypokalaemia and hyponatraemia), gout and renal dysfunction.[2] In patients with advanced heart failure, high doses of loop diuretics, and even the combination of a loop diuretic with a thiazide or thiazide-like diuretic (such as metolazone), may be needed to maintain dry weight.

Angiotensin-converting enzyme inhibitors

By reducing the production of angiotensin II (and, possibly, by increasing bradykinin), angiotensin-converting enzyme (ACE) inhibitors exert a myriad of biological effects that lead to symptom improvement, reduced admission to hospital and increased longevity in heart failure; as a consequence, they are recommended for all patients with systolic dysfunction (Fig 1).[3] The main causes of intolerance are cough, symptomatic hypotension and renal dysfunction (exacerbated by overdiuresis and non-steroidal anti-inflammatory drugs). Table 1 lists the specific agents shown to improve outcome in large randomised trials.

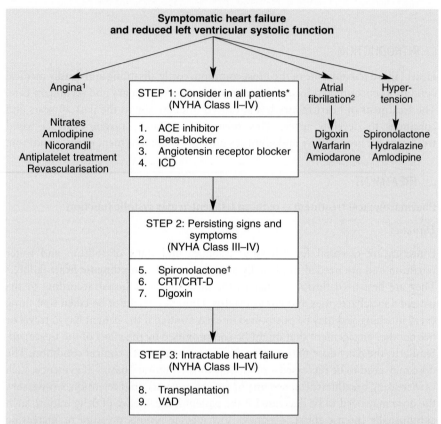

1   Amiodarone is safer than other antiarrhythmic drugs in heart failure and may help maintain sinus rhythm. If a beta blocker alone fails to control the ventricular rate (ideally <70 bpm at rest and <100 bpm during exercise), digoxin can be added (digoxin may be used first to control the ventricular rate when a beta blocker is being initiated or uptitrated). Patients with heart failure and atrial fibrillation are at high risk of thromboembolism and should be considered for anticoagulation.
2   Nitrates, amlodipine and, probably, nicorandil can be used safely to prevent and relieve symptoms in patients with heart failure and a reduced left ventricular ejection fraction who continue to have angina despite a beta blocker (or can be used while a beat blocker is being initiated or uptitrated). Antiplatelet treatment also should be considered. Revascularisation relieves symptoms and may improve prognosis in some patients.
3   In patients who remain hypertensive despite an ACE inhibitor and beta blocker, spironolactone or hydralazine should be considered. Amlodipine also is safe.

Fig 1 Treatment algorithm for patients with heart failure and reduced left ventricular systolic function. The starting and target doses of 'evidence-based' agents are given in Table 2. ACE = angiotensin-converting enzyme inhibitor; CRT = cardiac resynchronisation therapy; CRT-D = cardiac resynchronisation-defibrillator device; ICD = implantable cardioverter defibrillator; VAD = ventricular assist device; NYHA = New York Heart Association.
*These treatments usually are added to existing diuretic treatment dosed flexibly to maintain 'dry weight'; H-ISDN also can be considered in African-Americans. †Safety and efficacy of a combination of ACE inhibitor, angiotensin receptor blocker and aldosterone antagonist not known. Adapted from Ref 3.

Table 1 Evidence-based pharmacological treatment of heart failure[*]

Drug	Starting dose (mg)	Target total daily dose (mg)†	Doses per day†	Mean total daily dose in outcome studies (mg)
ACE inhibitors:				
Captopril	6.25	150	3	121
Enalapril	2.5	20–40	2	16.6
Lisinopril	2.5–5.0	20–35	1	–‡
Ramipril	2.5	10	1 or 2	8.7**
Trandolapril	1.0	4	1	3
Beta blockers:				
Bisoprolol	1.25	10	1	6.2
Carvedilol	3.125	50–100	2	37††
Metoprolol controlled release/extended release	12.5 or 25	200	1	159‡‡
Angiotensin receptor blockers:				
Candesartan	4	32	1	24***
Valsartan	40	320	2	254
Aldosterone blockers:				
Eplerenone	25	50	1	43
Spironolactone	25	50	1	26
Hydralazine–isosorbide dinitrate:†††				
Hydralazine	37.5	225	3	143
Isosorbide dinitrate	20	120	3	60

[*]Based on randomised controlled trials in patients with chronic heart failure or heart failure, left ventricular systolic dysfunction or both after myocardial infarction.
†Total daily dose taken once daily or split into two or three equal portions – for example, target total daily dose of captopril is 150 mg, taken as 50 mg three times a day (based on SAVE study).
‡The Assessment of Treatment with Lisinopril and Survival trial compared high-dose lisinopril (32·5–35 mg) with low-dose lisinopril (2·5–5·0 mg); guidelines recommend 20 mg daily as a single dose.
**Based on the Infarction Ramipril Efficacy Study, in which ramipril was prescribed twice daily (target total daily dose 10 mg).
††In the Carvedilol Prospective Randomized Cumulative Study, in which the target total daily dose was 50 mg.
‡‡Metoprolol succinate; the Carvedilol or Metoprolol European Trial showed that low doses of metoprolol tartrate are inferior to carvedilol. Metoprolol succinate is not currently available in the UK.
***In Candesartan in Heart Failure Assessment of Reduction in Mortality and Morbidity-Added.
†††Based on African-American Heart Failure Trial; this combination was given four times daily in Vasodilator Heart Failure Trial I.
Adapted from Ref 3.

Beta blockers

Beta blockers probably act to protect the heart from the harmful effects of the sympathetic nervous system mediated by norepinephrine and epinephrine. They represent the greatest advance in the treatment of heart failure since ACE inhibitors. Their addition to an ACE inhibitor leads to a further and substantial reduction in mortality (by about one-third) and morbidity (such as hospital admissions), as well as an improvement in symptoms and patients' wellbeing (as evidenced, for example, by improved New York Heart Association functional class and quality of life).[4,5] Consequently, the combination of an ACE inhibitor and beta blocker is now the cornerstone of the treatment of patients with reduced left ventricular systolic function (see Fig 1 and Table 2). A beta blocker should be initiated at a low dose and the dose carefully uptitrated – the so-called 'start low, go slow' approach. When used in this way, intolerance is infrequent and most commonly due to dizziness and bradycardia. Rarely, early worsening of heart failure may occur, but this usually can be managed by a reduction in the dose of the beta blocker and an increase in the dose of diuretic, which usually only needs to be temporary.[2]

Angiotensin receptor blockers (ARBs)

These drugs block angiotensin II binding to its type 1 receptor and have broadly similar effects to ACE inhibitors in terms of tolerability (with the exception of cough) and clinical outcomes in heart failure. [6,7] These conclusions are supported by similar findings from a study in patients with left ventricular systolic dysfunction, heart failure, or both after myocardial infarction. Consequently, an ARB should be substituted in a patient with an intolerable ACE inhibitor-induced cough. Although an ARB also has been shown to be of benefit in patients with other causes of ACE-inhibitor intolerance, the use of an ARB in patients with prior hypotension and, especially, hyperkalaemia or renal dysfunction mandates very careful monitoring.[2]

Of more importance, when ARBs are added to recommended doses of ACE inhibitors (and other treatments for heart failure), they lead to further neurohumoral suppression and greater reverse remodelling of the left ventricle, possibly because concentrations of angiotensin II in the blood often remain high or increase despite ACE inhibition.[6,7] The addition of an ARB to an ACE inhibitor also reduces cardiovascular mortality and hospital admissions for heart failure. The addition of an ARB to an ACE inhibitor also improves symptoms, signs and patient wellbeing. Consequently, an ARB is recommended to be added to treatment with an ACE inhibitor and beta blocker in patients with symptomatic heart failure (see Fig 1 and Table 2). Intolerance is infrequent and most commonly is the result of hypotension and renal dysfunction. The addition of an ARB to an ACE inhibitor mandates careful monitoring of blood chemistry.[2]

Aldosterone blockade

Aldosterone is the second effector hormone in the renin–angiotensin–aldosterone cascade and seems to have detrimental cardiac, vascular, renal and other actions when produced in excess in patients with heart failure. Whereas ACE inhibitors, beta blockers and ARBs have been studied across the spectrum of severity of heart failure (and ARBs have been added to background treatment with an ACE inhibitor and beta blocker across this spectrum), aldosterone blockade has been tested only in patients with severe symptomatic heart failure – most of whom were treated with an ACE inhibitor but few of whom were treated with a beta blocker (because the Randomized Aldactone Evaluation Study (RALES) was conducted before the evidence that supported use of beta blockers in patients of this type became available).[8] In those patients, spironolactone led to a substantial reduction in all-cause mortality and morbidity (heart failure and other hospital admissions) and improved symptoms.[8] These findings were supported by similar, but smaller, benefits with eplerenone in patients with heart failure and reduced left ventricular systolic function after acute myocardial infarction (most of whom were treated with an ACE inhibitor and beta blocker). Aldosterone blockade, therefore, is recommended for patients who remain in New York Heart Association classes III and IV despite treatment with an ACE inhibitor and beta blocker (see Fig 1 and Table 2). Whether aldosterone blockade is advantageous in milder heart failure is unknown. The main causes of intolerance are renal dysfunction, hyperkalaemia (mandating careful biochemical monitoring) and, with spironolactone, anti-androgenic side effects, especially gynaecomastia in men. Anti-androgenic side effects are thought to be less common with eplerenone.

In a stable patient with symptomatic heart failure and low left ventricular ejection fraction, an ARB or aldosterone blocker should be added, with the caveat that extra biochemical monitoring is essential. Whether an ARB *and* aldosterone blocker can and should be combined with an ACE inhibitor, that is three blockers of the renin–angiotensin–aldosterone system are used (in addition to a beta blocker), is unknown and carries a significant risk of renal dysfunction and hyperkalaemia.[9]

Hydralazine and isosorbide dinitrate (H-ISDN)

This vasodilator combination was the first treatment shown to improve survival in heart failure but was later shown to be less effective than an ACE inhibitor in a head-to-head comparison. Recently, a strategy of adding H-ISDN to conventional treatment, including an ACE inhibitor, beta blocker and spironolactone, was shown to reduce mortality (and admissions to hospital for heart failure) in African–Americans, although this conclusion was based on relatively small numbers of events.[10] Whether this drug combination is an effective addition in other patients is unknown. Intolerance usually is the result of headache and dizziness though hydralazine can rarely cause a lupus-like syndrome.

Digoxin

Although digoxin usually is considered to be an inotrope, it has autonomic, neurohumoral and diuretic actions. In patients with atrial fibrillation, digoxin, when added to a beta blocker, is useful for controlling the ventricular rate.[11] Digoxin, however, now has a limited role in patients in sinus rhythm. In one large clinical trial, digoxin added to an ACE inhibitor reduced the risk of admission to hospital with worsening heart failure, although it did not have a survival benefit; it may also have a modest symptom benefit.[12] Consequently, digoxin is recommended only in patients with persistent symptoms and signs despite the use of the more effective treatments mentioned above (see Fig 1). Evidence shows that withdrawal of digoxin can lead to worsening of heart failure. Intolerance usually is the result of nausea, although conduction disturbances and arrhythmias are also a concern. Toxicity is more likely with higher doses and is increased by hypokalaemia (careful biochemical monitoring is needed), and measurement of concentrations of digoxin in the blood is advised.

Pharmacological treatment – preserved left ventricular systolic function

Unlike for heart failure with left ventricular systolic dysfunction, there are no generally agreed, evidence-based treatments for patients with heart failure and preserved systolic function. The following outlines possible empirical approaches.

Treat underlying condition

Treatment of underlying cardiovascular and other conditions that might be contributing to the development of heart failure, such as hypertension, myocardial ischaemia, atrial fibrillation and diabetes, is important.[13]

Diuretics

Diuretics are used empirically and according to the same principles as in heart failure with reduced systolic function.[2]

Angiotensin receptor blockers

In the Candesartan in Heart Failure Assessment of Reduction in Mortality and Morbidity (CHARM)-Preserved trial, treatment with candesartan did not lead to a significant reduction in the risk of the primary composite endpoint (adjudicated death from cardiovascular causes or admission with heart failure), but it did bring about a substantial reduction in the risk of investigator-reported admissions for heart failure.[14] Another trial, Irbesartan in Heart Failure with Preserved Systolic Function (I-Preserve), is evaluating the effect of another ARB, irbesartan, on mortality and cardiovascular morbidity in these patients, as is a study with the ACE inhibitor perindopril.

Beta blockers

By reducing heart rate, beta blockers should increase the time for left ventricular filling, and by enhancing relaxation, they also should improve diastolic filling. The anti-ischaemic antihypertensive actions also might be beneficial in patients with heart failure and preserved systolic function. Study of Effects of Nebivolol Intervention on Outcomes and Rehospitalisation in Seniors with heart failure

(SENIORS) recently evaluated the effect of nebivolol in elderly patients with heart failure, a proportion of whom had preserved systolic function. A full analysis of outcomes in this subgroup is awaited.

Verapamil

Verapamil shares the above-mentioned pharmacological effects of beta blockers, which are theoretically attractive in patients with heart failure and preserved systolic function. Several small trials suggest that verapamil may improve symptoms and exercise tolerance in patients with heart failure and preserved systolic function.[15] No mortality–morbidity outcome trials have been undertaken with this drug in heart failure, although it generally has been safe and well tolerated in large trials in other cardiovascular disease areas.

Aldosterone blockade

Aldosterone is believed to promote extracellular matrix growth and ventricular hypertrophy – effects likely to reduce ventricular relaxation and diastolic filling. A large outcome trial (Trial of Aldosterone Antagonist Therapy in Adults with Preserved Ejection Fraction Congestive Heart Failure (TOPCAT)) is planned with spironolactone in patients with heart failure and preserved systolic function.

Other pharmacological treatments

Vaccination against influenza and pneumococcal infection is recommended in vulnerable people, including patients with heart failure in whom these infections can often precipitate worsening and lead to hospital admission. Some patients with heart failure may have thiamine deficiency. The choice of treatment for comorbidity may be influenced by heart failure (see Fig 1). Antiplatelet treatment generally is recommended in patients with arterial disease, although the role of aspirin is under debate.[16] Prior trials with statins generally excluded patients with symptomatic heart failure, and two morbidity–mortality outcome studies in heart failure are underway. Many drugs should be avoided in heart failure, including most antiarrhythmic agents, calcium channel blockers, antipsychotics, antihistamines and corticosteroids, as should non-steroidal anti-inflammatory drugs, where possible.[17] Metformin and thiazolidinediones (glitazones) should be used with caution in patients with heart failure and diabetes. Some salt substitutes are rich in potassium and can cause hyperkalaemia. Dietary supplements are becoming more widely used, and some of these can interact with drugs taken by patients with heart failure, such as St John's Wort with warfarin and digoxin. Interest is growing in the use of erythropoietic agents to treat anaemia in patients with heart failure, and outcome trials are planned.

Non-pharmacological, non-device, non-surgical treatments

Although no evidence shows that sodium and fluid restriction are of benefit in heart failure, these are advocated widely. No evidence shows that alcohol, in moderation, is harmful, although patients with alcoholic cardiomyopathy should abstain. Smoking and obesity should be avoided by all, although significant involuntary weight loss indicates a bad prognosis. We do not know how to treat cachexia. Regular exercise seems to improve well-being; its effect on prognosis is unclear but is under study. The optimum exercise regimen for patients with heart failure is unknown. The role of psychological interventions also is uncertain.

Acute 'decompensated' heart failure

The management of this heterogeneous group of patients is complex and changing and cannot be reviewed in detail. New guidelines have been published.[18] The major goal of treatment is relief of symptoms (usually extreme dyspnoea) and, in more critically ill patients, pharmacological or mechanical haemodynamic support either to recovery or an operative procedure (such as transplantation). For most patients, some combination of oxygen and intravenous opiate, diuretic and nitrate is sufficient. Continuous positive airways pressure (CPAP) also may be helpful. Hypotension or other severe systemic underperfusion may necessitate an inotropic agent (usually a catecholamine such as dobutamine). Phosphodiesterase inhibitors do not improve, and may worsen, outcome. Similar concerns exist about dobutamine. The calcium-sensitising 'inodilator' levosimendan and the B-type natriuretic peptide nesiritide have shown some promise, but more convincing efficacy and safety data are needed. Arginine vasopressin receptor antagonists also are under evaluation. Discharge planning and subsequent management to reduce the risk of readmission is important.

Organisation of care

A substantial number of studies have shown that organised, usually specialist nurse-led, multidisciplinary care can improve outcomes in patients with heart failure, particularly by reducing recurrent admission to hospital.[19] The most successful approach seems to involve education of the patients and carers about heart failure and its treatment (including flexible diuretic dosing and reinforcing the importance of adherence), recognising (and acting on) early deterioration and optimising proven pharmacological treatments. A home-based rather than clinic-based approach may be best, although trials are needed to directly compare types of intervention.

Devices and surgery

Implantable cardioverter defibrillator (ICDs)

About half of patients with heart failure die suddenly, mainly, it is believed, because of a ventricular arrhythmia. Antiarrhythmic drugs do not improve survival in heart failure. Recently, the Sudden Cardiac Death in Heart Failure Trial showed that an ICD reduced the risk of death by 23% in optimally medically treated patients with mild-to-severe symptomatic heart failure and a reduced left ventricular ejection fraction.[20] These findings are supported by similarly large reductions in death with a cardiac resynchronisation-defibrillator device (CRT-D) in patients with severe symptomatic heart failure and a low left ventricular ejection fraction in the Comparison of Medical Therapy, Pacing, and Defibrillation In Heart Failure (COMPANION) trial (see below)[21] and with an ICD in survivors of myocardial infarction with a reduced left ventricular ejection fraction in the second Multicenter Automatic Defibrillator Trial (MADIT-2). Consequently, ICDs will become more widely used in heart failure (see Fig 1). Currently, much debate surrounds the selection of suitable recipients and recognition that patients with truly advanced heart failure will die despite having an ICD.

Cardiac resynchronisation therapy (CRT)

About 25% of patients with heart failure often have abnormal electrical activation of the left ventricle (usually reflected by a prolonged QRS duration on a surface electrocardiogram), which leads to dyssynchronous contraction between the walls of the left ventricle and results in less efficient ventricular emptying and, often, mitral regurgitation.[21,22] Atrioventricular coupling also may be abnormal (reflected by a prolonged PR interval), as may interventricular synchrony. Atriobiventricular or multisite pacing resynchronises cardiac contraction, improves pump function, reduces symptoms and increases exercise tolerance in patients with severe heart failure. Two morbidity–mortality outcome trials have completed recently. In COMPANION, CRT reduced the composite of death or hospital admission (for any cause and for heart failure) in patients with severe heart failure (Table 2).[21] There was a strong trend to a reduction in death alone. In CARE-HF, CRT not only reduced the risk of the primary outcome of death or hospital admission for a cardiovascular reason by 37% but also reduced the risk of death from any cause by 36% (Table 2).[22] The absolute risk reductions were large and these were obtained despite excellent evidence-based background medical treatment (Table 2). Many other outcome measures, including quality of life, also improved. Debate remains about how best to select patients for CRT. Most existing trials did this by using marked prolongation of the QRS duration, usually manifest as left bundle branch block (BBB) and a QRS duration of >120 msec; the Cardiac Resynchronization in Heart Failure (CARE-HF) study used additional echocardiographic criteria for patients with a QRS duration of 120–149 msec. Tissue Doppler echocardiography and other imaging techniques may be better at identifying those likely to benefit, although this remains to be proved and the approach used in the large outcome trials mentioned above remains the only evidence-based one. Whether patients with right BBB, atrial fibrillation, dyssynchrony without marked QRS prolongation and milder heart failure are helped by CRT is uncertain. No consensus has yet been agreed on whether (or in whom) CRT alone or a CRT-D device should be used.

Surgery

Table 3 outlines surgical treatments for heart failure. Few of these are of proved benefit, and none is used widely in patients with heart failure, with the exception of

Table 2 Controlled trials* in symptomatic heart failure with reduced systolic function.

Trial	n	Severity of heart failure	Estimated first year placebo/control group mortality	Background treatment†	Treatment added	Trial duration (years)	Primary endpoint	Relative risk reduction (%)‡	Events prevented per 1,000 patients treated**		
									Death	Hospitalisation for heart failure††	Death or hospitalisation for heart failure
ACE inhibitors:											
CONSENSUS, 1987	253	End stage	52	Spironolactone	Enalapril 20 mg twice daily	0.54‡‡	Death	40	146	–	–
SOLVD-T, 1991	2,569	Mild–severe	15.7	None	Enalapril 20 mg twice daily	3.5	Death	16	45	96	108
Beta blockers:											
CIBIS-2, 1999	2,647	Moderate–severe	13.2	ACE inhibitor	Bisoprolol 10 mg once daily	1.3‡‡	Death	34	55	56	–
MERIT-HF, 1999	3,991	Mild–severe	11.0	ACE inhibitor	Metoprolol controlled release/extended release 200 mg once daily‡‡‡	1.0‡‡	Death	34	36	46	63
COPERNICUS, 2001	2,289	Severe	19.7	ACE inhibitor	Carvedilol 25 mg twice daily	0.87‡‡	Death	35	55	65	81
Angiotensin receptor blockers:											
Val-HeFT, 2001	5,010	Mild–severe	About 8.0	ACE inhibitor	Valsartan 160 mg twice daily	1.9	Cardiovascular death or morbidity***	13	0	35	33***

Study	n	Severity		Background therapy	Intervention		Endpoint				
CHARM-Alternative, 2003	2,028	Mild–severe	12.6	Beta blocker	Candesartan 32 mg once daily	2.8	Cardiovascular death or hospitalisation for heart failure	23	30	78	60
CHARM-Added, 2003	2,548	Moderate–severe	10.6	ACE inhibitor + beta blocker	Candesartan 32 mg once daily	3.4	Cardiovascular death or hospitalisation for heart failure	15	28	47	39
Aldosterone blockade:											
RALES, 1999	1,663	Severe	~25	ACE inhibitor	Spironolactone 25–50 mg once daily	2.0‡‡	Death	30	113	95	–
H-ISDN:											
V-HeFT-1, 1986	459	Mild–severe	26.4	–	Hydralazine 75 mg three–four times daily Isosorbide dinitrate 40 mg four times daily	2.3	Death	34	52	0	–
A-HeFT, 2004	1,050	Moderate–severe	~9.0	ACE inhibitor + beta blocker + spironolactone	Hydralazine 75 mg three times daily Isosorbide dinitrate 40 mg four times daily	0.83‡‡	Composite	–	40	80	–
Digitalis glycosides:											
DIG, 1997	6,800	Mild–severe	~11.0	ACE inhibitor	digoxin	3.1	Death	0	0	79	73
Cardiac resynchronisation therapy (biventricular pacing):											
COMPANION, 2004	925	Moderate–severe	19.0	ACE inhibitor + beta blocker + spironolactone	CRT	1.35‡‡	Death or hospitalisation for any reason	19	38	–	87

continued over

Table 2 Controlled trials* in symptomatic heart failure with reduced systolic function – *continued*.

Trial	n	Severity of heart failure	Estimated first year placebo/control group mortality	Background treatment†	Treatment added	Trial duration (years)	Primary endpoint	Relative risk reduction (%)‡	Events prevented per 1,000 patients treated**		
									Death	Hospitalisation for heart failure††	Death or hospitalisation for heart failure
CARE-HF, 2005	813	Moderate–severe	12.6	ACE inhibitor + beta blocker + spironolactone	CRT	2.45	Death or hospitalisation for a cardiovascular reason	37	97	151	184
Defibrillating cardiac resynchronisation therapy:											
COMPANION, 2004	903	Moderate–severe	19.0	ACE inhibitor + beta blocker + spironolactone	CRT-ICD	1.35‡‡	Death or hospitalisation for any reason	20	74	–	–
Implantable cardioverter defibrillator:											
SCD-HeFT, 2005	1,676	Mild–severe	~7.0	ACE inhibitor + beta blocker	ICD	3.8	Death	23	–	–	–
Ventricular assist device:											
REMATCH, 2001	129	End-stage	75	ACE inhibitor + spironolactone	LVAD	1.8	Death	48	282	–	–

CHARM = Candesartan in Heart Failure Assessment of Reduction in Mortality and Morbidity; CIBIS-2 = Cardiac Insufficiency Bisoprolol Study II; CONSENSUS = Cooperative North Scandinavian Enalapril Survival Study; COPERNICUS = Carvedilol Prospective Randomized Cumulative Survival study; MERIT-HF = Metoprolol CR/XL Randomized Intervention Trial in congestive Heart Failure; RALES = Randomized Aldactone Evaluation Study; SOLVD-T = studies of left ventricular dysfunction treatment arm; Val-HeFT = Valsartan Heart Failure Trial.
*Excluding active-controlled trials.
†In more than one-third of patients: ACE inhibitor + beta blocker means ACE inhibitors used in almost all patients and beta blockers in the majority. Most patients also took diuretics and many took digoxin (except in the DIG trial). Spironolactone was used at baseline in 5% of patients in Val-HeFT, 8% in MERIT-HF, 17% in CHARM-Added, 19% in SCD-HeFT, 20% in COPERNICUS and 24% in CHARM-Alternative.
‡Relative risk reduction in primary endpoint.
**Individual trials may not have been designed or powered to evaluate effect of treatment on these outcomes.
††Patients with at least one hospital admission for worsening heart failure; some patients had multiple admissions.
‡‡Stopped early for benefit
***Primary endpoint, which also included treatment of heart failure with intravenous drugs for four hours or more without admission and resuscitated cardiac arrest (both added small numbers).
‡‡‡Not currently available in the UK.
Adapted from Ref 3.

Table 3 Surgical and other interventional treatments for heart failure.

Conventional	• Surgical coronary revascularisation
	• Percutaneous coronary revascularisation
	• Mitral valve repair/annuloplasty
	• Surgical left ventricular remodelling (eg Dor procedure)
Transplantation	• Orthotopic/heterotopic
	• Xenotransplantation
Ventricular assist devices/ mechanical pumps	• Bridge to transplantation
	• Destination therapy
Other left ventricular surgery	• External compression
	• Splinting
Total artificial heart	
Cell and gene therapy*	• Skeletal muscle myoblasts
	• Stem cells
	– Bone marrow
	– Embryonic
	• Gene delivery[†]

*Can be delivered at time of conventional surgery.
†Can also be delivered percutaneously.
Adapted from Ref 3.

coronary revascularisation (much of which is carried out percutaneously). Two large outcome trials are evaluating the value of conventional surgery, including coronary bypass grafting, mitral valve or annulus repair and reconstruction of the left ventricle.[23] The role of revascularisation in patients without angina but with ischaemia, viability or 'hibernation', or both, is of particular interest, but identifying appropriate patients continues to challenge. Orthotopic (or heterotopic) transplantation remains the treatment of last resort in selected patients, but, because of the limited supply of donor organs, xenotransplantation continues to be of interest. Ventricular assist devices can be used as a 'bridge to transplantation' but interest in (and evidence for (see Table 2)) is also growing in their use as 'destination therapy'.[24] Development of total artificial hearts also continues, as does that of novel ventricular splinting and compressive devices.[25] Cell and gene therapy, delivered at the time of conventional surgery, as a primary surgical procedure or percutaneously, also are under evaluation.

Palliative care

The treatments discussed may not be tolerated by, or may be inappropriate for, the often very elderly patients with multiple comorbidities who present with, or progress to, end-stage heart failure. End-of-life care has not been evaluated adequately in patients with advanced heart failure, as it has for other terminal disorders.

Future challenges and directions

Despite the impressive number of effective treatments discussed, patients with heart failure continue to experience progression of their disease – that is, worsening of symptoms, frequent admission to hospital and premature death. Better treatments are needed. Polypharmacy is a growing problem, and interest is growing in finding better alternatives than simply adding extra drugs. Comorbidity seems to be an increasing problem that often limits the use of proven treatments – for example, renal dysfunction preventing the use of ACE inhibitors, ARBs and aldosterone blockers. Indeed, comorbidities are now a therapeutic target in their own right – such as erythropoietic agents for anaemia, selective A_1 adenosine agonists for patients with 'cardio–renal syndrome', various treatments for atrial fibrillation and continuous positive airway pressure (CPAP) for ventilatory abnormalities. *Tailoring* pharmacological treatment – for example, to normalise natriuretic peptide concentrations – and *targeting* treatment on the basis of biological mechanisms or genetic make up are attractive but unproved approaches. Other experimental approaches to treatment are exploring completely novel pathophysiological processes. Another area that remains remarkably under-researched is that of monitoring patients during follow up to detect deterioration in the hope of reversing this and preventing an adverse outcome. Current approaches such as asking the patient to measure their weight daily are crude, and intriguing new approaches use home telemonitoring and devices (such as implantable devices that measure right heart pressures and devices that use bioimpedance to make serial measurements of cardiac function and detect fluid overload). There is also interest in using natriuretic peptides for this purpose. Technological and surgical advances will lead to more widespread use of cardiac mechanical support – for example, ventricular assist devices – although these treatments are likely to remain restricted to selected, younger, patients with little comorbidity. The 'holy grail' of repairing or replacing dead or damaged heart muscle seems hypothetically possible with cell and gene therapy, but only time will tell if it is really attainable.

REFERENCES

1 Faris R, Flather M, Purcell H, Henein M *et al.* Current evidence supporting the role of diuretics in heart failure: a meta analysis of randomised controlled trials. *Int J Cardiol* 2002;**82**:149–58.

2 McMurray J, Cohen-Solal A, Dietz R, Eichhorn E *et al.* Practical recommendations for the use of ACE inhibitors, beta-blockers, aldosterone antagonists and angiotensin receptor blockers in heart failure: Putting guidelines into practice. *Eur J Heart Fail* 2005;**7**:710–21.

3 McMurray JJ, Pfeffer MA. Heart failure. *Lancet* 2005;**365**:1877–89.

4 Shibata MC, Flather MD, Wang D. Systematic review of the impact of beta-blockers on mortality and hospital admissions in heart failure. *Eur J Heart Fail* 2001;**3**:351–7.

5 Flather MD, Shibata MC, Coats AJ, Van Veldhuisen DJ *et al.* Randomized trial to determine the effect of nebivolol on mortality and cardiovascular hospital admission in elderly patients with heart failure (SENIORS). *Eur Heart J* 2005;**26**:215–25.

6 Pfeffer MA, Swedberg K, Granger CB, Held P *et al.* Effect of candesartan on mortality and morbidity in patients with chronic heart failure: the CHARM-Overall programme. *Lancet* 2003;**362**:759–66.

7 Cohn J, Tognoni G, the Valsartan Heart Failure Trial Investigators. A randomized trial of the angiotensin-receptor blocker valsartan in chronic heart failure. *N Engl J Med* 2001;**345**:1667–75.

8   Pitt B, Zannad F, Remme WJ, Cody R *et al.* The effect of spironolactone on morbidity and mortality in patients with severe heart failure. Randomized Aldactone Evaluation Study Investigators. *N Engl J Med* 1999;**341**:709–17.

9   McMurray JJ, Pfeffer MA, Swedberg K, Dzau VJ. Which inhibitor of the renin-angiotensin system should be used in chronic heart failure and acute myocardial infarction? *Circulation* 2004;**110**:3281–8.

10   Taylor AL, Ziesche S, Yancy C, Carson P *et al.* Combination of isosorbide dinitrate and hydralazine in blacks with heart failure. *N Engl J Med* 2004;**351**:2049–57.

11   The Digitalis Investigation Group. The effect of digoxin on mortality and morbidity in patients with heart failure. *N Engl J Med* 1997;**336**:525–33.

12   Hood WB Jr, Dans AL, Guyatt GH, Jaeschke R *et al.* Digitalis for treatment of congestive heart failure in patients in sinus rhythm: a systematic review and meta-analysis. *J Card Fail* 2004; **10**:155–64.

13   Zile MR, Brutsaert DL. New concepts in diastolic dysfunction and diastolic heart failure: Part II: causal mechanisms and treatment. *Circulation* 2002;**105**:1503–8.

14   Yusuf S, Pfeffer MA, Swedberg K, Granger CB *et al.* Effects of candesartan in patients with chronic heart failure and preserved left-ventricular ejection fraction: the CHARM-Preserved Trial. *Lancet* 2003;**362**:777–81.

15   Setaro JF, Zaret BL, Schulman DS, Black HR *et al.* Usefulness of verapamil for congestive heart failure associated with abnormal left ventricular diastolic filling and normal left ventricular systolic performance. *Am J Cardiol* 1990;**66**:981–6.

16   Cleland JG, Findlay I, Jafri S, Sutton G *et al.* The Warfarin/Aspirin Study in Heart failure (WASH): a randomized trial comparing antithrombotic strategies for patients with heart failure. *Am Heart J* 2004;**148**:157–64.

17   Amabile CM, Spencer AP. Keeping your patient with heart failure safe: a review of potentially dangerous medications. *Arch Intern Med* 2004;**164**:709–20.

18   Nieminen MS, Böhm M, Cowie MR, Drexler H *et al.* Executive summary of the guidelines on the diagnosis and treatment of acute heart failure. *Eur Heart J* 2005;**26**:384–416.

19   McAlister FA, Stewart S, Ferrua S, McMurray JJ. Multidisciplinary strategies for the management of heart failure patients at high risk for admission: a systematic review of randomized trials. *J Am Coll Cardiol* 2004;**44**:810–9.

20   Bardy GH, Lee KL, Mark DB, Poole JE *et al.* Amiodarone or an implantable cardioverter-defibrillator for congestive heart failure. *N Engl J Med* 2005;**352**:225–37.

21   Bristow MR, Saxon LA, Boehmer J, Krueger S *et al.* Cardiac-resynchronization therapy with or without an implantable defibrillator in advanced chronic heart failure. *N Engl J Med* 2004; **350**:2140–50.

22   Cleland JGF, Daubert JC, Erdmann E, Freemantle N *et al.* The effect of cardiac resynchronization on morbidity and mortality in heart failure. *N Engl J Med* 2005;**352**:1539–49.

23   Jones RH. Is it time for a randomized trial of surgical treatment of ischemic heart failure? *J Am Coll Cardiol* 2001;**37**:1210–3.

24   Rose EA, Gelijns AC, Moskowitz AJ, Heitjan DF *et al.* Long-term mechanical left ventricular assistance for end-stage heart failure. *N Engl J Med* 2001;**345**:1435–43.

25   Copeland JG, Smith RG, Arabia FA, Nolan PE *et al.* Cardiac replacement with a total artificial heart as a bridge to transplantation. *N Engl J Med* 2004;**351**:859–67.

□ CARDIOLOGY SELF ASSESSMENT QUESTIONS

Genetics of cardiomyopathy

1   The following are characteristic of the inherited cardiomyopathies:
(a) Multifactorial inheritance
(b) Autosomal dominant transmission
(c) Near-complete penetrance in all gene carriers
(d) Variable expressivity
(e) Genetic anticipation

2   Mutations in sarcomeric proteins have been identified in patients with the following conditions:
(a) Dilated cardiomyopathy
(b) Arrhythmogenic right ventricular cardiomyopathy
(c) Hypertrophic cardiomyopathy
(d) Restrictive cardiomyopathy
(e) Muscular dystrophy

3   The following genotype–phenotype associations are recognised:
(a) Troponin T mutations and marked left ventricular hypertrophy
(b) Mutations in lamin A/C and dilated cardiomyopathy with conduction system disease
(c) Mutations in myosin binding protein C and late-onset hypertrophic cardiomyopathy
(d) Mutations in troponin I and restrictive physiology
(e) Mutations in adenosine 5'-phosphate (AMP)-activated protein kinase and hypertrophic cardiomyopathy with pre-excitation

4   Arrhythmogenic right ventricular cardiomyopathy:
(a) Exclusively affects the right ventricle
(b) Is caused by mutations in desmosomal proteins
(c) Commonly arises in childhood
(d) Typically manifests as heart failure
(e) Occurs in association with cutaneous disease in syndromic forms

5   Regarding familial assessment for diseases of the heart muscle:
(a) Asymptomatic relatives are unlikely to be affected
(b) A single normal evaluation in adulthood offers a lifetime of reassurance
(c) Dilated cardiomyopathy and arrhythmogenic right ventricular cardiomyopathy may seem to 'skip' a generation
(d) Mutations with low penetrance are identified easily
(e) A thorough history and physical examination are adequate

Pulmonary hypertension

1   Pulmonary arterial hypertension is caused by:
(a) High altitude
(b) Sickle cell disease
(c) A mutation of nitric oxide synthase
(d) Sarcoidosis
(e) Infection with human immunodeficiency virus

2   In the investigation of pulmonary hypertension:
(a) Spirometry usually reveals significant abnormality in patients with idiopathic pulmonary arterial hypertension
(b) Pulmonary hypertension is defined by a systolic pulmonary arterial pressure ≥25 mmHg
(c) Echocardiography is the best screening investigation
(d) Pulmonary hypertension reliably is associated with raised brain natriuretic peptide
(e) Left atrial enlargement is expected in patients with pulmonary arterial hypertension

3   In the treatment of pulmonary hypertension:
(a) Randomised trials have shown a survival advantage for all of the disease-modifying therapies
(b) Calcium antagonists are first-line treatment for idiopathic pulmonary arterial hypertension
(c) Lung transplantation normally is indicated if disease-modifying therapies are failing
(d) The evidence for bosentan in idiopathic pulmonary arterial hypertension is mainly for patients with New York Heart Association functional class III
(e) All three classes of disease-modifying therapies for pulmonary arterial hypertension have antiproliferative effects on vascular smooth muscle

Advances in cardiovascular imaging

Magnetic resonance imaging

Stefan Neubauer

☐ INTRODUCTION

The physical phenomenon of magnetic resonance (MR), or nuclear magnetic resonance (NMR), was discovered independently by two American physicists in 1946: Felix Bloch at Stanford University and Edward Purcell at Harvard. They shared the 1952 Nobel Prize in Physics for this discovery. Compared with the physics of X-rays or ultrasound, the physics of magnetic resonance are substantially more complex. In short, atomic nuclei with an uneven number of protons or neutrons, or both, have the property of a nuclear spin. When these nuclei are exposed to an external magnetic field and are excited by radiofrequency waves, they send out a signal in return, termed the free induction decay (FID). These weak radiofrequency signals can be detected by MR coils, recorded by a computer and used to construct an MR image.

The second important discovery in the development of magnetic resonance imaging was made by Paul Lauterbur in the United States and Peter Mansfield in the United Kingdom, who shared the 2003 Nobel Prize in Medicine in recognition of their findings. They reported that application of a magnetic field strength gradient allows imaging of the spatial distribution of the nuclear spins. The original publication on this phenomenon shows the first MR image ever reported – that of a water-filled glass vial.[1] The contrast of an MR image depends, in short, on spin density (the number of nuclei susceptible to MR imaging in the tissue), the relaxation parameters (T_1 and T_2), the effects of flow and the type of pulse sequence used. A pulse sequence is a pattern of radiofrequency waves used to excite the nuclear spins.

The major advantage of cardiac MR (CMR) is that it is an extremely versatile technique. The ultimate goal for a comprehensive CMR examination would be to obtain, within less than 30 minutes of acquisition time and less than 10 minutes of post-processing time, information on: cardiac and great vessel anatomy; cardiac volumes and mass; global and regional contractile function; regional myocardial tissue perfusion; regional tissue characteristics (such as viability, inflammation, fibrosis and metabolism); the coronary artery lumen, wall and blood flow; and finally heart valves.

The University of Oxford Centre for Clinical Magnetic Resonance Research has been in operation since February 2002. It is a centre for clinical research (see www.cardiov.ox.ac.uk/ocmr/trackrec.htm) but also provides an NHS clinical CMR service, with 1.5 Tesla and 3 Tesla human MR systems from Siemens.

Indications for clinical CMR scanning based on referrals to our centre over the past year include the investigation of cardiomyopathy (hypertrophic and dilated cardiomyopathy, arrhythmogenic right ventricular cardiomyopathy, sarcoidosis and so on: 36% in total); aorta and valves (26%); viability imaging (16%); congenital heart disease (8%); and, less frequently, the pericardium, perfusion measurements, cardiac masses and anomalous coronaries.

□ IMAGING CARDIAC ANATOMY AND FUNCTIONS

Cardiac MR is considered the gold standard for the high-resolution investigation of cardiac and thoracic anatomy and for measurement of global and regional myocardial function.[2-4] To depict anatomy, we obtain stacks of coronal, transverse and sagittal plane images in the so-called conventional planes. To arrive at the four-chamber and two-chamber views of the heart, which are more familiar from echocardiography, requires double-angulated planes that can be obtained through a series of well-defined pilot images. For anatomic imaging, turbospin echo or HASTE sequences typically are used, where blood appears dark and the myocardium bright. For imaging of cardiac function, True-FISP cine sequences (alternative names: steady-state free precession, balanced FFE, FIESTA) are used. Here, blood in the chambers is bright (bright blood imaging) and the myocardium dark. Such images show information on global and regional function with unprecedented detail.

Unlike in echocardiography, MRI is not limited by acoustic windows and can always view the entire heart. The contrast between blood in the chambers and the myocardium is extremely high and allows for accurate and reliable determination of the subendocardial and subepicardial borders. Right ventricular global and regional function also can be assessed, and, in addition, we are free to select any imaging plane that might give additional functional information.

Typical cine imaging planes include the horizontal long axis (four-chamber), vertical long axis (two-chamber) and short axis views. A stack of short axis cine images is obtained, typically using 1-cm slices from the base of the heart to the apex of the heart. Each slice then is quantified for myocardial chamber volumes and mass – both in systole and diastole. Using Simpson's rule, slice volumes are added up to give extremely reproducible and accurate measurements of myocardial mass, ejection fraction, end-diastolic and end-systolic volumes – for the left and right ventricles.

Measurements are accurate even when the left ventricle has lost its symmetry, such as when a large anterior myocardial infarction leads to formation of an aneurysm; this is unlike two-dimensional echocardiography, for example, in which volume calculations assume an eliptoid shape of the left ventricle. Bellenger *et al* showed that if a given change of left ventricular volumes, ejection fraction or left ventricular mass is to be demonstrated with a set statistical power level in clinical research studies, CMR can achieve this with a fraction of the number of patients required compared with the use of echocardiography for such a study (typically reducing patient numbers by 80–97%).[2] Thus, the size of clinical trials can be reduced substantially. A large number of current clinical trials on heart failure therefore have chosen CMR as the imaging modality to monitor changes in left ventricular function and mass.

Other imaging planes are unique to CMR, such as the right ventricular outflow tract and the right ventricular inflow plane or transverse planes that are used to investigate right ventricular global and segmental function – and these are of major importance in the diagnosis of arrythmogenic right ventricular cardiomyopathy. Stress testing with CMR also is feasible, and for this, a protocol analogous to stress echocardiography is used, where the heart is stimulated with increasing dosages of dobutamine (10–40 µg/kg/min). Stress-induced wall motion abnormalities indicate territories supplied by stenosed coronary arteries. Nagel *et al* showed that dobutamine stress MR has significantly higher sensitivities, specificities and predictive values than dobutamine stress echocardiography; this is exclusively because MR is superior in patients with poor image quality from echocardiograms.[5] Thus, dobutamine stress MR may be indicated in patients referred for dobutamine stress echocardiography who show inadequate acoustic windows for ultrasound imaging.

☐ REGIONAL MYOCARDIAL PERFUSION

Cardiac MR allows the assessment of regional myocardial perfusion with unprecedented resolution.[6] Typically, this is performed as a so-called first-pass perfusion study with the MR contrast agent gadolinium diethylenetriamine pentaacetic acid (GdDTPA). This contrast agent shortens T_1 relaxation time and thus markedly brightens T_1-weighted MR images. A bolus of MR contrast agent is flushed into a peripheral vein, and the passage of the contrast agent through the heart is observed with high spatial and temporal resolution. The contrast agent first appears in the right ventricle, then passes through the lungs and then through the left ventricular cavity. Finally, the contrast agent arrives in the left ventricular tissue, which therefore becomes brighter ('enhances'). Areas in which contrast arrival is delayed because of an associated coronary stenosis will appear darker on perfusion images, thus allowing the diagnosis of a perfusion deficit. Typically, this is performed before and after vasodilator stress (adenosine or dipyridamole), acquiring three to five short-axis slices. Each slice is then divided into six or eight segments, and perfusion is evaluated for each segment. This can be achieved qualitatively (eyeballing), semi-quantitatively (perfusion reserve) or by absolute quantification. Future studies will have to show which quantification approach is the most appropriate for clinical practice. Three clinical studies (one single centre and two multicentre), each including close to 100 patients, have been published in the past year (for example, see 'Myocardial first-pass perfusion magnetic resonance imaging: a multicenter dose-ranging study'[7]) and showed a diagnostic accuracy with MR perfusion imaging for the diagnosis of significant coronary artery stenosis (typically defined as >70% on angiography) in the order of 85–90%. Compared with the traditional approach of imaging myocardial perfusion by nuclear scintigraphy, the MR method has the following advantages: much higher spatial resolution (including analysis of the transmural extent of perfusion deficits), radiation free, much faster (about 15 minutes in duration) and can be part of a comprehensive CMR examination. Current limitations are the lack of large trials that evaluate the prognostic power of perfusion CMR, lack of a uniformly accepted approach to quantification and time-consuming data processing.

☐ DELAYED-ENHANCEMENT CMR

Over the past few years, delayed-enhancement CMR has been established as the golden standard method for assessment of myocardial viability.[8] Alternative current methods, such as positron emission tomography, nuclear scintigraphy and dobutamine stress echocardiography, all have limitations related to resolution, radiation, patient discomfort, availability and requirements for appropriate acoustic windows. Delayed-enhancement CMR is performed 10–20 minutes after injection of a bolus of GdDTPA with an inversion recovery sequence. On such images, acutely necrotic and chronically scarred myocardium appears bright, while normal, stunned and hibernating myocardium is black.

Experimental studies have shown excellent agreement of the area of late enhancement with histological scar sizes. This technique allows *in vivo* infarct imaging in humans with previously unprecedented resolution. Such images give information on the three-dimensional nature of a myocardial infarction, often revealing islands of normal myocardium interspersed with scar tissue. Planimetry allows accurate quantification of infarct size in terms of percentage of total left ventricular mass, and this information is very useful in clinical practice. Late-enhancement CMR is highly superior to single photon emission computed tomography for the detection of subendocardial infarction, which easily can be missed by the substantially lower resolution nuclear technique but can be depicted accurately with CMR. The clinical relevance of this finding and the prognostic implications of detecting small subendocardial infarcts remain to be determined.

We and others have shown that the transmural extent of hyperenhancement strongly predicts the likelihood of improvement of regional myocardial contractility after revascularisation: most dysfunctional segments without any hyperenhancement have improved contractility at six months, while segments with three quarters to full thickness hyperenhancement do not recover.[8,9] We recently showed the value of delayed-enhancement CMR for studying irreversible myocardial damage induced by coronary artery bypass surgery or complex percutaneous coronary intervention.[10] For example, we showed that after complex percutaneous coronary intervention, 29% of patients show areas of new hyperenhancement, equalling about 5 g of myocardial tissue.

Importantly, the late enhancement phenomenon cannot distinguish between acute myocardial necrosis and chronic scarring and, furthermore, it is not specific for ischaemic injury. Multiple small spots of hyperenhancement can be shown in patients with acute myocarditis, the extent of myocardial fibrosis in patients with hypertrophic cardiomyopathy,[11] and midwall streaks of hyperenhancement – again representing fibrosis – in some patients with dilated cardiomyopathy. Thus, while we may be able to provide diagnostic information derived from the regional distribution pattern of hyperenhancement, thereby greatly aiding the diagnosis of various forms of cardiomyopathy, a specific diagnosis cannot be made on the basis of the hyperenhancement phenomenon alone.

The advantages of viability imaging by MR imaging compared with echo-cardiography or nuclear methods are that delayed enhancement provides by far the highest spatial resolution (including analysis of the transmural extent), is radiation free, does not need to stress the heart, and can use one contrast agent bolus for analysis of perfusion and viability imaging.

☐ ANGIOGRAPHY

Contrast-enhanced MR angiography is a technique with enormous success in clinical practice, and it can depict almost every vascular territory with superb resolution, with the exception of the coronaries. This technique is in routine use, for example, for leg or renal arteriography or depiction of the complex anatomy of the large thoracic arteries (such as in aortic coarctation). Another important new application of this technique is pulmonary vein and left atrial angiography, which is of major use to electrophysiologists when performing ablation for atrial flutter or fibrillation.

One area in which CMR has not yet fulfilled expectations is MR coronary angiography. Fundamental challenges are that coronary arteries are small structures (1–4 mm in diameter), that move rapidly with the cardiac cycle and with respiration (the right coronary artery by as much as 10 cm), so three-dimensional resolution is needed. Current MR coronary angiography is not a real-time technique – data from several cardiac cycles have to be averaged – and electrocardiography triggering and breath hold or navigator imaging are also needed. The current spatial resolution of this technique is limited to approximately 0.7 × 1 × 1.5 mm. The largest multicentre study into MR coronary angiography showed a sensitivity for the detection of coronary artery disease of 83%, but only 84% of images were interpretable.[12] Clearly, at the present time, MR coronary angiography is not ready for clinical prime time, and substantial further development is needed to achieve this. The great potential of vascular MR for the future, however, lies in the fact that it can go beyond pure luminography and also can yield information on the structure of vessel walls, including qualitative and quantitative analysis of atherosclerotic plaques (fibrous cap, lipid core, and so on). Furthermore, vessel function can be analysed, and flow velocity and arterial distensibility can be determined. Functional vascular measurements likely can serve as a more sensitive indicator of early vascular damage than structural images.

☐ VALVE STENOSIS AND REGURGITATION

Cardiac MR is the most accurate technique for quantification of valve stenosis and regurgitation, although it is inferior to echocardiography with regard to depiction of valve morphology. Valve regurgitation is quantified by measuring the antegrade and retrograde flow through the valve in an orthogonal plane, using flow-sensitive MR sequences ('velocity encoding'). For example, to quantify regurgitation, the forward stroke volume and regurgitation volume are measured from the flow curve, and from this the regurgitant fraction is calculated. Alternatively, valve incompetence can be estimated by comparing the left and right ventricular stroke volumes determined from planimetry – although this method is valid only when a single valve shows significant regurgitation. For quantification of stenosis, the maximum flow velocity is measured through MR velocity encoding, and from this the stenosis gradient can be calculated directly. An alternative method is to obtain a cine image through the valve plane and determine the maximum valve opening area by direct planimetry.

☐ FUTURE TECHNIQUES

A number of CMR techniques on the horizon have not made it into clinical practice yet but may well do so in coming years. Tagging or tissue phase mapping is used to measure regional myocardial strain. Arterial spin labelling techniques may allow assessment of myocardial perfusion without the use of MR contrast agent. Blood oxygenation level-dependent imaging allows the assessment of regional myocardial oxygenation. With ^{23}Na-imaging, regional myocardial sodium concentrations, which are increased in scar tissue, can be determined. Magnetic resonance spectroscopy opens a window into the non-invasive determination of cardiac metabolism. Higher field magnets (such as 3 Tesla) may allow unprecedented resolution. Finally, the highly promising field of molecular imaging should, in the future, allow imaging of myocardial and vascular proteins with molecular specificity.

ACKNOWLEDGEMENTS

I would like to thank my co-workers from the University of Oxford Centre for Clinical Magnetic Resonance Research, Adrian Cheng, Jane Francis, Lucy Hudsmith, Justin Lee, Saul Myerson, Steffen Petersen, Monique Robinson, Matthew Robson, Joseph Selvanayagam, Michaela Scheuermann-Freestone, Juergen Schneider, Cheerag Shirodaria, and Damian Tyler, for their excellent contributions and hard work.

REFERENCES

1   Lauterbur P. Image formation by induced local interactions: examples employing nuclear magnetic resonance. *Nature* 1973;**242**:190–1.

2   Bellenger NG, Davies LC, Francis JM, Coats AJ *et al.* Reduction in sample size for studies of remodeling in heart failure by the use of cardiovascular magnetic resonance. *J Cardiovasc Magn Reson* 2000;**2**:271–8.

3   Pennell DJ. Cardiovascular magnetic resonance: twenty-first century solutions in cardiology. *Clin Med* 2003;**3**:273–8.

4   Neubauer S. MRI and CT. *Medicine* 2002;**30**:40–45.

5   Nagel E, Lehmkuhl HB, Bocksch W, Klein C *et al.* Noninvasive diagnosis of ischemia-induced wall motion abnormalities with the use of high-dose dobutamine stress MRI: comparison with dobutamine stress echocardiography. *Circulation* 1999;**99**:763–70.

6   Jerosch-Herold M, Wilke N. MR first pass imaging: quantitative assessment of transmural perfusion and collateral flow. *Int J Card Imaging* 1997;**13**:205–18.

7   Wolff SD, Schwitter J, Coulden R, Friedrich MG *et al.* Myocardial first-pass perfusion magnetic resonance imaging: a multicenter dose-ranging study. *Circulation* 2004;**110**:732–7.

8   Kim RJ, Wu E, Rafael A, Chen EL *et al.* The use of contrast-enhanced magnetic resonance imaging to identify reversible myocardial dysfunction. *N Engl J Med* 2000;**343**:1445–53.

9   Selvanayagam JB, Kardos A, Francis JM, Wiesmann F *et al.* Value of delayed-enhancement cardiovascular magnetic resonance imaging in predicting myocardial viability after surgical revascularization. *Circulation* 2004;**110**:1535–41.

10 Selvanayagam JB, Petersen SE, Francis JM, Robson MD *et al.* Effects of off-pump versus on-pump coronary surgery on reversible and irreversible myocardial injury: a randomized trial using cardiovascular magnetic resonance imaging and biochemical markers. *Circulation* 2004;**109**:345–50.

11 Moon JC, McKenna WJ, McCrohon JA, Elliott PM *et al.* Toward clinical risk assessment in hypertrophic cardiomyopathy with gadolinium cardiovascular magnetic resonance. *J Am Coll Cardiol* 2003;**41**:1561–7.

12 Kim WY, Danias PG, Stuber M, Flamm SD *et al.* Coronary magnetic resonance angiography for the detection of coronary stenoses. *N Engl J Med* 2001;**345**:1863–9.

Echocardiography

Petros Nihoyannopoulos

This chapter reviews the position of echocardiography today. It also provides information about a number of the new applications, some of which are being performed today, while others, it is hoped, will be performed in the future.

Echocardiography has seen a rapid evolution from single crystal M-mode to two-dimensional echocardiography, Doppler and now colour-flow imaging. Clinical use of echocardiography now extends from the operating room, in both transesophageal and intraoperative echocardiography, to the community. In patients with known or suspected coronary artery disease, echocardiography has become a pivotal first-line investigation for the differential diagnosis of acute chest pain syndromes, assessment of global and regional left ventricular function at rest and during stress and evaluation of the complications of myocardial infarction.

One of the biggest advantages of echocardiography is its ability to obtain the fastest frame rates of all imaging modalities, maintaining a spatial resolution of about 1 mm. This obviously is important when looking at global and regional ventricular function as well as valvular morphology and function.

Another great advantage of echocardiography is its ability to quantify everything in the heart, including dimensions, ventricular function, volumes and pressures, non-invasively and with great accuracy. For an imaging modality to be really useful clinically, however, it needs to:

☐ be feasible in the vast majority of patients

☐ be cost effective

☐ be able to be performed and analysed during normal working hours

☐ be reproducible

☐ have measurements linked to clinical outcomes.

This has been achieved today mainly because of the following developments.

☐ New ultrasound transducers capable of imaging the heart in the second and subharmonic range of the returning beam.

☐ Intravenous contrast agents capable of crossing the cardiopulmonary barrier and opacifying the left ventricular cavity, so that the endocardial border can be defined more accurately.

☐ Real-time, three-dimensional transducers, which have been a reality since 2004 and are routinely used in many echocardiographic departments. These currently are available from two ultrasound companies and are improving rapidly. The major advantage of real-time, three-dimensional echocardiography is the assessment of left ventricular volumes without geometric assumptions.

☐ Use of low-amplitude Doppler signals to measure parameters of myocardial deformation, such as myocardial velocities, myocardial strain and stain rate imaging.

☐ CURRENT DEVELOPMENTS OF ECHOCARDIOGRAPHY

New transducers

New developments mean transducers are now capable of harmonic imaging. Cardiac ultrasound is a tomographic imaging modality of the heart. Unlike computed tomography, echocardiography produces sequential sections of the heart in real time with the use of ultrasound. Its greatest advantage therefore is the total absence of radiation despite production of the highest frame rate of all imaging modalities.

Two-dimensional echocardiography remains the standard technique for ultrasound imaging and evolved from the original single-crystal M-mode echocardiography. Transducers used for echocardiography typically generate frequencies in the range 1.5–7 MHz. Although M-mode echocardiography used a single crystal, two-dimensional echocardiography uses up to about 256 crystals in one transducer. This produces a slice of the heart less than 1 mm thick. The use of several such slices imaged from different positions around the chest wall allows the entire heart to be visualised.

Clear visualisation of the ventricular walls, and particularly the endocardial border, is vital for the accurate assessment of the regional function of the wall. About 15% of patients may have poor endocardial definition on conventional echocardiographic imaging. This may be the result of a variety of reasons, including large body habitus, lung disease or distorted architecture of the left ventricle. New methods and transducers have been developed to help overcome these limitations and improve left ventricular delineation.

Conventional (or fundamental) echocardiography uses a transducer to emit and receive ultrasound waves at the same frequency. Not all signals reflected back to the transducer from myocardial tissue are of the original frequency, however, and some may reflect back at twice or even three times the original frequency. These are known as harmonic frequencies.

Harmonic imaging uses broadband transducers capable of receiving reflected signals of twice (second harmonic) or three times (ultraharmonics) the original frequency and thus improves image quality. This method reduces the number of spurious echoes detected within the left ventricle and allows clearer definition of the endocardial border. Harmonic imaging is well validated and is being used routinely.

Contrast echocardiography

Despite improvements in imaging, some patients' endocardial definition remains a problem. This may be overcome by the use of intravenous ultrasound contrast agents.

Contrast enhancement is used extensively in diagnostic radiology. Methods such as X-ray, computed tomography, magnetic resonance imaging and nuclear scintigraphy regularly rely on the introduction of foreign material to tissue to improve the image resolution. Contrast agents consist of gas-filled microbubbles in a protein shell, which reflect ultrasound, generate harmonic backscatter and, therefore, enhance information on ultrasound images. The development of gas-filled microbubbles that can be injected intravenously and remain stable through the pulmonary circulation until they reach the left ventricular cavity has been a major advance in contrast technology. Only recently, transpulmonary contrast agents became readily available for clinical use. The primary indication for the use of contrast echocardiography today is to improve endocardial border delineation in patients in whom adequate imaging is difficult. In patients with coronary artery disease, in whom particular attention should be focused on regional myocardial contraction, clear endocardial definition is crucial. The combination of harmonic transducers with contrast enhancement should not preclude any myocardial region from being assessed in any patient. Several studies have shown that measurement of left ventricular volumes and mass with such echocardiographic machines provides reproducible values similar to those obtained with cardiac magnetic resonance imaging. Patients who are difficult to image should belong to the past.

Stress echocardiography

Stress echocardiography is performed routinely now for clinical purposes. This is not a new technique and has been used around the world for more than 20 years. What is now new, however, is the wealth of data on outcome. Data from several thousands of patients with evidence of ischaemia and scarring on stress echocardiography show that such patients will not do well over a period of 10 years, whereas the outcome of patients who have a negative stress exercise echocardiograph is excellent. These patients can be told that a normal dobutamine stress echocardiograph (which means normal wall motion at stress) carries an excellent prognosis, with an annual event rate of 1.3%. The advent of harmonic imaging and contrast echocardiography means that stress echocardiography can be performed accurately in all patients.

Three-dimensional echocardiography

The clinical use of three-dimensional echocardiography previously was hindered by the prolonged and tedious nature of data acquisition. The recent introduction of real-time, three-dimensional echocardiographic imaging techniques has revolutionised echocardiography, as images are obtained in just one beat. This has been achieved by the development of a full-matrix array transducer (X4, Phillips Medical Systems, Andover, Massachusetts), which uses 3000 elements. This leads into a volume of data acquisition from a single projection in the shape of a pyramid.

The major advantage of real-time, three-dimensional echocardiography is that, for the first time, volumetric analysis does not rely on geometric assumptions (as is the case with two-dimensional echocardiography). Quantification of left ventricular volumes and mass with real-time 3D echocardiography can be performed from an apical wide-angled acquisition with the use of different methods. Since a dataset comprises the entire left ventricular volume, multiple slices may be obtained from the base to the apex of the heart to evaluate wall motion. This acquisition then can be combined with the use of an infusion of contrast agents, particularly in patients with difficult acoustic windows in whom further improvements in the delineation of the endocardial border might be of benefit. Early studies convincingly showed that volume calculations are similar to those obtained with cardiac magnetic resonance imaging.

Tissue Doppler imaging

All moving objects intersected by the ultrasound beam generate Doppler shifts, including the fastest moving blood cells and the slower moving structures, such as valves and muscle. For the study of blood flow, Doppler signals from the slower moving heart structures, such as valve leaflets, are filtered out. The filtering is possible because the characteristics of Doppler signals from blood and tissue differ markedly: blood generally has high velocities and relatively low signal amplitude, while muscle and valve tissue have much slower velocities and higher signal amplitudes.

If the low velocities are filtered in and the high velocity signals from blood filtered out, Doppler signals from tissue motions can be recorded as pulse-wave spectral displays or in colour (2-D or M-mode). Tissue Doppler imaging allows regional assessment of myocardial function and deformation in very high frame rates (100–200 Hz).

Major applications of tissue Doppler imaging are assessment of diastolic left ventricular function and the early detection of cardiomyopathies, particularly in patients with familial hypertrophic cardiomyopathy and dilated cardiomyopathy.

□ FUTURE DEVELOPMENTS OF ECHOCARDIOGRAPHY

Myocardial perfusion

This is almost a current application of echocardiography: microbubbles injected after opacification of the left ventricular cavity will move on and enter the capillary circulation; they are true flow tracers. The ability to assess myocardial perfusion has revolutionised echocardiography.

Myocardial perfusion is assessed by injecting tiny microbubbles the size of the blood cells that can trace myocardial blood flow into the smallest capillaries. When these microbubbles vibrate, and eventually break up, when subjected to an ultrasound field, they emit a strong echo signal that can be detected by modern transducers (second harmonic imaging). Myocardial perfusion thus can be assessed at rest and during stress, so the sensitivity for a positive stress echocardiograph will be higher, without any loss of specificity. Myocardial perfusion also can be quantified with commercially available software.

Tissue targeting

In the future, loading or conjugation of drugs within the microbubbles, which may be transferred to a specific myocardial region, might be possible and would enable the microbubbles to deliver the drug in a more selective manner. Similarly, microbubbles can be conjugated with specific ligands, such as antibodies, which will then target selective tissues.

☐ SUMMARY

Echocardiography today is a global imaging modality for cardiac function and perfusion. Cardiac ultrasound has evolved from one- to two- to three-dimensional imaging and the benefits are clear. Tomorrow, it may be possible to move on to molecular imaging and tissue targeting.

☐ ADVANCES IN CARDIOVASCULAR IMAGING SELF ASSESSMENT QUESTIONS

Magnetic resonance imaging

1 The following are involved in magnetic resonance image generation:
   (a) X-rays
   (b) Radiofrequency waves
   (c) Ultrasound waves
   (d) Radioisotopes
   (e) All of the above

2 The following are domains of cardiac magnetic resonance imaging:
   (a) Cardiac function
   (b) Myocardial viability
   (c) Valve morphology
   (d) Thoracic anatomy
   (e) Myocardial perfusion

3 The following are typical cardiac magnetic resonance imaging planes for assessment of cardiac function:
   (a) Horizontal long axis plane
   (b) Vertical long axis plane
   (c) Coronal plane
   (d) Short axis plane
   (e) Right ventricular outflow tract plane

4 The following are true statements about cardiac magnetic resonance imaging:
   (a) Cardiac magnetic resonance imaging is the most accurate technique for quantification of cardiac volumes and mass
   (b) Valvular stenosis and regurgitation can be assessed accurately with cardiac magnetic resonance imaging
   (c) Cardiac magnetic resonance provides insufficient resolution for coronary imaging in coronary artery disease
   (d) The late enhancement phenomenon is specific for detection of irreversible ischaemic damage
   (e) Large multicentre trials are needed to establish the prognostic value of cardiac magnetic resonance imaging-derived parameters

Rheumatology

Changing scene of therapy for rheumatoid arthritis

Duncan Porter

☐ INTRODUCTION

The last 25 years have seen dramatic changes in the therapy of rheumatoid arthritis, and the pace of change is quickening. Twenty-five years ago, the only drugs in the rheumatologist's armamentarium were corticosteroids, antimalarial drugs, gold salts, immunosuppressant drugs and penicillamine. Very little robust evidence came from well-designed, randomised controlled trials, and widespread doubts were expressed about the efficacy of so-called 'second line' or 'slow-acting' antirheumatic drug therapy. In the 1980s, the drugs that have proved to be the mainstay of disease-modifying antirheumatic drug (DMARD) therapy – namely, sulfasalazine and methotrexate – were proved to be effective. The 1990s saw the introduction of ciclosporin, minocycline and leflunomide and a proliferation of studies that proved unequivocally that conventional DMARD therapy is effective both clinically and in reducing the rate of radiographic progression. Arguably, however, the most important developments over the past decade have been the evolution of new strategies for the utilisation of the available drugs, which will be the focus of this review. These strategies have echoes of other disciplines of medicine, and the new strategies will be illustrated through comparison with the treatment of other diseases.

☐ THE PROBLEM

The advent of trials that confirmed the efficacy of conventional DMARDs was welcomed within the rheumatological community – and rightly so. Improved measures of disease activity (for example, the disease activity score) and agreed measures of outcome (such as the American College of Rheumatology response criteria) allowed trials to show clear superiority of DMARDs over placebo. These advances in the measurement of disease activity also provided a less welcome observation, however – namely, that while patients undoubtedly were better, they also, as a general rule, had evidence of ongoing disease activity. For example, Eberhardt and colleagues followed up 183 patients with early rheumatoid arthritis for five years. Encouragingly, more than half the patients had an episode of remission; however, this remission was sustained only for more than six months in 20% of patients and, overall, remission was seen in only 7% of follow-up visits.[1] Persistent disease activity is the norm in the vast majority of patients, and this translates into slowly deteriorating physical function, joint damage and impaired quality of life. Consequently, long-term follow-up trials have shown that about 40% of patients are work disabled as a result of their rheumatoid arthritis after 10 years of the disease;[2] 25% of patients require joint replacement surgery within 20 years;[3] and long-term mortality studies show that patients with rheumatoid arthritis have a reduced life expectancy. What could be done to remedy this depressing situation?

☐ STRATEGY 1 – COMBINATION DMARD THERAPY (OR 'TREAT RHEUMATOID ARTHRITIS LIKE TUBERCULOSIS')

It long has been known that multiple antibiotics should be used to treat active tuberculosis because otherwise there is a serious risk of incomplete cure (and so a risk of subsequent recrudescence) or the emergence of antibiotic resistance. Of course, similar strategies have been employed successfully in the treatment of many haematological malignancies, for which 'combination chemotherapy' has become the standard treatment. Would the use of conventional DMARDs be more effective if drugs were used in combination? No doubt exists over whether this is the case, and evidence from randomised controlled trials is proliferating. The seminal trial from O'Dell *et al* showed that triple therapy (with methotrexate, sulfasalazine and hydroxychloroquine) was more effective than dual therapy (sulfasalazine and hydroxychloroquine) or methotrexate monotherapy in established disease.[4] Similarly, in patients with early rheumatoid arthritis, Calguneri *et al* have shown that three drugs are better than two, which are better than one.[5] Nonetheless, uncertainties remain about the role of combination therapy: few trials have compared directly different drug combinations, and, moreover, some patients respond very well to drug monotherapy, so is it wise to delay the introduction of combination therapy until it becomes apparent which patients require it?

☐ STRATEGY 2 – WINDOW OF OPPORTUNITY (OR 'TREAT RHEUMATOID ARTHRITIS LIKE ACUTE MYOCARDIAL INFARCTION')

The trials of acute thrombolysis in the treatment of acute myocardial infarction show clearly that the longer the delay between symptom onset and the administration of thrombolysis, the smaller the benefit in terms of reduced mortality. Is it possible that there is a window of opportunity in the treatment of rheumatoid arthritis? The timescale involved clearly is different, being measured in terms of weeks and months rather than hours, but intriguing data suggests that early, aggressive intervention yields long-term benefits in the treatment of rheumatoid arthritis. In the *Combinatietherapie Bij Reumatoide Artritis* (COBRA) trial, patients were randomised to receive sulfasalazine monotherapy or a combination of high-dose oral corticosteroids, sulfasalazine and methotrexate. The patients who received combination therapy had their treatment tapered, such that after nine months, both groups were receiving sulfasalazine monotherapy. After 12 months, no significant differences were seen between the groups in terms of clinical disease activity. However, less radiographic disease progression was seen in the combination group.

After 12 months, all patients were treated in the same way, but the remarkable finding was that the differences in joint damage scores not only persisted but increased over the next five years.[6] The implication is that even relatively brief, intensive, early interventions can in some way 'set the thermostat' for future disease progression. Other trials have resulted in similar findings: for example, a Finnish trial that compared sulfasalazine monotherapy with triple therapy in patients with early rheumatoid arthritis found that the rate of remission was approximately double in the triple therapy group (40% vs 18%), and this was mirrored by a reduction in radiographic disease progression. The clinical advantage was lost after the end of the trial (when all patients could be treated in the same way), such that the remission rates in patients randomised to the two groups were similar after five years of follow up (28% vs 22%, $p = NS$). The differences in radiographic disease progression rates persisted.[7]

☐ STRATEGY 3 – ZERO TOLERANCE (OR 'TREAT RHEUMATOID ARTHRITIS LIKE DIABETES MELLITUS')

The poor long-term outcome of rheumatoid arthritis already has been argued to be related to persistent, low-grade disease activity. Diabetes is another autoimmune disease that results in substantial morbidity and increased mortality from complications that arise insidiously over many years, and parallels have been drawn between it and rheumatoid arthritis. Tight glycaemic control (however achieved) has become established to be associated with a reduction in serious diabetic complications, such as retinopathy and nephropathy.[8] It was mooted, therefore, that 'zero tolerance' towards synovitis, and treatment strategies that target persistent disease activity in rheumatoid arthritis, might reap similar benefits in terms of outcome. The Tight Control for Rheumatoid Arthritis (TICORA) trial aimed to study this by randomising patients to 'routine' or 'intensive' treatment of early rheumatoid arthritis. The intensive management comprised regular review, objective assessment of disease activity, liberal use of intra-articular corticosteroid injections into swollen joints and the escalation of oral DMARD therapy, according to a protocol, in patients who exhibited persistent disease activity. The results showed that startling improvements in the rate of remission can be achieved, and this is mirrored by marked improvements in physical function and health related quality of life.[9] Whether the results can be replicated and whether the strategy will deliver similar reductions in long-term outcomes, such as the need for joint replacement surgery, remains to be seen.

☐ STRATEGY 4 – NEW THERAPIES

The new millennium has seen the emergence of targeted biologic therapies. In rheumatoid arthritis, the most important are the anti-tumour necrosis factor (TNF) α drugs, but, in all probability, drugs directed against other targets will become available over the next five years. Although much remains unknown about the long-term use of anti-TNF therapy, particularly with respect to any long-term toxicity, they have proved remarkably safe and effective drugs. The drugs are expensive (costing approximately £9,000 per patient per year), so their use has been restricted to patients with severe disease who have proved resistant to conventional DMARD therapy. Even in such patients, in whom response to treatment is difficult to achieve, a proportion of patients have a dramatic response to anti-TNF therapy. The drugs clearly do not represent a panacea, however, with some patients not responding to therapy at all and others having only modest benefit. The most exciting findings, however, have been in the realm of radiographic progression. Studies of conventional DMARDs (like the TICORA trials) have shown that progression of radiographic joint damage continues to be seen even when excellent clinical outcomes are achieved. With the use of anti-TNF therapies in patients with established rheumatoid arthritis, further progression of radiographic damage seems to be abolished, with zero (or even negative) increases in joint damage scores over 12 months of therapy.[10] The results from trials that studied patients with early rheumatoid arthritis have not (by and large) been so dramatic, with some continuing radiographic disease progression – albeit at a reduced rate.

☐ THE FUTURE

The progress made in our understanding of what constitutes 'best practice' in the treatment of rheumatoid arthritis has been encouraging, but many uncertainties remain. Clearly, early intervention, combination therapy and biologic therapies all have a role to play, and emphasis should be given to targeting persistent disease activity. But which combination or combinations will prove to be the most effective? When should anti-TNF drugs (and their successors) be used in the disease process? Is it possible to identify patients who will do well on monotherapy, thereby allowing clinicians to target patients with a poor prognosis? If not, is it sensible to use a 'step-up' strategy, whereby patients have their treatment escalated if they have a suboptimal response to treatment? Or should the standard treatment involve triple therapy from the outset – 'stepping down' therapy in patients who are in persistent remission? These questions indicate that clinical scientists have a busy programme of research ahead of them!

REFERENCES

1 Eberhardt K, Fex E. Clinical course and remission rate in patients with early rheumatoid arthritis: relationship to outcome after 5 years. *Br J Rheumatol* 1998;**37**:1324–9.

2 Sokka T, Kautiainen H, Mottonen T, Hannonen P. Work disability in rheumatoid arthritis 10 years after the diagnosis. *J Rheumatol* 1999;**26**:1681–5.

3 Wolfe F, Zwillich SH. The long-term outcomes of rheumatoid arthritis: a 23-year prospective, longitudinal study of total joint replacement and its predictors in 1,600 patients with rheumatoid arthritis. *Arthritis Rheum* 1998;**41**:1072–82.

4 O'Dell JR, Haire CE, Erikson N, Drymalski W *et al.* Treatment of rheumatoid arthritis with methotrexate alone, sulfasalazine and hydroxychloroquine, or a combination of all three medications. *N Engl J Med* 1996;**334**:1287–91.

5 Calguneri M, Pay S, Caliskaner Z, Apras S *et al.* Combination therapy versus monotherapy for the treatment of patients with rheumatoid arthritis. *Clin Exp Rheumatol* 1999;**17**:699–704.

6   Boers M, Verhoeven A, Markusse HM, van de Laar MA *et al.* Randomised comparison of combined step-down prednisolone, methotrexate and sulphasalazine with sulphasalazine alone in early rheumatoid arthritis. *Lancet* 1997;**350**:309–18.

7   Korpela M, Laasonen L, Hannonen P, Kautiainen H *et al.* Retardation of joint damage in patients with early rheumatoid arthritis by initial aggressive treatment with disease-modifying antirheumatic drugs: five-year experience from the FIN-RACo study. *Arthritis Rheum* 2004;**50**:2072–81.

8   The Diabetes Control and Complications Trial Research Group. The effect of intensive treatment of diabetes on the development and progression of long-term complications in insulin-dependent diabetes mellitus. *N Engl J Med* 1993;**329**:977–86.

9   Grigor C, Capell H, Stirling A, McMahon AD *et al.* Effect of a treatment strategy of tight control for rheumatoid arthritis (the TICORA study): a single-blind randomised controlled trial. *Lancet* 2004;**364**:263–9.

10 Klareskog L, van der Heijde D, de Jager JP, Gough A *et al.* Therapeutic effect of the combination of etanercept and methotrexate compared with each treatment alone in patients with rheumatoid arthritis: double-blind randomised controlled trial. *Lancet* 2004;**363**:675–81.

5.

6.

7.

8.

9.

10.

Seronegative spondyloarthopathies

Andrew Keat

☐ INTRODUCTION

Spondyloarthopathies may occur at any age but most commonly present in young adult life. Together they are as prevalent in the United Kingdom as rheumatoid arthritis. The spondyloarthopathy family of conditions shares a range of characteristic articular and extra-articular lesions, including oligoarticular peripheral arthritis, sacroiliitis, enthesitis and sometimes also inflammatory eye disease, inflammatory bowel disease or psoriasis. The dissimilarity with rheumatoid arthritis, including the absence of immunoglobulin M rheumatoid factor and the predilection for spinal involvement, has led to the designation seronegative spondyloarthopathy. The identification of common genetic factors, especially human leucocyte antigen (HLA)-B27, has confirmed that it is appropriate to regard this group of conditions as an inter-related family, potentially with common aetiological and pathogenetic factors.[1]

The principal differentiated forms of spondyloarthropathy are ankylosing spondylitis, psoriatic arthritis, enteropathic arthritis and reactive arthritis, but undifferentiated forms occur in adults and children.[2]

☐ HOW TO RECOGNISE SPONDYLOARTHOPATHIES

The diagnosis may be made and appreciated at three levels:

- ☐ presenting features
- ☐ associated disorders
- ☐ enthesitis connection.

Presenting features

Patients with spondyloarthopathy most commonly present with monoarthritis or oligoarthritis, spinal pain and stiffness, dactylitis or peripheral enthesitis, especially at the heel. Pain and swelling at a single knee or at one of a group of small joints, such as a metatarsophalanageal joint at one foot, is common and contrasts with the picture of rheumatoid disease. Buttock pain and stiffness in a young adult may indicate sacroiliitis, although pain over the sacroiliac region, even with local tenderness, should not be assumed to necessarily indicate sacroiliitis. X-ray evidence of sacroiliitis is notoriously slow to develop; characteristic appearances on magnetic resonance images, along with a response to anti-inflammatory medication, may contribute usefully to early diagnosis. Dactylitis at one toe – sausage toe – is characteristic of spondyloarthopathies, although dactylitis may also affect fingers in the presence of psoriasis. Enthesopathies may occur at many sites, but most typically affect the calcaneal attachments of the Achilles' tendon and/or plantar fascia, giving rise to highly characteristic Achilles' tendon bursitis and heel pain.

Associated disorders

In ankylosing spondylitis and undifferentiated spondyloarthopathy, features may be restricted to spinal pain, stiffness and fatigue or peripheral inflammatory joint or enthesis lesions. However, 60% of people with ankylosing spondylitis have asymptomatic, low-grade inflammatory bowel disease; conversely, approximately 6% of people with ulcerative colitis or Crohn's disease have peripheral arthritis – either large joint oligoarthritis (type 1) or polyarthritis (type 2) – and 1% have typical ankylosing spondylitis. Similarly, 5–8% of people with psoriasis also have peripheral arthritis or spondylitis. The arthritis that follows within a month of sexually transmitted infection or specific bacterial gut infections (which may be mild) constitutes reactive arthritis. The typical features of Reiter's syndrome may be present. Many other causative infections have been implicated in recent years, including streptococcal infection in adults, but the exact link between infections and arthritis remains obscure.

Anterior uveitis may complicate any of the above conditions, although it frequently occurs alone, especially in people positive for HLA-B27. Many patients who attend with isolated acute anterior uveitis will have sacroiliitis, spondylitis or another feature of a spondyloarthopathy.

Enthesitis connection

The term enthesitis (or enthesopathy) refers to inflammation at the attachments to bone of tendon, ligament or joint capsule.[3] Although some lesions are apparent clinically and are highly characteristic of spondyloarthopathies (for example, Achilles tendonitis and plantar fasciitis), it is becoming clear that inflammation at enthesial sites is fundamental to the spondyloarthopathies as a group. Entheses may be relatively simple insertions, while others are linked intricately with surrounding structures, including the synovium and subchondral bone, which gives rise to the notion of a complex 'enthesis organ'.[4]

Biopsy studies and modern imaging techniques have shown that enthesitis lesions often are associated with pronounced osteitis of underlying bone, as well as adjacent synovitis, so even peripheral joint arthritis may be linked intimately with underlying enthesitis. The same is likely to be true of the many enthesial attachments in the digits, which underpin the characteristic spondyloarthopathic lesion of dactylitis.

Within the pelvis, inflammatory change at the capsular enthesis of the sacroiliac joints leads to formation of new bone around the sacroiliac joint and eventual apparent obliteration of the joints on X-ray, while adjacent osteitis accounts for many of the changes seen on magnetic resonance images. Synovitis within the synovial (lower) portion of the sacroiliac joint and enchondral ossification in the joint cartilage make up a complex set of changes that underpin eventual sacroiliac fusion. Higher up in the spine, similar changes of capsular enthesitis combined with adjacent synovitis affect the apophyseal joints. Eventually, the inflammatory lesions lead to ossification within the capsular enthesis, ankylosing the joint. Similar changes, which are easier to see on spinal X-rays, affect the margins of the discovertebral joints. Initial lesions may appear radiographically as 'erosions', although osteitis is probably the underlying lesion. Subsequently, ossification of these inflammatory enthesial lesion leads to the development of 'shiny corners' or Romanus lesions, then to syndesmophytes and ultimately to ankylosis.

□ ANKYLOSING SPONDYLITIS – A NEGLECTED DISEASE

Although the classic features of severe ankylosing spondylitis are familiar to doctors, the activity, severity and personal impact of this condition only recently became amenable to analysis. Several composite measures of disease activity and severity have emerged just in time to provide some objective means of judging the appropriateness and effectiveness of new treatments.

Numerous measures have been introduced, and consensus as to which are best has not been reached yet. Among the most useful indicators of activity and severity of ankylosing spondylitis, however, are the Bath ankylosing spondylitis disease activity index (BASDAI) and Bath ankylosing spondylitis functional index (BASFI).[5] The short-form questionnaire (SF-36) and the ankylosing spondylitis quality of life (ASQOL) instrument are used widely to assess quality of life; the former allows some comparisons with other disabling conditions. These provide essential tools for assessing the impact of and justification for new forms of treatment. Assessment of psoriatic arthritis is more problematic, although psoriatic arthritis response criteria (PsARC) have been established. For patients with polyarticular disease, the assessments used for rheumatoid disease may be appropriate.

These measures include some other important aspects of this neglected disease only tangentially, or not at all. Osteoporosis that affects the axial skeleton develops early on and leads to an excess of vertebral fractures in patients with longstanding disease. These, in turn, contribute to morbidity and mortality, as well as an enhanced need for treatment. Excess mortality in people with ankylosing spondylitis probably applies only to patients with severe disease in whom premature death is attributable to amyloidosis, cardiac disease, trauma and surgical complications. Work disability is an under-recognised aspect of ankylosing spondylitis. Fatigue, pain and hip involvement lead many patients to reduce working hours, give up physically demanding jobs and fail to progress up their career path as might be expected. Data on early retirement on health grounds is comparable with employment data for people with rheumatoid arthritis, although figures vary from one country to another as a result of significant differences in social security arrangements. Ankylosing spondylitis and other spondyloarthopathies thus are associated with considerable socioeconomic consequences that have to be added to the balance when considering potentially hazardous and expensive forms of treatment.

□ TREATMENT

Although the treatment of peripheral joint lesions of spondyloarthopathies is very similar to that of rheumatoid arthritis (with the use of local and systemic anti-inflammatory drugs and disease-modifying agents), few useful treatments exist for spondylitis *per se*. For spondylitis, exercise – whether physiotherapy or recreational – and non-steroidal anti-inflammatory drugs (NSAIDs) remain crucial. So too are means of maintaining motivation, self-esteem and hope in the face of a progressive, lifelong, painful disorder. Conventional treatment also now should be extended to include assessment of bone mineral density at the earliest opportunity, so that calcium and vitamin D supplementation and/or treatment with appropriate agents such as bisphosphonates can be introduced.[6] The evidence base for such interventions is emerging, but it is by no means complete.

The introduction of treatments for ankylosing spondylitis and psoriatic arthritis that block tumour necrosis factor (TNF) seems set to revolutionise the treatment of these conditions and related forms of arthritis. It now is clear that treatment with infliximab and etanercept provides rapid and sustained symptomatic relief for patients with severe ankylosing spondylitis, with dramatic improvements in well-being and quality of life.[7,8] Treatment with TNF blockers also provides comparable benefits for patients with psoriatic arthritis, undifferentiated spondyloarthopathy and enteropathic arthritis. Other forms of spondyloarthopathy also are likely to benefit, although the response of acute anterior uveitis to TNF blockers is unpredictable. Current evidence does not show a disease-modifying effect, although early indicators are of rapid resolution of osteitis and reversal of the osteoporosis seen early in ankylosing spondylitis.

The decision to use TNF blockade rests on the balance between currently recognised benefits and short- and long-term risks of treatment, tempered by financial and regulatory considerations.[9] Although the licensed use of these agents in rheumatoid arthritis in the United Kingdom is guided by national guidelines supported by data that show disease modification and is sanctioned by the National Institute for Health and Clinical Excellence (NICE), treatment of spondyloarthopathy currently has not been shown to modify disease and has not yet been addressed by NICE. National guidelines exist for the use of infliximab and etanercept for ankylosing spondylitis and psoriatic arthritis,[10,11] but considerable variations exist between trusts and different regions of the United Kingdom as to the availability of treatment. Other biologic agents, including adalimumab and anakinra, are under trial.

In ankylosing spondylitis, the effects of TNF blockade on pain, quality of life and well-being are demonstrated clearly. So too are the financial costs and short-term risks; longer-term risks may yet emerge. Thus, balancing the overall costs and benefits of treatment requires very substantial data that include other medical costs and prolongation of the working life, as well as symptom control. Attempts to provide such data are emerging, driven by the need to justify expensive biologic therapies,[12] but inevitably current cost estimates will change as treatment regimens become refined and newer agents are introduced.

REFERENCES

1   Khan MA, Ball EJ. Genetic aspects of ankylosing spondylitis. *Best Pract Res Clin Rheumatol* 2002;**16**:675–90.

2   Dougados M, Hochberg MC. Why is the concept of spondyloarthopathies important? *Best Pract Res Clin Rheumatol* 2002;**16**:495–505.

3   McGonagle D, Marzo-Ortega H, Benjamin M, Emery P. Report on the Second international Enthesitis Workshop. *Arthritis Rheum* 2003;**48**:896–905.

4   Benjamin M, Moriggl B, Brenner E, Emery P *et al*. The "enthesis organ" concept: why enthesopathies may not present as focal insertional disorders. *Arthritis Rheum* 2004;**50**: 3306–13.

5   van der Heijde D, Braun J, McGonagle D, Siegel J. Treatment trials in ankylosing spondylitis: current and future considerations. *Ann Rheum Dis* 2002;**61**(Suppl. 3):iii24–32.

6   Bessant R, Keat A. How should clinicians manage osteoporosis in ankylosing spondylitis? *J Rheumatol* 2002;**29**:1511–9.

7   Braun J, Brandt J, Listing J, Zink A *et al*. Two year maintenance of efficacy and safety of infliximab in the treatment of ankylosing spondylitis. *Ann Rheum Dis* 2005;**64**:229–34.

8   Davis JC Jr, Van Der Heijde D, Braun J, Dougados M *et al* Recombinant human tumour necrosis factor receptor (etanercept) for treating ankylosing spondylitis: a randomized, controlled trial. *Arthritis Rheum* 2003;**48**:3230–6.

9   Paul S, Keat A. Assessment of patients with spondyloarthopathies for treatment with tumour necrosis factor alpha blockade. *Rheumatology (Oxford)* 2005;**44**:17–23.

10 Keat A, Barkham N, Bhalla A, Gaffney K *et al*. BSR guidelines for prescribing TNF-alpha blockers in adults with ankylosing spondylitis. Report of a working party of the British Society for Rheumatology. *Rheumatology (Oxford)* 2005;**44**:939–47. www.rheumatology.org.uk/guidelines/clinicalguidelines/bsrguideankspond (accessed 19 July 2005).

11 Kyle S, Chandler D, Griffiths CEM, Helliwell P *et al*. Guideline for anti-TNF therapy in psoriatic arthritis. *Rheumatology* 2005;**44**:390–7.

12 Kobelt G, Andlin-Sobocki P, Brophy S, Jonsson L *et al*. The burden of ankylosing spondylitis and the cost effectiveness of treatment with infliximab (Remicade). *Rheumatology* 2004;**43**:1158–66.

Fibromyalgia

Michael Doherty

☐ BACKGROUND

As doctors, we generally are well trained and confident in dealing with patients who have symptoms that result from identifiable disease. When we have accompanying clinical signs, abnormal tests and definable pathology, we can give the patient a specific diagnosis that explains their problem and readily can devise a logical management plan to counter, and possibly cure, the underlying cause. Unfortunately, however, we can apply this traditional biomedical model to only a minority of patients who consult with symptoms (Fig 1). More often, we are faced with people who have disabling symptoms but no accompanying clinical signs, normal investigations and no definable disease.[1] To appropriately advise and manage such people with medically unexplained symptoms is a common but challenging requirement for many healthcare professionals. Unexplained symptoms can affect any body system, but when the major problem is chronic widespread musculoskeletal pain, the term 'fibromyalgia' often is used. Although this is an unsatisfactory term, it remains in common use and is more acceptable to many patients than 'medically unexplained symptoms'.

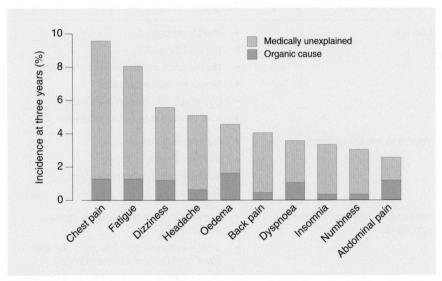

Fig 1 Incidence of common symptoms that present in general practice, showing the relatively low proportion of those that eventually are explained by definable medical conditions. Adapted from Ref 1.

☐ CLINICAL FEATURES

The main presenting feature is multiple regional pain, often with a central focus on the neck and back (Table 1). At presentation, just one or a few regions may dominate the picture, but over the preceding months, pain will have affected all quadrants of the body – both arms, both legs and the neck and/or back. Characteristically, the pain shows a poor response to traditional measures such as analgesics, non-steroidal anti-inflammatory drugs and weak opioids, and physiotherapy often makes it worse. Additional locomotor symptoms may include widespread often prolonged early morning stiffness, subjective swelling of the hands (with uncomfortable tightness wearing rings) and numbness or tingling of all fingers of both hands.

Marked fatigability, particularly in the morning, is the usual second major problem. This often is associated with poor concentration and forgetfulness. The person inevitably recognises that they sleep badly, with poor latency (difficulty getting off to sleep), waking frequently through the night and feeling completely unrefreshed in the morning. Pain and sleeplessness usually are given as reasons for the irritability, low affect and weepiness that patients often have. Reported disability often is marked. Although patients usually can dress, feed and groom themselves, they may be unable to do daily tasks such as shopping, housework or gardening. They may have experienced major difficulties at work or even stopped employment because of pain and fatigue.

Table 1 Symptoms of fibromyalgia.

Frequency and type of symptoms	Symptom
Common	• Multiple regional pain
	• Marked fatiguability
	• Marked functional impairment or disability
	• Broken non-restorative sleep
	• Low affect, irritability and weepiness
	• Poor concentration and forgetfulness
Variable locomotor symptoms	• Early morning stiffness
	• Swelling of hands or fingers
	• Numbness and tingling of all fingers
	• Temporomandibular joint pain (atypical facial pain)
Additional, variable, non-locomotor symptoms	• Non-throbbing bifrontal headache ('tension headache')
	• Colicky abdominal pain, bloating or variable bowel habit ('irritable bowel syndrome')
	• Bladder fullness, nocturnal frequency ('irritable bladder' or 'interstitial cystitis')
	• Hyperacusis, dyspareunia or discomfort when touched (allodynia)
	• Common side effects with drugs ('multiple chemical sensitivity')

Symptoms in other systems may be present to varying degrees. For example, frequent bifrontal non-throbbing headache, colicky abdominal pain relieved by defecation, and fullness of the bladder at night, with the need to frequently empty the bladder (but with only small volumes passed). Several symptoms may reflect allodynia (when normally non-noxious stimuli become painful): for example, dyspareunia, marked discomfort on being caressed or discomfort with normal noise levels – the person often turns down the television volume while their partner keeps turning it up. The person often experiences distressing side effects (recognised, not atypical or bizarre side effects) from any tablets and medicines that they try.

Examination usually is unremarkable, with no joint inflammation or damage, no muscle wasting and no neurological signs. Older patients especially may show signs of osteoarthritis or other prevalent musculoskeletal conditions, but these are of insufficient severity to explain such widespread symptoms and severe disability. The principal finding is hyperalgesia at recognised natural tender sites in the body (Fig 2). Moderate digital pressure at each site may be uncomfortable in a normal person, but in a patient with fibromyalgia it produces a wince or withdrawal response. The amount of applied pressure clearly is relevant. Metered dolorimeters are available for research purposes, but moderate digital pressure – enough to just blanch the nail – is sufficient for clinical diagnosis.

To fulfil clinical criteria for fibromyalgia, the person first needs to show the appropriate symptoms, including pain that affects all body quadrants, and second to show positive hyperalgesic tender sites axially and in each arm and each leg.

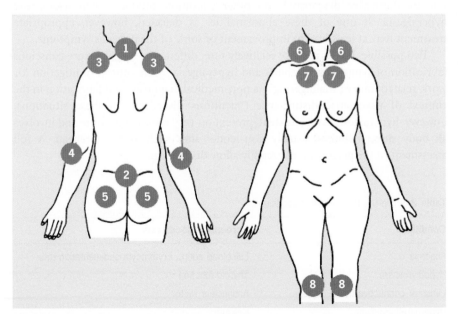

Fig 2 The main tender sites to examine for hyperalgesia. 1 = interspinous ligaments lower cervical spine; 2 = interspinous ligaments lower lumbar spine; 3 = midsupraspinatus belly; 4 = 1–2 cm distal to lateral epicondyle; 5 = mid-gluteal region; 6 = skin fold rolling over mid-trapezius; 7 = second to third anterior costochondral junctions; 8 = medial fat pad (upper medial tibia).

Although different numbers of hyperalgesic tender sites have been specified in different diagnostic criteria (for example, at least 11 of 18 specified sites), the key feature is the widespread nature of the pain and the hyperalgesia. It is not an all-or-none phenomenon, and, in practice, a spectrum of severity is encountered.

□ DIFFERENTIAL DIAGNOSIS AND INVESTIGATIONS

Localised hyperalgesia is found commonly in areas of referred pain from single or pauci-articular regional syndromes, such as cervical or lumbar spondylosis, or a rotator cuff injury. In common practice, however, widespread four-quadrant hyperalgesia is characteristic only of fibromyalgia.

People with recognised musculoskeletal or other disease (for example, rheumatoid arthritis, lupus or cancer) are not exempt from developing fibromyalgia. Assessment of someone with coexistent rheumatoid arthritis or lupus may prove challenging, as many of the symptoms could relate to activity of their multisystem disease. Marked discordance between the severity of reported and observed abnormality, however, is an important feature to suggest fibromyalgia, and widespread hyperalgesic tender sites are not explained by polyarticular disease.

Fibromyalgia is a diagnosis based solely on a full clinical assessment. It does not associate with any abnormality of routine testing. It is important, however, to screen for certain conditions that do not always produce overt clinical signs but that may, in part, account for some of the symptoms, such as tiredness, weakness, myalgia or arthralgia (Table 2). Should one of these conditions be detected, it is an additional not an alternative diagnosis – no other condition produces such widespread hyperalgesia. If one of these abnormalities is detected, however, appropriate treatment may at least lead to improvement of some of the patient's symptoms.

Two possible, but in practice relatively rare, differential diagnoses are conscious fabrication of symptoms, disability and hyperalgesia in the context of litigation for work-related injury ('malingering' – a non-medical diagnosis) and fabrication in the context of psychiatric disturbance ('factitious disorder'). In these situations, however, hyperalgesia is inconsistent, present on very minimal pressure and involves all body sites, including usually non-tender sites such as the forehead. A full assessment of the person should readily allow distinction.

Table 2 Screening for coexisting conditions.

Conditions	Screening blood tests
Anaemia	Full blood count; Erythrocyte sedimentation rate
Hypothyroidism	Thyroid function
Lupus or connective tissue disease	Antinuclear factor
Hyperparathyroidism	Calcium
Osteomalacia	Alkaline phosphatase
Inflammatory myositis	Creatine kinase

☐ EPIDEMIOLOGY

Population surveys have confirmed the clustering of poor sleep, multiple regional pain, widespread hyperalgesia and increased measures of anxiety and depression,[2] giving credence to the clinical condition described as 'fibromyalgia'. Furthermore, population surveys and cohort studies confirm frequent concurrence and overlap of the unexplained clinical conditions listed in Table 1, which suggests that they are varying manifestations of a similar functional disorder.[4]

The crude unadjusted prevalence of people with fibromyalgia in adult communities in the United Kingdom and United States is about 2–3% (Fig 3).[2,3] The female predominance is strong (around 10:1). Although fibromyalgia can occur at any age, including in teenagers, it shows a progressive increase with age, reaching a maximum prevalence of 7% in women older than 70 years (see Fig 3). The condition seems ubiquitous and is reported in a wide variety of racial groups and cultural settings, although it always predominates in women.

In cross-sectional studies, apart from ageing and female sex, other associations include a wide variety of life events that cause psychological distress[2,3] – for example, divorce; marital disharmony; bereavement; alcoholism in the family; traumatic injury or assault; low income; and prior childhood events, such as hospitalisation, operations and self-reported childhood abuse. People with chronic widespread pain also show increased measures of anxiety and depression and an increased tendency to focus on bodily symptoms ('somatisation'). These psychological factors, of course, could be secondary to stressful events and chronic pain. Prospective studies,

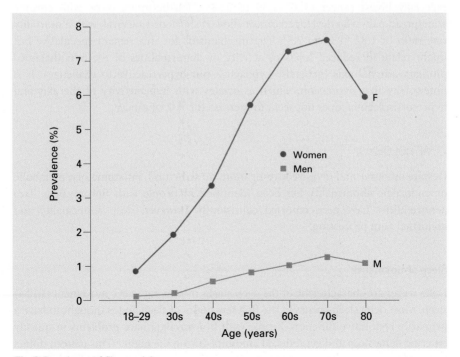

Fig 3 Prevalence of fibromyalgia.

however, suggest that the indicators of somatisation (reporting somatic symptoms and patterns of illness behaviour), rather than the presence of psychological distress itself, are the key risk factors for future development of chronic widespread pain.[5]

A number of studies suggest that fibromyalgia occurs more commonly in patients with other recognised chronic painful conditions. For example, up to 20% of patients with defined chronic rheumatic disease seen in hospital clinics are reported to have coexistent fibromyalgia. This has led to the suggestion that chronic regional pain may predispose to development of more widespread chronic pain ('pain amplification'), and some support for this now comes from prospective community studies.

□ NATURAL HISTORY

The prognosis of fibromyalgia is very poor in all series of hospital cases, with more than 90% of people being expected to retain diagnostic criteria at follow-up of five years. A better outcome has been reported in patients identified through community surveys, with approximately 60% still experiencing widespread pain at two years and 33% at seven years.[6] In such people, the risk factors for worse outcome are female sex, older age and having marked fatigue and additional functional symptoms.

One prospective population study of eight years' duration suggested shortened survival in those with chronic widespread pain, with an incidence rate ratio for mortality from all causes of 1.31 (95% confidence interval 1.05 to 1.65).[7] This was accounted for almost entirely by an increase in cancers (2.07 (1.37 to 3.13)), especially breast cancer (3.67 (1.39 to 9.68)). Furthermore, those with chronic widespread pain who developed cancer showed shortened survival, with a mortality rate ratio of 1.82 (1.18 to 2.8). The mechanisms for this remain speculative but might relate to reduced levels of activity or abnormalities of the hypothalamo-pituitary-adrenal axis (generally hypoactive but hyperreactive to challenge). It is noteworthy that depression, which associates with hyperactivity of the axis and hypercortisolaemia, does not seem to increase the risk of cancer.

□ AETIOLOGY

Despite intensive and invasive investigation, no structural, inflammatory, metabolic or endocrine abnormality has been identified in people with fibromyalgia. Two abnormalities have been reported consistently, however: sleep abnormality and abnormal pain processing.

Sleep abnormality

Delta waves are characteristic of the deep stages of non-rapid eye movement (REM) sleep. Most delta sleep occurs in the first few hours of sleep and is thought to have a primarily restorative function. People with fibromyalgia have problems in quickly entering delta sleep and get reduced amounts during the night.[8] This pattern differs from sleep abnormalities associated with clinical depression alone. Furthermore, deprivation of delta but not REM sleep in normal volunteers produces the symptoms and signs of fibromyalgia.[9] Such observations support a central role for non-restorative sleep in this condition.

Abnormal pain processing

A reduced threshold to pain perception and pain tolerance at characteristic sites throughout the body is a central clinical feature of fibromyalgia. Affected people also have peripheral sensitisation and spinal cord 'wind-up' (temporal summation of second pain), as evidenced by an exaggerated skin flare and pain in response to topically applied capsaicin and frequent occurrence of dermatographism and allodynia. Other observations to support abnormal pain processing include:[10]

- □ increased levels of substance P in the cerebrospinal fluid

- □ reduced levels of serotonin in the cerebrospinal fluid

- □ decreased regional cerebral blood flow in the caudate and thalamus at rest

- □ augmented responses to painful stimuli seen on functional magnetic resonance imaging

- □ abnormalities of the hypothalamo-pituitary-adrenal axis, with low basal levels of free cortisol, reduced suppression by dexamethasone, raised evening trough levels of (salivary) cortisol and altered levels of somatomedin

- □ abnormalities of the autonomic nervous system.

The observed abnormalities of sleep and pain processing may interrelate. Poor sleep may impair the descending noxious inhibitory control system, reducing the normal descending inhibition to the spinal cord centres that moderate ascending excitation. Equally, chronic pain may interrupt sleep. The strong association with distressing life events also might explain initial disruption of normal sleep and restoration. A working hypothesis to explain these interrelations is outlined in Fig 4.

□ MANAGEMENT

The aims of management are education about the nature of the problem, pain control and improvement of sleep. Table 3 summarises the key elements of management. Some of these have a base of research evidence, while others are more pragmatic, being based predominantly on expert consensus.[11]

Education is central. Wherever possible, discussion should include the spouse, family or carer, so that the same information is shared. The fact that the person's chronic pain does not reflect inflammation, damage or disease is a vital but difficult concept to explain. Repeated or drawn-out investigation may reinforce the patient's belief in the presence of occult serious pathology and should be avoided. The central importance of sleep and the fact that selective sleep deprivation can cause these symptoms in anyone deserves emphasis. Ascribing the symptoms to a cause for

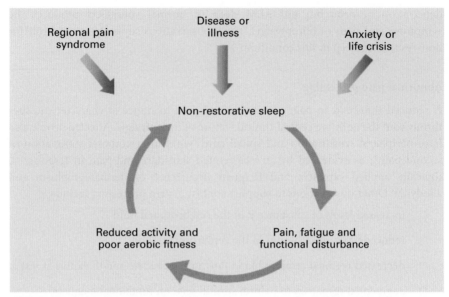

Fig 4 Simple suggested mechanism to explain some aspects of fibromyalgia.

which the patient cannot be blamed, and knowing that it is very common, often helps. It should be admitted that although we recognise fibromyalgia, we currently do not understand it fully. The model of a self-perpetuating cycle of poor sleep that causes body pain, limits activity, then worsens sleep and then makes pain worse is often accepted readily (see Fig 3) and is a useful framework for a problem-based management strategy. Any recognised generator of peripheral pain that is present (for example, osteoarthritis of the knee or rheumatoid arthritis) should be treated as effectively as possible.

The two main evidence-based interventions that can help some individuals are:

☐   Low-dose amitriptyline (25–75 mg at night) for a limited trial of 2–3 weeks, continuing if pain and fatigue are improved. Combination with fluoxetine (20 mg in the morning) may increase the benefit. Many people with fibromyalgia, however, are intolerant of even small doses of amitriptyline.

☐   Graded increase in aerobic exercise to improve well being and sleep quality.[10,12] This often requires regular supervision if it is to succeed.

The use of self-help strategies should be encouraged. A cognitive behavioural approach, with relaxation techniques and other coping strategies may help the person better deal with their symptoms. Many people with chronic pain 'from no obvious cause' adopt maladaptive illness behaviour patterns, which sometimes can be modified, with resultant improved coping. Although access to formal cognitive behavioural therapy often is limited, practitioners readily can learn and apply a reattribution model to help patients better come to terms with their symptoms. Sublimated anxiety that relates to distressing life events should be explored and

---

Box 1 Key elements of management.

- Acknowledge reality of symptoms or distress
- Offer some explanation
- 'No blame' causation
- Explore possible psychosocial stressors
- Involve family or carer
- Undertake no further investigations
- Define problems and set realistic goals
- Treat generators of peripheral pain wherever possible
- Encourage activity and graded increase in aerobic fitness
- Encourage self-help strategies
- Try amitriptyline at night (with or without fluoxetine in morning)
- Stop ineffective drugs
- Consider cognitive behavioural therapy (or simpler reattribution model)

---

addressed specifically by appropriate counselling. Additional information and support can be obtained from literature and patient organisations.

Although many people retain their symptoms and diagnostic criteria in the long term, appropriate management may reduce some of their symptoms and improve quality of life.

ACKNOWLEDGEMENT

I am grateful to Arthritis Research Campaign for infrastructure support (ICAC grant 14851; staff grant 14802).

REFERENCES

1   Kroenke K, Mangelsdorff AD. Common symptoms in ambulatory care: incidence, evaluation, therapy, and outcome. *Am J Med* 1989;**86**:262–6.

2   Croft P, Schollum J, Silman A. Population study of tender point counts and pain as evidence of fibromyalgia. *BMJ* 1994;**309**:696–9.

3   Wolfe F, Ross K, Anderson J, Russell IJ *et al*. The prevalence and characteristics of fibromyalgia in the general population. *Arthritis Rheum* 1995;**38**:19–28.

4   Aaron LA, Buchwald D. A review of the evidence for overlap among unexplained clinical conditions. *Ann Intern Med* 2001;**134**:868–81.

5   McBeth J, Macfarlane GJ, Benjamin S, Silman AJ. Features of somatization predict the onset of chronic widespread pain: results of a large population-based study. *Arthritis Rheum* 2001;**44**:940–6.

6   Papageorgiou AC, Silman AJ, Macfarlane GJ. Chronic widespread pain in the population: a seven year follow up study. *Ann Rheum Dis* 2002;**61**:1071–4.

7   McBeth J, Silman AJ, Macfarlane GJ. Association of widespread body pain with an increased risk of cancer and reduced cancer survival: a prospective, population-based study. *Arthritis Rheum* 2003;**48**:1686–92.

8   Drewes AM, Nielsen KD, Taagholt SJ, Bjerregard K *et al*. Sleep intensity in fibromyalgia: focus on the microstructure of the sleep process. *Br J Rheumatol* 1995;**34**:629–35.

9   Lentz MJ, Landis CA, Rothermel J, Shaver JL. Effects of selective slow wave sleep disruption on musculoskeletal pain and fatigue in middle aged women. *J Rheumatol* 1999;26:1586–92.

10 Crofford LJ, Clauw DJ. Fibromyalgia: where are we a decade after the American College of Rheumatology classification criteria were developed? *Arthritis Rheum* 2002:46:1136–8.

11 Anonymous. What to do about medically unexplained symptoms. *Drug Ther Bull* 2001;39:5–8.

12 Gowans SE, Dehueck A, Voss S, Silaj A *et al.* Six-month and one-year followup of 23 weeks of aerobic exercise for individuals with fibromyalgia. *Arthritis Care Res* 2004;51:890–8.

☐ RHEUMATOLOGY SELF ASSESSMENT QUESTIONS

Rheumatoid arthritis

1   Anti-tumour necrosis factor therapy:
   (a) Is cheap and effective
   (b) Abolishes all radiographic progression if used early in patients with rheumatoid arthritis
   (c) Can be very effective in patients who have failed conventional disease-modifying antirheumatic drug therapy
   (d) Is proved to be the first-line treatment in early rheumatoid arthritis
   (e) Is at least partially effective in all patients with rheumatoid arthritis

2   Combination disease-modifying antirheumatic drug therapy:
   (a) Is associated with too much toxicity for routine clinical use
   (b) Has been studied only in patients with late rheumatoid arthritis
   (c) Is associated with sustained clinical benefits, even after it is discontinued
   (d) Is associated with improved rates of remission in patients with early rheumatoid arthritis when compared with monotherapy
   (e) Consisting of methotrexate, sulfasalazine and hydroxychloroquine is more effective than methotrexate alone

3   Optimal conventional disease-modifying antirheumatic drug therapy in rheumatoid arthritis:
   (a) Has yet to be established
   (b) Involves delaying disease-modifying antirheumatic drug therapy for 6–12 months to see if patients respond to non-steroidal anti-inflammatory drugs
   (c) Should target persistent disease activity
   (d) Achieves remission in almost all patients
   (e) Abolishes radiographic disease progression

Seronegative spondyloarthropathies

1   Enthesitis (enthesopathy):
   (a) May lead to ankylosis
   (b) Occurs at the junction between a tendon and a bone
   (c) Occurs at the junction between a joint capsule and a bone
   (d) Occurs in the spine in patients with ankylosing spondylitis
   (e) Frequently causes heel pain in patients with spondyloarthropathies

2   In ankylosing spondylitis:
   (a) The disease always 'burns out' eventually
   (b) A third of patients give up work prematurely
   (c) Spinal bone strength gradually increases
   (d) Life expectancy is normal
   (e) Knee swelling may be the first indicator of the diagnosis

3   Spondyloarthritides are characterised by:
    (a) Symmetrical metacarpophalangeal joint arthritis
    (b) Buttock pain
    (c) Raynaud's phenomenon
    (d) Immunoglobulin M rheumatoid factor in the blood
    (e) Episodic eye disease, which may cause blindness

4   Spinal symptoms in ankylosing spondylitis may be improved by treatment
    with:
    (a) Sulphasalazine
    (b) Methotrexate
    (c) Non-steroidal anti-inflammatory drugs
    (d) Prednisolone
    (e) Infliximab

5   Disease activity in ankylosing spondylitis is best reflected by:
    (a) Psoriatic activity severity index
    (b) Bath ankylosing spondylitis disease activity index
    (c) Erythrocyte sedimentation rate
    (d) Short-form questionnaire (SF-36)
    (e) C-reactive protein

Fibromyalgia

1   The following clinical features should lead to consideration of fibromyalgia:
    (a) Objective swelling of painful joints
    (b) Occipital headache and diplopia
    (c) Good response to analgesics and non-steroidal anti-inflammatory drugs
    (d) Marked disparity between degree of reported disability and objective
        impairment
    (e) Marked fatigue, especially in the morning

2   The following associations are reported in fibromyalgia:
    (a) Increased prevalence with age
    (b) Obesity, insulin resistance and hyperuricaemia
    (c) Raynaud's phenomenon
    (d) Increased risk of cancer and reduced survival from cancer
    (e) Hospitalisation in childhood and self-reported child abuse

3   The following abnormalities are reported in people with fibromyalgia:
    (a) Reduced rapid eye movement sleep
    (b) Increased activity of the diffuse noxious inhibitory controls system
    (c) Peripheral and central pain sensitisation
    (d) Lymphopaenia and positive antinuclear factor
    (e) Abnormality of the hypothalamo-pituitary-adrenal axis

4   The following sites are naturally tender sites to examine for hyperalgesia in someone suspected of having fibromyalgia:
   (a) Middle of the infraspinatus belly
   (b) Interspinous ligaments of the lower cervical spine
   (c) Forehead
   (d) Medial fat pad at the knee
   (e) 1–2 cm distal to the medial epicondyle

5   The following treatments and interventions should be considered for a person with fibromyalgia:
   (a) Amitriptyline at night (25–75 mg)
   (b) Graded increase in aerobic activity
   (c) Topical capsaicin cream applied to hyperalgesic tender sites
   (d) Injection of hyperalgesic tender sites with local anaesthetic
   (e) Access to information about fibromyalgia

Endocrinology

Vitamin D deficiency

Niamh M Martin and Graham R Williams

☐ INTRODUCTION

Homeostatic regulation of calcium balance and mineralisation of the skeleton is achieved largely by complex interactions between vitamin D and parathyroid hormone (PTH) (Fig 1). The major roles of vitamin D are to increase the efficiency of intestinal absorption of dietary calcium and phosphate and to mobilise calcium and phosphate stores from bone. In addition, vitamin D inhibits PTH gene expression, as well as inhibiting parathyroid cell growth and the synthesis and secretion of PTH from the parathyroid glands. Like vitamin D, PTH also stimulates release of calcium and phosphate from bone; however, PTH potently stimulates renal calcium reabsorption and increases renal phosphate excretion. Parathyroid hormone also stimulates conversion of stored $25(OH)$-vitamin D_3 prohormone to the active vitamin D metabolite, $1\alpha,25$-dihydroxyvitamin D_3 (calcitriol; $1\alpha,25(OH)_2D_3$), by

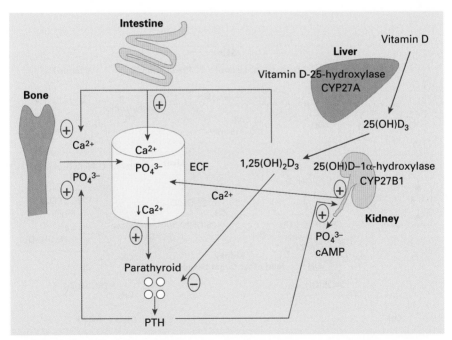

Fig 1 Physiological regulation of calcium and phosphate homeostasis by vitamin D and parathyroid hormone (PTH) (+ = stimulatory action of vitamin D or PTH; – = inhibitory action of vitamin D or PTH; ECF = extracellular fluid; cAMP = cyclic adenosine monophosphate).

increasing activity of the renal 1α-hydroxylase enzyme. The net consequences of these interactions are that excess PTH tends to deplete vitamin D stores, while vitamin D deficiency tends to increase production and secretion of PTH, which leads to an exacerbating situation of positive feedback.[1]

☐ VITAMIN D METABOLISM

The D vitamins are secosteroids that are synthesised in the skin or obtained from the diet. Dietary sources of vitamin D_3 (cholecalciferol) include fatty fish and dairy products, while vitamin D_2 (ergocalciferol) is obtained from plants and yeast. Vitamin D_2 differs from vitamin D_3 only because of its double bond between carbon atoms C_{22} and C_{23} and its methyl group at position C_{24}. Vitamin D_2 and D_3 both are modified by the same metabolic pathways and have similar biological potencies when given to humans, although $1\alpha,25(OH)_2D_3$ is the active metabolite. Vitamin D is biologically inert and must undergo two sequential hydroxylation modifications in the liver and kidney to become biologically active.[1]

Vitamin D_3 is synthesised in the skin from 7-dehydrocholesterol (7-DHC) by a photochemical reaction involving high-energy ultraviolet B (UVB) photons derived from sunlight and a subsequent temperature-sensitive isomerisation step (Fig 2).

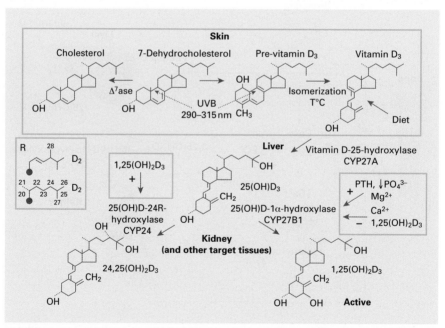

Fig 2 Vitamin D metabolic pathways. Vitamin D_3 is synthesised in skin by a photochemical reaction involving ultraviolet B radiation (UVB) and a temperature sensitive isomerisation step (T°C). The box on the left shows the structural difference between the vitamin D_2 and vitamin D_3 side chains that are attached to the secosteroid ring structure (black circle). The middle and right boxes show the factors that regulate activities of the CYP24 and CYP27B1 enzymes, respectively (+ = factor that stimulates enzymes; – = factor that inhibits enzymes).

Vitamin D_3 is lipophilic and must be transported in blood almost entirely bound to vitamin D-binding protein (VDBP). When vitamin D_3 reaches the liver, its first hydroxylation occurs in an efficient first-pass metabolism reaction that involves the cytochrome P450 enzyme, 25-hydroxylase (CYP27A). This results in synthesis of 25-hydroxyvitamin D_3 ($25(OH)D_3$) – the major circulating form of vitamin D – which redistributes into fat, from where it is released slowly with a half life of up to two months. Biologically inert $25(OH)D_3$ is activated by further hydroxylation at the 1α position by renal 1α-hydroxylase (CYP27B1), which is responsible for most circulating $1\alpha,25(OH)_2D_3$. Nevertheless, it has been appreciated recently that 1α-hydroxylation also occurs normally in vitamin D target tissues, including skin, bone, cartilage, placenta and monocytes, as well as pathologically in granulomas and activated macrophages. Circulating levels of $1\alpha,25(OH)_2D_3$ are very low (around 40–100 pmol/l) – approximately 1,000-fold lower than those of $25(OH)D_3$. The biological half-life of $1\alpha,25(OH)_2D_3$ circulating in blood is short: 6–8 hours.[1,2]

An additional hydroxylation at the C_{24} position inactivates $25(OH)D_3$ and $1\alpha,25(OH)_2D_3$ in peripheral tissues. Catalysis of this reaction by the enzyme 24-hydroxylase (CYP24) generates the inactive metabolites $24,25(OH)_2D_3$ and $1\alpha,24,25(OH)_3D_3$ in the kidney, cartilage, bone, intestine, liver and other vitamin D-responsive sites. The relative activities of the activating CYP27B1 and inactivating CYP24 enzymes are thought to determine the intracellular concentration of $1\alpha,25(OH)_2D_3$ that is available to bind and stimulate the vitamin D receptor (VDR) in target cell nuclei (Fig 3).[3] This is a highly regulated process because activation of $25(OH)D_3$ by CYP27B1 – the rate limiting step in vitamin D metabolism – is inhibited by vitamin D and calcium in a negative feedback loop, whereas CYP24 inactivation is stimulated by vitamin D and the levels of available active hormone are maintained in homeostasis.[1,2]

☐ VITAMIN D DEFICIENCY

Vitamin D deficiency results from insufficient synthesis of vitamin D in the skin or from inadequate dietary vitamin D intake.[1] The photochemical synthetic reaction in the skin requires UVB light in the 290–315 nm wavelength range. The reaction is effectively prevented by reduced UVB exposure, and vitamin D synthesis ceases. Table 1 gives the causes of reduced UVB exposure. In non-Caucasian people with darker skin pigmentation, melanin competes with dehydrocholesterol for UVB photons, so a longer exposure to the sun – that correlates with the degree of pigmentation – is needed for an equivalent amount of vitamin D synthesis. In ethnic groups resident in the United Kingdom and other countries in the northern hemisphere, the situation is exacerbated. During winter, sunlight must pass over a longer distance through the atmosphere, and most UV light is absorbed before it reaches the earth. A distinct seasonal variation in vitamin D levels thus exists in the northern latitudes. In northern America, Canada and north-western Europe, for example, vitamin D synthesis virtually is absent between October and March. In contrast, in Los Angeles, which is situated at lower latitude, cutaneous production of vitamin D_3 occurs throughout the year. In people from certain cultures, who wear

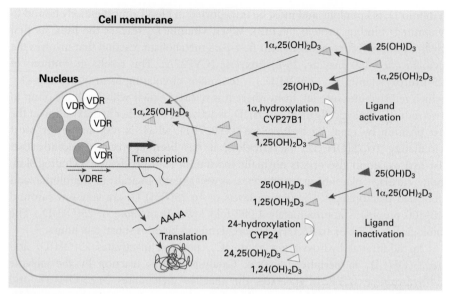

Fig 3 Intranuclear mechanism of action of vitamin D. The extracellular vitamin D metabolites, $25(OH)D_3$ and $1\alpha,25(OH)_2D_3$, enter the cell and are substrates for inactivation by 24-hydroxylation (performed by CYP24) or activation by 1α-hydroxylation (performed by CYP27B1). The active $1\alpha,25(OH)_2D_3$ metabolite passes into the cell nucleus, where it binds to the nuclear vitamin D receptor (VDR) with high affinity. The VDR binds to vitamin D response elements (VDRE), situated within promoters of vitamin D-responsive target genes, in a heterodimer complexed with a retinoid X receptor (black circles). Interaction of the ligand-bound VDR with the transcriptional machinery of the target gene promoter results in transcriptional activation of the target gene in response to vitamin D, synthesis of mRNA and, ultimately, translation of protein. Vitamin D thus acts via specific nuclear receptors to increase expression of vitamin D-inducible target genes.

extensive concealment clothing or have dietary customs that preclude adequate intake of vitamin D, these additional factors increase the risk of vitamin D deficiency. In older people, susceptibility to vitamin D deficiency from insufficient sunlight exposure is compounded by the fact that cutaneous vitamin D synthesis is impaired because of reduced concentrations of unesterified 7-DHC in ageing skin. In addition, institutionalised and housebound people are further susceptible, because window glass absorbs UVB radiation very efficiently. Where exposure to sunlight is suboptimal, dietary sources of vitamin D become important. In the United States, but not in the United Kingdom, milk is fortified with vitamin D; these dietary contributions are particularly relevant in young children and older people. Little vitamin D is present in breast milk, although infant formulas and some weaning foods are fortified with vitamin D. In older people, vitamin D deficiency is a significant risk factor for fracture, and oral vitamin D and calcium supplementation may be a cost-effective measure for preventing hip fractures. Vitamin D deficiency in infants and young children may be exacerbated further by concerns about the negative effects of exposure to sunlight, which lead to increased use of sunscreens. In older people, reduced activity of renal 1α-hydroxylase is a further concern because renal function declines with age, and this may also contribute to vitamin D deficiency.[4–6]

Table 1 Risk factors for vitamin D deficiency.

Vitamin D synthesis and metabolism

Reduced sun exposure
- Concealment clothing
- Older age
- Ethnicity
- Excessive use of sunblocks
- Housebound and indoor living (childcare/residential homes)
- Northern latitudes
- Seasonal variations

Chronic renal disease
- Impaired 1α-hydroxylation

P450 enzyme-inducing drugs
- Rifampicin
- Phenytoin

Chronic liver disease
- Impaired 25-hydroxylation

Dietary insufficiency

Prolonged breastfeeding
- Minimal vitamin D in breast milk

Elderly
- Generally poor diet

Ethnicity
- Vegetarianism and ingestion of phytates

Malabsorption

Coeliac disease

Crohn's disease

Chronic liver disease and jaundice

☐ MEASUREMENT OF VITAMIN D STATUS

Measurement of concentrations of 25(OH)D and $1\alpha,25(OH)_2D$ in serum is difficult, and assays can be unreliable. The first assays for 25(OH)D relied on high-performance liquid chromatography and the quantitative detection of 25(OH)D and related metabolites by UV light. In the 1980s, specific antibodies to 25(OH)D became available, and current radioimmunoassays use an antibody that recognises $25(OH)D_2$ and $25(OH)D_3$ equally efficiently. The assay also detects other inactive vitamin D_2 and D_3 metabolites that comprise about 6% of all circulating D_2 and D_3 derivatives. Nevertheless, this apparent lack of specificity is not important clinically, because 25(OH)D is biologically stable in serum and levels are relatively high in the nmol/l range: being present at 1,000-fold higher concentrations than the 1α-hydroxylated active metabolites. The 25(OH)D assay thus reflects the measurement of total vitamin D stores, and samples do not need special handling other than a centrifugation step before storage and analysis.[1] Nevertheless, problems can be associated with interpretation of this assay, which is most useful in the diagnosis of vitamin D deficiency. Firstly, variation in assay methods between laboratories leads to a lack of standardisation. Secondly, the assay measures free and VDBP-bound 25(OH)D, and values must be interpreted cautiously in patients with protein-deficient states, such as nephrotic syndrome and liver failure. Thirdly, the seasonal variation in cutaneous vitamin D production is reflected by a peak vitamin D concentration that occurs in autumn and a seasonal minimum in spring: interpretation of 25(OH)D measurements should take this into account. A 25(OH)D concentration measured in autumn at the lower end of the reference range thus may be considered suboptimal and insufficient to sustain adequate vitamin D levels throughout the winter months. Fourthly, in view of ethnic differences in vitamin D synthesis, use of the same reference ranges for 25(OH)D in Caucasian and non-Caucasians within the United Kingdom might be inappropriate. Finally, normal reference ranges for concentrations of circulating 25(OH)D can vary significantly between countries as a result of causes such as lack of assay standardisation, variations in latitude (this can also result in problems within a country that spans a large range of latitude such as the United States), ethnicity and dietary supplementation.[4,5,7] In light of these considerations, 25(OH)D levels should be measured in combination with determination of concentrations of PTH. This is a physiological marker of the functional concentration of vitamin D and, therefore, in patients with vitamin D deficiency, PTH levels increase, while vitamin D supplementation causes PTH levels to fall. Interpretation of abnormal vitamin D concentrations thus is facilitated greatly by consideration of their physiological effects on PTH secretion.

Measurement of $1\alpha,25(OH)_2D$ is much more problematic.[1] The first radioreceptor assays in 1974 were expensive, technically difficult and relatively non-specific. In the 1990s, specific antibodies for $1\alpha,25(OH)_2D$ metabolites were obtained, and the current radioimmunoassay is approximately 99.9% specific, with only 0.1% cross-reactivity for 25(OH)D metabolites. Nevertheless, because 25(OH)D metabolites circulate at 1,000-fold higher concentrations than $1\alpha,25(OH)_2D$ itself, the measured concentration of $1\alpha,25(OH)_2D$ actually includes at least a 10% error because of this cross-reaction. The $1\alpha,25(OH)_2D$ assay reflects 1α-hydroxylase status and can be useful for assessing patients with vitamin D resistance or suspected 1α-hydroxylase deficiency, although this should be viewed as a specialist test that is unnecessary in everyday clinical practice. Even in situations in which measurement of $1\alpha,25(OH)_2D$ can be justified, practical problems exist. Metabolites of $1\alpha,25(OH)_2D$ have a short half-life and they are unstable at room temperature and light sensitive. Blood must be taken on ice, the sample should be separated immediately, and the serum should be frozen on dry ice. Frozen samples must be transported on dry ice for analysis in one of the few laboratories that offers this service, and assays usually are performed in batches, as few measurements are requested. In many instances, therefore, samples are taken or stored incorrectly, rendering the assay measurements unreliable. Furthermore, assay results often are not received for several weeks, because of the practical limitations described, and may have no influence on clinical management. For these reasons, measurement of $1\alpha,25(OH)_2D$ should be restricted to specialist centres.

☐ PRACTICAL CONSEQUENCES OF INTERACTIONS BETWEEN VITAMIN D AND PTH

The main consequences of vitamin D deficiency result from the reduced stores of $25(OH)D_3$, decreased concentrations of circulating $1\alpha,25(OH)_2D_3$ and impaired calcium absorption. The combination of vitamin D deficiency and a falling serum calcium concentration causes secondary hyperparathyroidism, with a resulting increase in osteoclast activity and release of calcium and phosphate from bone. Established vitamin D deficiency causes rickets in children and osteomalacia in adults, although in modern clinical practice frank bone disease is encountered only rarely because of improvements in diet, prevention and diagnosis.[8] Nevertheless, vitamin D deficiency is common in the United Kingdom and its early diagnosis and treatment is important but often problematic.

The most relevant issues to consider are how to interpret the biochemical finding of a level of 25(OH)D at the lower end of, or just below, the quoted reference range and how to interpret a modestly raised concentration of PTH.[9–11] This is a common problem, which frequently occurs in the presence of normal calcium and alkaline phosphatase concentrations. Its management requires clinical judgement, and patients in whom vitamin D deficiency is especially deleterious must be identified. The only way to interpret these issues is to ensure that vitamin D status is always considered in the context of PTH status and vice versa . Measurement of PTH in the context of a 25(OH)D level at the lower end of the reference range thus provides information about whether there is a coexistent functional vitamin D deficiency, in which case the PTH concentration would be elevated. Similarly, the presence of an elevated PTH must be considered in the context of the 25(OH)D level to determine whether the raised PTH level results from primary or secondary hyperpara-thyroidism. Consideration of the physiological relation between vitamin D and PTH, as described previously, suggests the possibility that chronic vitamin D deficiency may fuel the emergence of hyperparathyroidism or that chronic early primary hyperparathyroidism may precipitate vitamin D deficiency. This has led to the hypothesis that symptomatic hyperparathyroidism results from coexistent vitamin D deficiency – a suggestion supported by studies that showed that patients with overt primary hyperparathyroidism in Brazil, China and India invariably were deficient in vitamin D. Similarly, in the United States, patients with primary hyperparathyroidism and 25(OH)D levels in the lowest tertile of the normal reference range had evidence of bone disease determined by biochemical measures, evaluation of bone mineral density and dynamic histomorphometry.[9–11]

These considerations indicate that early treatment of vitamin D deficiencies is likely to be advantageous. However, it is important to recognise that this can be hazardous in patients with hyperparathyroidism, as replenishment of vitamin D stores needs treatment with a long-acting vitamin D analogue that, in turn, may precipitate hypercalcaemia. A solution to this is to treat patients with vitamin D deficiency, in whom coexistent primary hyperparathyroidism is suspected, with a short-acting vitamin D analogue such as calcitriol ($1\alpha,25(OH)_2D_3$) and to measure the calcium and PTH response regularly over 2–3 weeks. If treatment with $1\alpha,25(OH)_2D_3$ does not precipitate hypercalcaemia and results in suppression of PTH levels to within the reference range, a diagnosis of vitamin D deficiency with secondary hyperparathyroidism can be made and replacement of vitamin D stores may proceed safely. If treatment with $1\alpha,25(OH)_2D_3$ fails to suppress PTH or results in hypercalcaemia, or both, however, a diagnosis of primary hyperparathyroidism is very likely. If confirmed, the coexistent vitamin D deficiency is particularly deleterious and will worsen the hyperparathyroid state. In these circumstances, early parathyroidectomy is recommended.[11]

☐ CONCLUSIONS

Vitamin D deficiency is increasingly encountered in the United Kingdom, and the physiological interactions between vitamin D and PTH are important clinically. Diagnosis of vitamin D deficiency is best made through determination of circulating 25(OH)D levels. Measurement of $1\alpha,25(OH)_2D$ should be reserved for specialist centres. It is important to recognise that measurement of 25(OH)D is not precise and that the quoted reference ranges are variable. This flexibility must be understood when interpreting vitamin D status, and measurement of PTH should be performed along with determination of 25(OH)D concentrations in order to assess the vitamin D/PTH axis. Replacement of vitamin D stores in normocalcaemic patients with raised PTH levels should proceed only after primary hyperparathyroidism has been excluded. In patients with primary hyperparathyroidism, coexistent vitamin D deficiency markedly worsens the condition and should be viewed as an indication for early surgical intervention.

REFERENCES

1   Favus MJ. *Primer on the metabolic bone diseases and disorders of mineral metabolism.* Philadelphia, PA: Lippincott Williams and Wilkins, 2004.

2   DeLuca HF. Overview of general physiologic features and functions of vitamin D. *Am J Clin Nutr* 2004;**80**(6 Suppl):1689S–96S.

3   Haussler MR, Haussler CA, Jurutka PW, Thompson PD, *et al.* The vitamin D hormone and its nuclear receptor: molecular actions and disease states. *J Endocrinol* 1997;**154**(Suppl):S57–73.

4   Holick MF. Environmental factors that influence the cutaneous production of vitamin D. *Am J Clin Nutr* 1995;**61**(3 Suppl):638S–45S.

5   Dawson-Hughes B. Racial/ethnic considerations in making recommendations for vitamin D for adult and elderly men and women. *Am J Clin Nutr* 2004;**80**(6 Suppl):1763S–6S.

6   Weaver CM, Fleet JC. Vitamin D requirements: current and future. *Am J Clin Nutr* 2004;**80**(6 Suppl):1735S–9S.

7   Heaney RP. Functional indices of vitamin D status and ramifications of vitamin D deficiency. *Am J Clin Nutr* 2004;**80**(6 Suppl):1706S–9S.

8   Bilezikian JP, Silverberg SJ. Clinical spectrum of primary hyperparathyroidism. *Rev Endocr Metab Disord* 2000;**1**(4):237–45.

9   Silverberg SJ, Shane E, Dempster DW, Bilezikian JP. The effects of vitamin D insufficiency in patients with primary hyperparathyroidism. *Am J Med* 1999;**107**:561–7.

10 Rao DS, Agarwal G, Talpos GB, Phillips ER, *et al.* Role of vitamin D and calcium nutrition in disease expression and parathyroid tumor growth in primary hyperparathyroidism: a global perspective. *J Bone Miner Res* 2002;**17**(Suppl 2):N75–80.

11 Bilezikian JP, Brandi ML, Rubin M, Silverberg SJ. Primary hyperparathyroidism: new concepts in clinical, densitometric and biochemical features. *J Intern Med* 2005;**257**:6–17.

Genetics of endocrine cancer syndromes

Rajesh V Thakker

☐ INTRODUCTION

Endocrine cancers are uncommon when compared with the incidences of lung, breast, colorectal and prostate cancers (Table 1).[1] For example, only ovarian cancer features in estimates of the worldwide incidence of the 18 major cancers, where it ranks as the sixth most frequent cancer in women.[1] It is important to note, however, that parathyroid tumours that give rise to primary hyperparathyroidism are more common, but as these tumours rarely are malignant, they often are not considered in the cancer registries.

Table 1 Incidence of some common cancers, endocrine cancers, and familial endocrine cancer syndromes.

Cancer	Annual incidence (per 100,000 population)		
	Men	**Women**	**Both sexes**
Non-endocrine:			
Breast		54	
Colorectal			40
Lung	72	19	
Prostate	20–30		
Endocrine:			
Neuroendocrine			0.7 (to 8.4)
Ovary		11	
Parathyroid			28
Testis	3.3		
Thyroid			1.5

Familial endocrine cancer syndromes, which generally are inherited as autosomal dominant traits (Table 2) with high penetrance, are rare,[2] but their recognition is important for two main reasons. Firstly, affected patients may be at risk from multiple tumours that may arise in different glands, and regular screening for these, together with earlier treatment, is likely to improve the prognosis. Secondly, the relatives of an affected patient are at 50% risk of having inherited the mutation and thus developing tumours. Identification of these people, together with screening for the early development of tumours, also is likely to improve the prognosis. These syndromes include:

- ☐ multiple endocrine neoplasia type 1

- ☐ multiple endocrine neoplasia type 2

- ☐ familial isolated primary hyperparathyroidism

- ☐ hyperparathyroidism–jaw tumour syndrome

- ☐ familial benign hypocalciuric hypercalcaemia and neonatal primary hyperparathyroidism

- ☐ Von Hippel–Lindau disease

- ☐ neurofibromatosis type 1

- ☐ Carney complex

- ☐ Cowden syndrome

- ☐ familial breast–ovarian cancer syndrome.

The clinical features and molecular genetics of each of these syndromes will be reviewed briefly.

Table 2 Familial endocrine cancer syndromes and their chromosomal locations.

Disorder	Chromosomal location (gene or protein)
Breast–ovarian cancer	17q21 (BRCA1)
Carney complex	2p16, 17q22-q23 (PPKARIA)
Cowden syndrome	10q23.3 (PTEN)
Familial benign hypercalcaemia, neonatal primary hyperparathyroidism	3q21 (CaSR)
Familial isolated primary hyperparathyroidism	11q13 (MENIN), 1p32-pter, 1q25
Hyperparathyroidism–jaw tumour syndrome	1q31.2
Multiple endocrine neoplasia type 1	11q13 (MENIN)
Multiple endocrine neoplasia type 2	10q11.2 (RET)
Neurofibromatosis type 1	17q11.2 (Neuro-fibromin)
Phaeochromocytoma	1p, 17p, 22q
Von Hippel–Lindau disease	3p26-p25 (pVHL, elongin)

☐ MULTIPLE ENDOCRINE NEOPLASIA

Multiple endocrine neoplasia (MEN) is characterised by the occurrence of tumours that involve two or more endocrine glands within a single patient.[2] The disorder has been referred to previously as multiple endocrine adenopathy (MEA) or pluriglandular syndrome. Glandular hyperplasia and malignancy also may occur in some patients, however, so the term multiple endocrine neoplasia is now preferred. Two major forms of multiple endocrine neoplasia exist, and these are referred to as type 1 and type 2. Each form is characterised by the development of tumours within specific endocrine glands (Table 3). Thus the combined occurrence of tumours of the parathyroid glands, the pancreatic islet cells and the anterior pituitary is characteristic of MEN1, which is also referred to as Wermer's syndrome.[2,3] In MEN2 (which is also called Sipple's syndrome[4]), however, medullary thyroid carcinoma (MTC) occurs in association with phaeochromocytoma, and three clinical variants, referred to as MEN2a, MEN2b, and MTC-only, are recognised (see below). Although MEN1 and MEN2 usually occur as distinct and separate syndromes, some patients occasionally develop tumours that are associated with MEN1 and MEN2. For

Table 3 Multiple endocrine neoplasia (MEN) syndromes, their characteristic tumours and associated biochemical abnormalities.*

Type	Tumour	Biochemical features
MEN1	Parathyroids	Hypercalcaemia and increased parathyroid hormone
	Pancreatic islets:	
	Gastrinoma	Increased gastrin and increased basal gastric acid output
	Insulinoma	Hypoglycaemia and increased insulin
	Glucagonoma	Glucose intolerance and increased glucagon
	VIPoma	Increased vasoactive intestinal peptide and watery diarrhoea, hypokalaemia and achlorhydria
	PPoma	Increased pancreatic polypeptide
	Pituitary (anterior):	
	Prolactinoma	Hyperprolactinaemia
	Growth hormone-secreting	Increased growth hormone
	Adrenocorticotrophin-secreting	Hypercortisolaemia and increased adrenocorticotrophin
	Non-functioning	Nil or α subunit
	Associated tumours:	
	Adrenal cortical	Hypercortisolaemia or primary hyperaldosteronism
	Carcinoid	Increased 5-hydroxyindoleacetic acid
	Lipoma	Nil
MEN2a	Medullary thyroid carcinoma	Hypercalcitoninaemia[†]
	Phaeochromocytoma	Increased catecholamines
	Parathyroid	Hypercalcaemia and increased parathyroid hormone
MEN2b	Medullary thyroid carcinoma	Hypercalcitoninaemia
	Phaeochromocytoma	Increased catecholamines
	Associated abnormalities:	
	Mucosal neuromas	
	Marfanoid habitus	
	Medullated corneal nerve fibres	
	Megacolon	

*Autosomal dominant inheritance of the MEN syndromes has been established.
[†]In some patients, basal concentrations of serum calcitonin may be normal but may show an abnormal rise one minute and five minutes after stimulation with 0.5 mcg/kg pentagastrin.

example, patients with islet cell tumours of the pancreas and pheochromocytomas or with acromegaly and pheochromocytoma have been described, and in these patients, MEN may represent an 'overlap' syndrome.

Multiple endocrine neoplasia type 1

Clinical features

Parathyroid, pancreatic and pituitary tumours constitute the major components of MEN1.[2] In addition to these tumours, adrenal cortical, carcinoid, facial angiofibromas, collagenomas and lipomatous tumours also may occur in some patients.[3]

Parathyroid tumours

Primary hyperparathyroidism is the most common feature of MEN1 and occurs in more than 95% of all patients with this condition.[3] Patients may present with asymptomatic hypercalcaemia, nephrolithiasis, osteitis fibrosa cystica or vague symptoms associated with hypercalcaemia – for example, polyuria, polydipsia, constipation, malaise or occasionally peptic ulcers. Biochemical investigations show hypercalcaemia, usually in association with increased circulating concentrations of parathyroid hormone (PTH). The hypercalcaemia usually is mild, and severe hypercalcaemia that results in crisis or parathyroid carcinoma is a rare occurrence. Additional differences between the primary hyperparathyroidism of patients with MEN1 and those without MEN1 include an earlier age of onset (20–25 years v 55 years) and an equal male:female ratio (1:1 v 1:3). Primary hyperparathyroidism in patients with MEN1 is unusual before the age of 15 years, and the age of conversion from being unaffected to being affected has been observed as between 20 and 21 years in some people.

No effective medical treatment for primary hyperparathyroidism generally is available, and surgical removal of the abnormally overactive parathyroid glands is the definitive treatment. All four parathyroid glands usually are affected with multiple adenomas or hyperplasia, although this histological distinction may be difficult, and partial or total parathyroidectomy has been proposed as a treatment for primary hyperparathyroidism in MEN1. If a total parathyroidectomy is undertaken, the resultant lifelong hypocalcaemia is treated with oral calcitriol (1,25-dihydroxy vitamin D_3). It has been suggested that parathyroidectomy should be reserved for symptomatic, hypercalcaemic patients with MEN1 and that asymptomatic, hypercalcaemic patients with MEN1 should not have parathyroid surgery but should instead have regular assessments for the onset of symptoms and complications, at which point total parathyroidectomy should be undertaken.

Pancreatic tumours

The incidence of pancreatic islet cell tumours in patients with MEN1 varies from 30% to 80% in different series. Most of these tumours produce excessive amounts of hormone, for example gastrin, insulin, glucagon or vasoactive intestinal polypeptide (VIP), and are associated with distinct clinical syndromes.[3]

Gastrinomas are gastrin-secreting tumours that represent more than 50% of all pancreatic islet cell tumours in MEN1, and approximately 20% of patients with gastrinomas will have MEN1.[3] Gastrinomas are the major cause of morbidity and mortality in patients with MEN1; this is the result of recurrent severe multiple peptic ulcers, which may perforate. This association of recurrent peptic ulceration, marked production of gastric acid and non β-islet cell tumours of the pancreas is referred to as Zollinger-Ellison syndrome. Additional prominent clinical features of this syndrome include diarrhoea and steatorrhoea. The diagnosis is established by an increased concentration of fasting serum gastrin in association with increased basal secretion of gastric acid. Medical treatment of patients with MEN1 and Zollinger-Ellison syndrome is directed to reducing basal acid output to less than 10 mmol/l, which may be achieved by the parietal cell H^+,K^+-ATPase inhibitor omeprazole. The ideal treatment for non-metastatic gastrinomas is surgical excision of the gastrinoma; however, in patients with MEN1, gastrinomas frequently are multiple or extra-pancreatic, and the role of surgery has been controversial. For example, in one study, only 16% of patients with MEN1 were free of disease immediately after surgery and at five years this had declined to 6%; the respective outcomes in patients without MEN1 were better – at 45% and 40%. The treatment of disseminated gastrinomas is difficult, and hormonal therapy with octreotide (a human somatostatin analogue), chemotherapy with streptozotocin and 5-fluorouracil, hepatic artery embolisation and removal of all resectable tumour all occasionally have been successful.

Insulinomas are β-islet cell tumours that secrete insulin and represent one-third of all pancreatic tumours in patients with MEN1.[3] Insulinomas also occur in association with gastrinomas in 10% of patients with MEN1, and the two tumours may arise at different times. Insulinomas occur more often in patients younger than 40 years with MEN1 and many arise in people younger than 20 years, whereas in patients without MEN1, insulinomas generally occur in those older than 40 years. Insulinomas may be the first manifestation of MEN1 in 10% of patients, and approximately 4% of patients who present with insulinoma will have MEN1. Patients with an insulinoma present with hypoglycaemic symptoms that develop after a fast or exertion and improve after glucose intake. Biochemical investigations show increased concentrations of plasma insulin in association with hypoglycaemia. Circulating concentrations of C-peptide and proinsulin, which also are increased, may be useful in establishing the diagnosis. Medical treatment, which consists of frequent carbohydrate feeds and diazoxide, is not always successful, and surgery often is needed. Most insulinomas are multiple and small; preoperative localisation with computed tomography scanning, coeliac axis angiography and pre- or perioperative percutaneous transhepatic portal venous sampling is difficult, and success rates have varied. Surgical treatment, which ranges from enucleation of a single tumour to distal or partial pancreatectomy, has been curative in some patients. Chemotherapy, which consists of streptozotocin or octreotide, is used for metastatic disease.

Glucagonomas are α-islet cell, glucagon-secreting pancreatic tumours that occur in <3% of patients with MEN1.[3] The characteristic clinical manifestations of skin rash (necrolytic migratory erythyema), weight loss, anaemia and stomatitis may be absent, and the presence of the tumour is indicated only by glucose intolerance and hyperglucagonaemia. The tail of the pancreas is the most frequent site for glucagonomas, and surgical removal of these is the treatment of choice. Treatment may be difficult, however, as 50% of patients have metastases at the time of diagnosis. Medical treatment of these with octreotide, or streptozotocin, has been successful in some patients.

VIPomas are vasoactive intestinal peptide (VIP)-secreting pancreatic tumours. Patients with VIPomas develop watery diarrhoea, hypokalaemia and achlorhydria, referred to as the WDHA syndrome.[3] This clinical syndrome also has been referred to as Verner–Morrison syndrome or VIPoma syndrome. VIPomas have been reported in only a few patients with MEN1, and the diagnosis is established by documenting markedly increased concentrations of VIP in plasma. Surgical management of VIPomas, which mostly are located in the tail of the pancreas, has been curative. In patients with unresectable tumours, however, treatment with streptozotocin, octreotide, corticosteroids, indomethacin, metoclopramide and lithium carbonate has proved beneficial.

PPomas, which secrete pancreatic polypeptide (PP), are found in a large number of patients with MEN1.[3] No pathological sequelae of excessive PP secretion are apparent, and the clinical significance of PP is unknown, although measurement of PP in the serum has been suggested for the detection of pancreatic tumours in patients with MEN1.

Pituitary tumours

The incidence of pituitary tumours in patients with MEN1 varies from 15% to 90% in different series.[3] About 60% of pituitary tumours associated with MEN1 secrete prolactin, <25% secrete growth hormone (GH), 5% secrete adenocorticotrophin (ACTH) and the remainder seem to be non-functioning. Prolactinomas may be the first manifestation of MEN1 in <10% of patients, and somatotrophinomas occur more often in patients older than 40 years. Fewer than 3% of patients with anterior pituitary tumours will have MEN1. The clinical manifestations depend on the size of the pituitary tumour and its product of secretion. Enlarging pituitary tumours may compress adjacent structures, such as the optic chiasm or normal pituitary tissue, and cause bitemporal hemianopia or hypopituitarism, respectively. The tumour size and extension are assessed radiologically by computed tomography scanning and nuclear magnetic resonance imaging. Treatment of pituitary tumours in patients with MEN1 is similar to that in patients without MEN1 and consists of medical therapy or selective hypophysectomy by the transphenoidal approach, if feasible, with radiotherapy reserved for residual unresectable tumours.

Associated tumours

Patients with MEN1 may have tumours that involve glands other than the parathyroid glands, pancreas and pituitary gland. Carcinoid, adrenal cortical, thyroid and lipomatous tumours, facial angiofibromas and collagenomas have been described in association with MEN1.[3]

Carcinoid tumours, which occur in >3% of patients with MEN1, may be inherited as an autosomal dominant trait in association with MEN1.[3] The carcinoid tumour may be located in the bronchi, gastrointestinal tract, pancreas or thymus. Bronchial carcinoid tumours in patients with MEN1 predominantly occur in women (male:female ratio = 1:4), whereas thymic carcinoids occur predominantly in men; cigarette smokers have a higher risk of developing tumours. Most patients are asymptomatic and do not suffer the flushing attacks and dyspnoea associated with carcinoid syndrome, which usually develops after the tumour has metastasised to the liver.

The incidence of asymptomatic *adrenal cortical tumours* in patients with MEN1 has been reported to be as high as 40%.[3] Most of these tumours are non-functioning; however, functioning adrenal cortical tumours in patients with MEN1 have been shown to cause hypercortisolaemia and Cushing's syndrome and primary hyperaldosteronism, as in Conn's syndrome.

Lipomas may occur in >33% of patients and frequently are multiple. In addition, pleural or retroperitoneal lipomas also may occur in patients with MEN1.[3]

Thyroid tumours, which consist of adenomas, colloid goitres and carcinomas, have been reported to occur in more than 25% of patients with MEN1.[3] The prevalence of thyroid disorders in the general population is high, however, so it has been suggested that the association of thyroid abnormalities in patients with MEN1 may be incidental and not significant.

Multiple *facial angiofibromas*, which are similar to those seen in patients with tuberous sclerosis, have been observed in 88% of patients with MEN1 and *collagenomas* in >70%.[3]

Genetics

The gene that causes MEN1 is located on chromosome 11q13. It consists of 10 exons, with a 1,830 base pair coding region that encodes a novel protein that contains 610 amino acids and is referred to as MENIN.[2,3] MENIN has a variety of functions, including regulation of transcription, genome stability and cell division.[3] Germline mutations of the MEN1 gene have been identified in patients with MEN1; most (75%) are inactivating, consistent with those expected in a tumour suppressor gene. Tumours from patients with MEN1 and those without have been seen to harbour the germline mutation, together with a somatic mutation or loss of heterozygosity involving chromosome 11q13, as expected from Knudson's model and the proposed role of the MEN1 gene as a tumour suppressor.[2] The mutations not only are diverse in type but also are scattered throughout the coding region of the MEN1 gene, with no evidence for the clustering seen in MEN2 (see below). In addition, correlations between the mutations behind MEN1 and the clinical manifestations of the disorder seem to be absent.[3] This lack of genotype–phenotype correlation, which contrasts with the situation in MEN2 (see below), together with the wide diversity of mutations in the 1,830 bp coding region of the MEN1 gene, has made mutational analysis for diagnostic purposes in MEN1 time consuming and expensive. Such DNA diagnostic testing is available, however (for example, at the Oxford Genetics Department, Churchill Hospital, Oxford, OX3 7LJ).

Multiple endocrine neoplasia type 2

Multiple endocrine neoplasia type 2 describes the association of medullary thyroid carcinoma (MTC), phaeochromocytomas and parathyroid tumours (Table 3). Three clinical variants of MEN2 are recognised: MEN2a, MEN2b and MTC-only.[2,4] The variant MEN2a is the most common, and the development of MTC is associated with phaeochromocytomas (50% of patients), which may be bilateral, and parathyroid tumours (20% of patients). Variant MEN2b, which represents 5% of all cases of MEN2, is characterised by the occurrence of MTC and phaeochromocytoma in association with a Marfanoid habitus, mucosal neuromas, medullated corneal fibres and intestinal autonomic ganglion dysfunction, which leads to multiple diverticulae and megacolon.[4] Parathyroid tumours do not usually occur in MEN2b. MTC-only is a variant in which medullary thyroid carcinoma is the sole manifestation of the syndrome.

Clinical features

Medullary thyroid carcinoma

Medullary thyroid carcinoma is the most common feature of MEN2a and occurs in almost all affected people. It represents 10% of all thyroid gland carcinomas, and 20% of patients with MTC have a family history of the disorder.[4] Patients with MTC may be asymptomatic, and the condition may have been identified by the presence of hypercalcitoninaemia during family screening. However, MTC also may present as a palpable mass in the neck, which may be asymptomatic or associated with symptoms of pressure or dysphagia in 16% of patients. Diarrhoea may occur in 30% of patients and is associated with increased circulating concentrations of calcitonin or with tumour-related secretion of serotonin and prostaglandins. Some patients also may have flushing. In addition, ectopic production of ACTH by MTC may cause Cushing's syndrome. Radionucleotide thyroid scans reveal MTC tumours as 'cold' nodules. The diagnosis of MTC relies on demonstration of hypercalcitoninaemia in the basal state (>90 pg/ml) or after stimulation with intravenous pentagastrin (0.5 mcg/kg) and/or infusion of calcium (2 mg/kg). Metastases of MTC in the early stages usually occur to the cervical lymph nodes and in later stages to the medistinal nodes, lungs, liver, trachea, adrenal gland, oesophagus and bone. Radiography may show dense irregular calcification within the involved portions of the thyroid gland and the lymph nodes involved with the metastases. The presence of metastases does not necessarily lead to a poor prognosis, however, and in 80% of patients the tumour or tumours pursue a relatively indolent course. Medullary thyroid carcinoma does pursue an aggressive course, with early metastases and death in <10% of patients, and a family history of such aggressive MTC or MEN2b may exist.

Treatment for MTC is total thyroidectomy, with central lymph node resection, followed by replacement thyroxine therapy.

Phaeochromocytoma

These noradrenaline- and adrenaline-secreting tumours occur in >50% of patients with MEN2a and are a major cause of morbidity and mortality.[4] Patients may have symptoms and signs of catecholamine secretion (eg headaches, palpitations, sweating and poorly controlled hypertension) or they may be asymptomatic and have been detected through biochemical screening because of a history of familial MEN2a or MTC. The biochemical and radiological investigation of phaeochromo-cytoma in patients with MEN2a is similar to that in patients without the condition and includes the estimation of urinary free catecholamines, computed tomography (or magnetic resonance image) scanning and radionuclide scanning with meta-iodo (^{123}I or ^{131}I)-benzyl guanidine (MIBG). An early biochemical abnormality in patients with MEN2a with phaeochromocytoma and medullary hyperplasia is an increase in the adrenaline: noradrenaline ratio to >0.15. Bilateral adrenomeduallary hyperplasia is the precursor to phaeochromocytoma in patients with MEN2. This is associated with expansion of the medullary tissue into the body and tail of the gland, with a decrease in corticomedullary ratio and nodular hyperplasia. Nodules that exceed 1 mm in diameter are designated phaeochromocytomas. The incidence of bilateral adrenal medullary tumours in patients with MEN2a is 70%, in contrast with the 10% incidence in patients without the condition. In addition, phaeo-chromocytoma in patients with MEN2a differ significantly in distribution when compared with those in patients without MEN2a. Thus, extra-adrenal phaeo-chromocytomas, which occur in 10% of patients without MEN2a, are observed rarely in patients with MEN2a, and, similarly, malignancy in patients with MEN2a and phaeochromocytoma is much less common.

A recommended treatment for phaeochromocytoma in patients with MEN2a is bilateral adrenalectomy, even in patients with MEN2a in whom only a unilateral tumour has been shown by radiology.

Parathyroid tumours

The incidence of parathyroid tumours in patients with MEN2a varies from 40% to 80% in different series.[4] More than 50% of these patients do not have hypercalcaemia, however, and the presence of abnormally enlarged para-thyroids, which are unusually hyperplastic, is seen in normocalcaemic patients undergoing thyroidectomy for MTC. The biochemical investigation and management of hypercalcaemic patients with MEN2a is similar to that of patients with MEN1.

Genetics

The gene that causes all three variants of MEN2 was mapped to chromosome 10cen-10q11.2 – a region that contains the *c-ret* proto-oncogene that encodes a tyrosine kinase receptor with cadherin-like and cysteine-rich extracellular domains and a tyrosine kinase intracellular domain.[4] Specific mutations of *c-ret* have been identified for each of the three MEN2 variants. In 95% of patients, therefore, MEN2a is associated with mutations of the cysteine-rich extracellular domain, and mutations in codon 634 (Cys→Arg) account for 85% of MEN2a mutations.[4] The MTC-only variant also is associated with missense mutations in the cysteine-rich extracellular domain, and most mutations are in codon 618. However, MEN2b is associated with mutations in codon 918 (Met→Thr) of the intracellular tyrosine kinase domain in 95% of patients. Interestingly, the *c-ret* proto-oncogene also is involved in the aetiology of papillary thyroid carcinomas and in Hirschsprung's disease.[4] Mutational analysis of *c-ret* to detect mutations in codons 609, 611, 618, 620, 634, 768 and 804 in MEN2a and MTC-only and in codon 918 in MEN2b has been used in the diagnosis and management of patients and families with these disorders. Such testing quickly and reliably identifies the 50% of family members who do not have the mutation and who therefore do not have to undergo further screening. For family members who have inherited the mutation and are at high risk of developing tumours, two clinical approaches exist.[4] In one approach, continued testing of calcitonin release after stimulation with pentagastrin is recommended, with total thyroidectomy being reserved until an abnormal pentagastrin test is seen. This usually delays total thyroidectomy until 10–13 years of age. In the alternative approach, a total thyroidectomy is recommended, on the sole basis of the abnormal genetic test, at the age of five years; this is the earliest age at which metastasis in MEN2a has been identified. In MEN2b, metastasis at two years of age has been reported, and total thyroidectomy at an earlier age has been recommended.[4] The advantages of this approach are that pentagastrin testing is avoided and a cure is more likely to be achieved before micrometastases develop. The management of affected families is complicated and requires careful coordination between the medical team (endocrinologists, geneticists, surgeons and general practitioners) and family.

☐ HYPERPARATHYROIDISM–JAW TUMOUR SYNDROME

Clinical features

Hyperparathyroidism–jaw tumour (HPT-JT) syndrome is an autosomal dominant disorder characterised by the development of parathyroid tumours and fibro-osseous jaw tumours.[5] In addition, some patients also may develop Wilms' tumours, renal cysts, renal hamartomas, renal cortical adenomas, papillary renal cell carcinomas, pancreatic adenocarcinomas, uterine tumours, testicular mixed germ cell tumours with a major seminoma component and Hurthle cell thyroid adenomas.[5] It is important to note that parathyroid tumours may occur in isolation and without any evidence of jaw tumours, and this may cause confusion with other hereditary hypercalcaemic disorders such as MEN1, familial benign hypercalcaemia, which is also referred to as familial hypocalciuric hypercalcaemia, and familial isolated primary hyperparathyroidism (see below). Hyperparathyroidism–jaw tumour syndrome can be distinguished from familial benign hypercalcaemia, because levels of calcium in serum in familial benign hypercalcaemia are increased from the early neonatal or infantile period, whereas such elevations in HPT-JT are uncommon in the first decade of life. In addition, patients with HPT-JT, unlike those with familial benign hypercalcaemia, will have associated hypercalciuria. The distinction between patients with HPT-JT and those with MEN1 who have only developed the usual first manifestation of hypercalcaemia (>90% of patients) is more difficult and is likely to be influenced by the operative and histological findings and the occurrence of other characteristic lesions in each disorder. It is important to note that patients with HPT-JT usually will have single adenomas or a carcinoma, while patients with MEN1 often will have multiglandular and hyperplastic parathyroid disease. The distinction between familial isolated primary hyperparathyroidism (see below) and HPT-JT in the absence of jaw tumours is difficult but important, because patients with HPT-JT may be at a higher risk of developing parathyroid carcinomas. These distinctions may be helped by the identification of additional features, and a search for jaw tumours and renal, pancreatic, thyroid and testicular abnormalities may help to identify patients with HPT-JT. The jaw tumours in HPT-JT are different to the brown tumours seen in some patients with primary hyperparathyroidism and do not resolve after parathyroidectomy. Indeed, ossifying fibromas of the jaw are an important feature that distinguishes HPT-JT from familial isolated primary hyperparathyroidism, and the occurrence of these occasionally may precede the development of hypercalcaemia in patients with HPT-JT by several decades.

Genetics

The gene that causes causing HPT-JT is located on chromosome 1q31.2 and encodes a protein that contains 531 amino acids,[5] PARAFIBROMIN, whose normal function remains to be elucidated.

☐ FAMILIAL ISOLATED PRIMARY HYPERPARATHYROIDISM

Clinical features

Primary hyperparathyroidism (HPT), which may result from parathyroid adenomas, hyperplasia or carcinoma, affects three in 1,000 adults and most frequently is encountered as a non-familial disorder.[3] However, about 10% of patients with primary HPT will have a hereditary form that may be part of the MEN1 or MEN2 syndromes or part of the HPT-JT syndrome (see above). In addition, hereditary primary HPT may develop as a solitary endocrinopathy, and this has also been referred to as familial isolated HPT (FIHP).

Genetics

Investigations of the hereditary and sporadic forms of primary HPT have helped to identify some of the genes and chromosomal regions involved in the aetiology of parathyroid tumours (see Table 2). Familial isolated primary hyperparathyroidism has been reported in several kindreds, and some have been shown to harbour mutations of the MEN1 or HPT-JT genes.[3,5]

☐ FAMILIAL BENIGN HYPERCALCAEMIA AND NEONATAL PRIMARY HYPERPARATHYROIDISM

Clinical features

Familial benign hypercalcaemia (FBH), which also is referred to as familial hypocalciuric hypercalcaemia (FHH), is an autosomal dominant disorder with a high degree of penetrance. It is characterised by lifelong asymptomatic hypercalcaemia in association with inappropriately low urinary calcium excretion (calcium clearance:creatinine clearance ratio <0.01).[6] A normal circulating concentration of parathyroid hormone (PTH) and mild hypermagnesaemia also typically are present. Although most patients with FBH are asymptomatic, chondrocalcinosis and acute pancreatitis occasionally have been seen in some patients. In addition, children of consanguineous marriages within FBH kindreds have been seen to have life-threatening hypercalcaemia as a result of neonatal primary hyperparathyroidism (NHPT) – symptomatic hypercalcaemia with skeletal manifestations of hyperparathyroidism in the first six months of life.[6] Children with NHPT often present in the first few days or weeks of life with failure to thrive, dehydration, hypotonia, constipation, ribcage deformities and multiple fractures as a result of bony undermineralisation. Children with NHPT often need urgent parathyroidectomy, which corrects the PTH-dependent hypercalcaemia and bone demineralisation.

The clinical importance of FBH lies in its differentiation from forms of primary hyperparathyroidism (see above), and 10% of patients in whom hypercalcaemia failed to respond to parathyroid surgery have been reported as having FBH. The diagnosis of FBH relies on the interpretation of urinary calcium clearance to creatinine clearance ratios (<0.01), together with a family history of hypercalcaemia and failed parathyroid surgery and identification of a mutation in the calcium-sensing receptor (CaSR). DNA diagnostic testing for CaSR mutations is now available (Oxford Genetics Department, address as above).

Genetics

Familial benign hypercalcaemia is the result of heterozygous inactivating mutations of CaSR, and NHPT often is associated with inactivating homozygous mutations of CaSR. However, NHPT also has been seen in children with only one parent with clinically apparent FBH, and many other cases of NHPT seem to be sporadic – that is, with both parents being normocalcaemic. In such patients with NHPT and heterozygous mutations of CaSR, the mutant CaSR may exert a dominant negative action on the normal CaSR. The human CaSR is a cell-surface protein with 1,078 amino acids that is expressed in the parathyroid glands, thyroid cells and kidney and is a member of the family of G-protein-coupled receptors.[6] The CaSR gene is located on chromosome 3q21.1. In addition to the loss of function CaSR mutations that result in FBH and NHPT, gain of function CaSR mutations that result in autosomal dominant hypocalcaemia with hypercalciuria also have been reported.[6]

☐ VON HIPPEL–LINDAU DISEASE

Clinical features

Von Hippel–Lindau (VHL) disease is an autosomal dominant disorder characterised by haemangioblastomas of the retina and central nervous system (CNS); cysts involving the kidneys, pancreas and epididymis; renal cell carcinomas; and phaeochromocytomas.[7] The retinal and CNS haemangioblastomas are benign vascular tumours that may be multiple and those in the CNS may cause symptoms by compression of adjacent structures and/or raised intracranial pressure. In the CNS, the cerebellum and spinal cord are the sites most frequently involved. The renal abnormalities consist of cysts and carcinomas, and it is important to note that the lifetime risk of a renal cell carcinoma in VHL is 70%. The endocrine tumours in VHL consist of phaeochromocytomas and pancreatic islet cell tumours. The clinical presentation of phaechromocytoma in VHL disease is similar to that in sporadic cases, except that the frequency of bilateral or multiple tumours, which may involve extra-adrenal sites, is higher in VHL disease. The most frequent pancreatic lesions in VHL disease are multiple cystadenomas, which rarely cause clinical disease. However, non-secreting pancreatic islet cell tumours occur in <10% of patients with VHL, who usually are asymptomatic, and the presence of the pancreatic tumour in these patients often is detected by regular screening with abdominal imaging. The pancreatic islet cell tumours frequently become malignant, so early surgery has been recommended.[7]

Genetics

The VHL gene, which is located on chromosome 3p26-p25, is expressed widely in human tissues and encodes a protein with 213 amino acids (pVHL). A wide variety of germline VHL mutations have been identified, and an analysis of the tumours indicates that VHL acts as a tumour suppressor gene.[7] A correlation seems to exist between the type of mutation and the phenotype, in that large deletions and protein-truncating mutations are associated with a low incidence of phaeochromocytomas, whereas some missense mutations in patients with VHL are associated with phaeochromocytoma (referred to as VHL type 2C). However, other missense mutations may be associated with haemangioblastomas and renal cell carcinomas but not phaeochromocytoma (referred to as VHL type 1), while other missense mutations are associated with haemanglioblastomas, renal cell carcinomas and phaeochromocytoma (VHL type 2B). The variant VLH type 2A, which refers to the occurrence of haemanglioblastomas and phaeochromocytoma without renal cell carcinomas, is associated with some rare missense mutations.[7] The basis for this complex genotype–phenotype relation remains to be elucidated. The functions of pVHL, which is also referred to as elongin, are being investigated; one major function is to downregulate the expression of vascular endothelial growth factor (VEGF) and other hypoxia-inducible mRNAs. Thus, pVHL in complex with other proteins regulates the expression of hypoxia-inducible factors (HIF-1 and HIF-2), such that loss of functional pVHL leads to a stabilisation of the HIF protein complexes, which results in overexpression of VEGF and tumour angiogenesis.

☐ NEUROFIBROMATOSIS

Clinical features

Neurofibromatosis type 1 (NF1), which is also referred to as von Recklinghausen's disease, is an autosomal dominant disorder characterised by the following manifestations:[8]

☐ neurological (eg peripheral and spinal neurofibromas)

☐ ophthalmological (eg optic gliomas and iris hamartomas such as Lisch nodules)

☐ dermatologial (eg café au lait macules)

☐ skeletal (eg scoliosis, macrocephaly, short stature and pseudoarthorosis)

☐ vascular (eg stenoses of renal and intracranial arteries)

☐ endocrine (eg phaeochromocytoma, carcinoid tumours and precocious puberty).

Neurofibromatosis type 2 (NF2) is also an autosomal dominant disorder but is characterised by the development of bilateral vestibular Schwannomas (acoustic neuromas) that lead to deafness, tinnitus or vertigo. Some patients with NF2 also develop meningiomas, spinal Schwannomas, peripheral nerve neurofibromas and café au lait macules.

Endocrine abnormalities are not found in NF2 and are associated solely with NF1. Thus, phaeochromocytomas, carcinoid tumours and precocious puberty occur in about 1% of patients with NF1, and growth hormone deficiency also has been reported occasionally. The features of phaeochromocytomas in patients with NF1 are similar to those in patients without the condition, with 90% of tumours located within the adrenal medulla and the remaining 10% at an extra-adrenal location, which often involves the para-aortic region.[8] Primary carcinoid tumours often are periampullary and also may occur in the ileum but rarely in the pancreas, thyroid or lungs. Hepatic metastases are associated with symptoms of the carcinoid syndrome, which include flushing, diarrhoea, broncho-constriction and tricuspid valve disease. Precocious puberty usually is associated with the extension of an optic glioma into the hypothalamus, with resultant increases in levels of gonadotrophins, but it also may arise rarely in the absence of chiasmal or hypothalamic involvement. Growth hormone deficiency also has been seen in some patients with NF1, who may or may not have optic chiasamal gliomas, but it is important to note that short stature in the absence of growth hormone deficiency is frequent in patients with NF1.

Genetics

The NF1 gene, which is located on chromosome 17q11.2 and acts as a tumour suppressor, consists of 60 exons that span more than 350 Kb of genomic DNA.[8] Mutations in NF1 are of diverse types and are scattered throughout the exons, thus making it difficult to implement mutational analysis in the clinical setting. The NF1 gene product is the protein neurofibromin, which has homologies to the p120GAP (GTPase activating protein), and it acts on p21ras by converting the active guanosine triphosphate bound form to its inactive guanosine diphosphate form. This down-regulates the p21ras signalling pathways, which, in turn, results in abnormal cell proliferation.[8]

☐ PHAEOCHROMOCYTOMAS AND PARAGANGLIOMA

Phaeochromocytomas occur as a part of several autosomal dominant syndromes that include MEN2, VHL and NF1 (see above). The same genes that cause these disorders, together with those that encode subunits B, C and D of succinate dehydrogenase (SDHB, SDHC and SDHD), frequently are involved in non-familial (that is, sporadic) forms of phaeochromocytomas and paragangliomas.[9] Thus, 24% of patients with sporadic phaeochromocytomas and paragangliomas were found to have germline mutations of VHL, RET, SDHB, SDHC and SDHD.

☐ CARNEY COMPLEX

Clinical features

Carney complex (CNC) is an autosomal dominant disorder characterised by spotty skin pigmentation (usually of the face, labia and conjunctiva), myxomas (usually of the eyelids and heart but also the tongue, palate, breast and skin), psammonatous melanotic schwannomas (usually of the sympathetic nerve chain and upper gastrointestinal tract) and endocrine tumours that involve the adrenals, Sertoli cells, somatotrophs, thyroid and ovary.[10]

Cushing's syndrome, the result of primary pigmented nodular adrenal disease (PPNAD), is the most common endocrine manifestation of CNC and may occur in one-third of patients. Patients with CNC and Cushing's syndrome often have an atypical appearance in being thin (as opposed to having truncal obesity). In addition, they may have short stature, muscle and skin wasting and osteoporosis. It is important to note that these patients may not have markedly increased levels of free cortisols in the urine but levels that are normal or increased only marginally. This pattern of normal cortisol production may be replaced periodically by days or weeks of hypercortisolism, however, and this variant is referred to as 'periodic Cushing's syndrome'. Patients with CNC and Cushing's syndrome usually have loss of the circadian rhythm of cortisol production.

Acromegaly, the result of a marco-somatotrophinoma, affects about 10% of patients with CNC. This may be detected early, through increases in 24-hour secretion of growth hormone.

Testicular tumours also may occur in one-third of patients with CNC. These may be large cell-calcifying Sertoli cell tumours, adrenocortical rests, or Leydig cell tumours. The large cell-calcifying Sertoli cell tumours occasionally may be oestrogen secreting and lead to precocious puberty or gynaecomastia. Some patients with CNC have been reported to develop thyroid follicular tumours, ovarian cysts and breast duct adenomas.

Genetics

Carney complex may be caused by one of two genes that have been mapped to chromosomes 2p16 and 17q22-q23. The CNC gene located on chromosome 17q22-q23, which is a tumour suppressor, has been identified to encode the protein kinase A (PKA) regulatory subunit 1 a(R1a) and is referred to as PPKARIA.[10] Germline mutations that would result in premature terminations, and hence truncated PPKARIA, have been identified in CNC kindreds, and an analysis of PKA activity in tumours has shown decreased basal activity. The CNC gene on chromosome 2p16 has not been identified yet, but it is interesting to note that some tumours do not show loss of heterozygosity of 2p16 but instead show genomic instability, which suggests that this CNC gene may not be a tumour suppressor.[10]

☐ COWDEN SYNDROME

Clinical features

Multiple hamartomatous lesions, especially of the skin, mucous membranes (eg buccal, intestinal and colonic), breast and thyroid, are characteristic of Cowden syndrome, which is an autosomal dominant disorder.[11] Thyroid abnormalities occur in two-thirds of patients with Cowden syndrome, and these usually consist of multinodular goitres or benign adenomas, although <10% of patients may have a follicular thyroid carcinoma. Breast abnormalities occur in >75% of patients and consist of fibrocystic disease or adenocarcinomas.

Genetics

The gene that causes Cowden syndrome is located on chromosome 10q23.3 and consists of nine exons that encode a protein of 403 amino acids referred to as PTEN (phosphate and tensin homologue deleted on chromosome ten).[11] This protein contains a thyrosine phosphatase domain that acts as a dual specificity phosphatase and, more specifically, as a lipid phosphatase. It may have roles in the apoptosis pathway and in cell migration and focal adhesion. Mutations that would lead to truncated, and hence inactive, forms of PTEN have been identified in kindreds with Cowden syndrome, and loss of heterozygosity has been detected in tumours, which suggests a role of PTEN as a tumour suppressor. One study indicates that the occurrences of malignant breast disease or multi-organ disease seem to correlate with two different mutations, but these preliminary observations need to be confirmed in a larger series.[11]

☐ OVARIAN CANCERS AND FAMILIAL BREAST–OVARIAN CANCER SYNDROME

Ovarian cancer affects >5% of women, and inherited mutations of the breast cancer genes (BRAC1 and BRAC2) and mismatch-repair genes (hMSH2 and hMLH1) are known to confer predisposition to ovarian cancer.[12] All of these genes have roles as tumour suppressors. The BRAC1 gene is considered to be involved in most families with breast–ovarian syndrome and in site-specific ovarian cancers. Approximately 5% of ovarian cancers that occur in women younger than 70 years are the result of germline mutations of BRAC1, which is located on chromosome 17q21. This gene encodes a 220-kDa protein that contains two zinc-finger DNA domains and localises to the nucleus, which suggests that it acts as a transcription factor.[12] The BRAC2 gene, which has only distant homology to BRAC1, is located on chromosome 13q13, and its function remains to be elucidated. The hMSH2 and hMLH1 genes, which are human homologues of the bacterial mutS and mutL genes, respectively, are located on chromosomes 2p22-p21 and 3p23-p22. These genes are involved in DNA repair mechanisms. One recent study that looked for germline mutations of BRAC1, BRAC2, hMSH2 and hMLH1 in women younger than 30 years with epithelial ovarian cancers found that only 2% of these cancers harboured a mutation in hMLH1, and none of the cancers had mutations of BRAC1, BRAC2 or hMSH2.[12] Thus, although BRAC1 mutations confer a high risk of breast and ovarian cancer in kindreds with familial breast–ovarian cancer syndrome, the roles of BRAC1, together with that of BRAC2, hMSH2 and hMLH1 and other genes, in the aetiology of other forms of ovarian cancers remain to be defined.

☐ ACKNOWLEDGEMENTS

I am grateful to the Medical Research Council (UK) for support and to Mrs Tracey Walker for expert secretarial assistance.

REFERENCES

1   Monson JP. The epidemiology of endocrine tumours. *Endocr Relat Cancer* 2000;7:29–36.

2   Thakker RV. Multiple endocrine neoplasia – syndromes of the twentieth century. *J Clin Endocrinol Metab* 1998;**83**:2617–20.

3   Thakker RV. Multiple endocrine neoplasia type 1. In: DeGroot LJ, Jameson JL (eds), *Endocrinology*. Philadelphia: WB Saunders, 2001:2503–17.

4   Gagel RF. Multiple endocrine neoplasia type 2. In: DeGroot LJ, Jameson JL (eds), *Endocrinology*. Philadelphia: WB Saunders, 2001: 2518–32.

5   Bradley KJ, Hobbs MR, Buley ID, Carpten JD *et al*. Uterine tumours are a phenotypic manifestation of the hyperparathyroidism-jaw tumour syndrome. *J Intern Med* 2005;**257**: 18–26.

6   Thakker RV. Diseases associated with the extracellular calcium-sensing receptor. *Cell Calcium* 2004;**35**:275–82.

7   Maher ER, Kaelin NG. Von Hippel-Lindau disease. *Medicine* 1997:76:381–91.

8   Huson SM. Neurofibromatosis 1: a clinical and genetic overview. In: Huson SM, Hughes RAC (eds), *The neurofibromatoses. A pathogenetic and clinical overview*. London: Chapman and Hall 1994: 160–203.

9   Neumann HP, Bausch B, McWhinney SR, Bender BU *et al*. Germ-line mutations in nonsyndromic phaeochromocytoma. *N Engl J Med* 2002;**346**:1459–66.

10 Kirscher LS, Carney IA, Pack SD, Taymans SE *et al*. Mutations of the gene encoding the protein kinase A type 1 a regulatory subunit in patients with the Carney Complex. *Nature Genetics* 2000:**26**:89–92.

11 Liaw D, Marsh DJ, Li J, Dahia PL *et al*. Germline mutations of the PTEN gene in Cowden disease, an inherited breast and thyroid cancer syndrome. *Nature Genetics* 1997:**16**:64–7.

12 Ford D, Easton DF. The genetics of breast and ovarian cancer. *Br J Cancer* 1995;**72**:805–12.

Molecular genetics goes to the diabetic clinic

Andrew T Hattersley

☐ INTRODUCTION

Diabetes has historically been thought of as a medical specialty which primarily deals with treatment rather than diagnosis. Molecular genetic testing can now be used to make a diagnosis of the 1–2% of all diabetic patients with monogenic diabetes. Making a diagnosis of monogenic diabetes is important as it can have a dramatic effect on the treatment a patient should receive: glucokinase MODY patients need no treatment; HNF1α MODY patients are very sensitive to low dose sulphonylureas; and patients with neonatal diabetes due to Kir6.2 mutations, despite being insulin dependent, can discontinue insulin and be well controlled on high dose sulphonylurea tablets. The challenge for diabetologists is to use clinical skills to detect these monogenic patients whose care will be greatly helped by the treatment changes that follow molecular genetic testing.

☐ DIAGNOSTIC DILEMMAS IN THE YOUNG ADULT WITH DIABETES

Diabetes has historically been thought of as a medical specialty which primarily deals with treatment rather than diagnosis. A diagnosis of diabetes is simply made by assessing if the patient has glycaemia levels above agreed standards defined by association with diabetes-specific complications in epidemiological studies. Subsequent division into the two largest diagnostic categories, type 1 and type 2, is usually made on the basis of simple clinical criteria such as age of onset, whether the patient is obese and the presence of ketoacidosis. Into which of these two categories a young adult is classified will make a fundamental difference to their management as they will either be treated with diet and exercise and then go on to metformin or they will immediately start on insulin. Despite the clear different therapeutic outcomes, there are limited clinical guidelines on how to diagnose these two major subgroups or how to recognise patients who have neither type 1 nor type 2 diabetes but have a defined genetic aetiology.

☐ MOLECULAR GENETICS AS A DIAGNOSTIC TEST IN DIABETES

Is there any role for molecular genetics in the difficult decisions about classification and treatment of children and young adults diagnosed with diabetes? Considerable advances have been made in our understanding of the genetics of type 1 and type 2 diabetes, but gene variants only *predispose* to these polygenic conditions and cannot be used in diagnostic testing. In contrast, in monogenic diabetes a mutation in a single gene *causes* diabetes, so genetic testing can potentially have an important role in the diagnosis. In these conditions a single base change often results in the diabetes phenotype, so it is possible to make a specific diagnosis by sequencing. This becomes important if it helps explain associated clinical features, anticipate the patient's prognosis and alter treatment decisions (Fig 1). The emphasis in this article will be on how a molecular genetic diagnosis can influence treatment decisions in maturity-onset diabetes of the young (MODY) and neonatal diabetes.

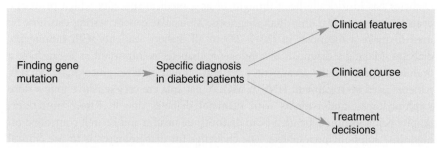

Fig 1 Finding a gene mutation can make a diagnosis of monogenic diabetes, with implications for clinical features, prognosis and treatment.

☐ MATURITY-ONSET DIABETES OF THE YOUNG: MOVING FROM CLINICAL DIAGNOSIS TO MOLECULAR CLASSIFICATION

With the advances in the last two decades in molecular genetic methodology it has been possible to define the underlying gene or genes in most clinically recognised subgroups of monogenic diabetes. In many cases this has altered the understanding of a clinically defined condition. One of the clearest and commonest examples is MODY, first recognised by Tattersall in 1974 as autosomal, dominantly inherited beta cell dysfunction resulting in early-onset, non-insulin dependent diabetes, typically before the age of 25.[1] Six different genes have now been identified:

- ☐ glycolytic enzyme glucokinase, and

- ☐ beta cell transcription factors: hepatic nuclear factor (HNF)1α, HNF4α, HNF1β, insulin promoter factor 1, and NeuroD1.[2,3]

There are marked differences between the diabetes caused by the different genes, but it was not recognised that there were discrete clinical entities until the genes were defined.[2,4] Patients with glucokinase mutations have mild fasting hyperglycaemia from birth; this deteriorates very little with age, pharmacological treatment is rarely required and it is only occasionally associated with microvascular complications (Fig 2).[4]

In contrast, patients with transcription factor mutations (most commonly HNF1α) are born normoglycaemic. There is then progressive hyperglycaemia – which results in diabetes being diagnosed in adolescence or young adult life –

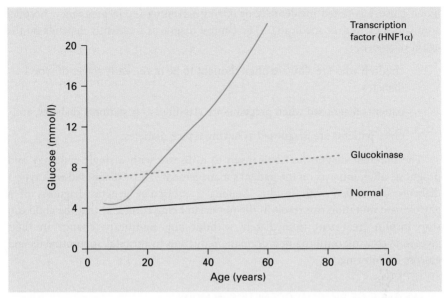

Fig 2 Diagram showing the variation of fasting glucose with age in normals and patients with glucokinase and transcription factor (usually hepatic nuclear factor (HNF)1α mutations.

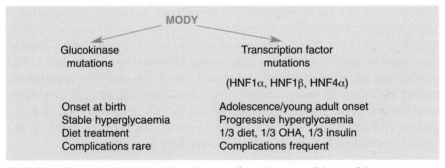

Fig 3 Clinical features of the two major subgroups of maturity onset diabetes of the young (MODY) (OHA = oral hypoglycaemic agent).

continuing thereafter to become more markedly severe (Fig 2).[4] Almost all patients will require pharmacological treatment. If hyperglycaemia is not adequately treated, complications are frequent.

The features of the two main subgroups of MODY are as marked as the differences between type 1 and type 2 diabetes (Fig 3).

☐ MAKING A MOLECULAR GENETIC DIAGNOSIS OF A GLUCOKINASE MUTATION
   CAN ALLOW TREATMENT TO BE DISCONTINUED

The stable, mild fasting hyperglycaemia in patients with glucokinase mutations rarely results in osmotic symptoms. These patients typically present when their blood glucose is tested incidentally or during screening (eg in pregnancy, hospital admissions or routine medicals).[5] The clinical diagnosis frequently depends on the age at diagnosis:

☐ children who are slim are often thought to be in the early stages of type 1 diabetes

☐ patients diagnosed when pregnant are classified as gestational diabetes, and

☐ older patients are diagnosed as having type 2 diabetes.

The different diagnostic labels given to a disease with a single aetiology and prognosis often impacts on the patient's management. Those diagnosed with type 1 diabetes are treated with insulin. Making a molecular genetic diagnosis of a glucokinase mutation can result in the physician being confident that the child can stop insulin treatment immediately without any significant change in their glycaemic control, resulting in a dramatic reduction in hospital appointments and glucose monitoring.

☐ EVIDENCE OF PHARMACOGENETICS IN MODY

HNF1α MODY is the most common form of monogenic diabetes and one of the commonest monogenic disorders, with over 20,000 people affected in the UK. Depending on the age of diagnosis, the subjects are frequently misdiagnosed as type 1 or type 2 diabetes. This is because it is uncommon to perform confirmatory tests for type 1 or type 2 diabetes (beta cell autoantibodies and C-peptide measurement) and the significance of the strong autosomal dominant family history is often not appreciated. It could be argued that if the patient is appropriately treated, the failure to make a diagnosis is only of academic interest. This clearly would be true if the patients responded to oral therapy in a similar way to type 2 patients and if glycaemic control achieved on insulin was better or similar to that achieved on tablets. Recent work has questioned both these assumptions.

Sulphonylureas in HNF1α MODY

HNF1α MODY patients can be extremely sensitive to the hypoglycaemic effects of sulphonylureas given in standard doses.[6] Their glycaemic control can markedly deteriorate when they are switched from a sulphonylurea to an equivalent dose of metformin, only to improve again on reintroducing the sulphonylurea (Fig 4).[6] This is in marked contrast to type 2 diabetes where meta-analysis showed sulphonylureas and metformin have a similar hypoglycaemic effect.

In a recent randomised crossover study, HNF1α patients had a four-fold greater response to the sulphonylurea gliclazide than body mass index and glycaemia matched type 2 diabetes patients (Fig 5).[7] Physiological tests showed that this pharmacogenetic response was not due to altered drug metabolism but to greater insulin secretion in response to the drug, this effect being amplified by increased insulin sensitivity.[7] Animal and cellular models with reduced HNF1α levels suggest the defects in the beta cell are early in glucose metabolism before the sulphonylurea

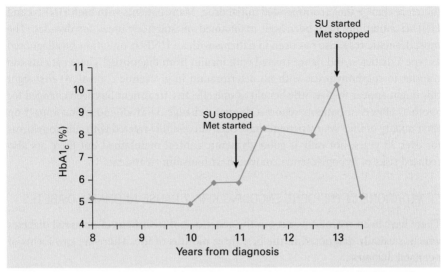

Fig 4 Sulphonylurea (SU) sensitivity in a patient with an hepatic nuclear factor (HNF)1a mutation shown by deterioration in glycosylated haemoglobin (HbA1$_c$) on stopping SUs and starting metformin (Met) and improvement of HbA1$_c$ on restarting SUs and discontinuing Met (adapted from Ref 6).

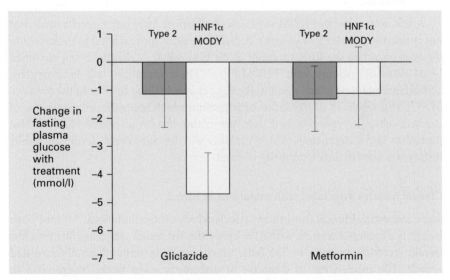

Fig 5 In a randomised crossover trial, hepatic nuclear factor (HNF)1α MODY patients had a four-fold greater fall in fasting glucose on gliclazide than body mass index and glycaemia matched type 2 patients (shown on the left), while the response to metformin was similar (shown on the right) (MODY = maturity-onset diabetes of the young) (adapted from Ref 7).

receptor in the K_{ATP} channel, explaining why the insulin secretion to sulphonylureas is relatively well preserved.[7]

This result has clear practical implications. Metformin has become the first-line pharmacological treatment for type 2 diabetes. Making a diagnosis of HNF1α will therefore change the recommended initial drug. Many patients with both HNF1α and HNF4α mutations have been well maintained on sulphonylureas for decades. The most dramatic response has been in patients with an HNF1α mutation misdiagnosed as type 1 diabetes, and hence treated with insulin from diagnosis.[8] These patients can transfer to sulphonylureas with no deterioration in glycaemic control. At first sight this might appear to give little benefit as one effective treatment has been changed for another. However, patients report a dramatic change, with an enormous impact on their quality of life.[9] Many patients have been successfully treated with sulphonylureas for over 25 years; not only is good glycaemic control maintained but there are also reduced risks of hypoglycaemia compared with insulin treatment.

☐ MUTATIONS IN THE GENE ENCODING KIR6.2 CAUSE NEONATAL DIABETES

There have been recent advances in the genetics and treatment of neonatal diabetes which is usually diagnosed in the first three months of life. There are two forms of neonatal diabetes:

- ☐ transient neonatal diabetes mellitus (TNDM) which resolves, usually within three months, and

- ☐ permanent neonatal diabetes mellitus (PNDM) which may require lifelong insulin.

A few rare causes of PNDM were described before 2004 but a genetic cause was not defined in over 90% of patients. A candidate gene approach led to mutations in the gene encoding the Kir6.2 subunit of the beta cell K_{ATP} channel being identified in 31–64% of patients with PNDM.[10,11,13] These mutations are heterozygous, activating mutations which result in the K_{ATP} channel failing to close in the presence of ATP. This results in a large influx of potassium which holds the cell membrane of the beta cell in a hyperpolarised state, preventing insulin secretion. Most of these mutations are spontaneous, which explains why an autosomal dominant family history was seen in only a minority of cases.

Clinical features associated with mutations in Kir6.2

Some interesting clinical features are associated with these mutations.[10,13] Low birth weight is a common feature, with 61% below the 3rd centile, reflecting the very low insulin secretion *in utero* by the fetus which results in reduced insulin-mediated growth. The median age of diagnosis of diabetes is seven weeks (range birth to six months). Most patients are markedly hyperglycaemic, some with ketoacidosis. Investigations and the insulin dose required are in keeping with no or minimal endogenous insulin secretion. These patients differ from type 1 diabetes in that pancreatic autoantibodies are not detectable and they are diagnosed before six months of age.

DEND syndrome

Although most patients with Kir6.2 mutations have isolated diabetes, some patients have multisystem disease, termed DEND syndrome (developmental delay, epilepsy and neonatal diabetes).[10,13] The developmental delay can be extremely severe, with patients unable to stand independently or speak even in early adulthood. Severe cases have generalised epilepsy diagnosed under the age of 12 months. These neurological features make the management of their diabetes with insulin extremely difficult. The pattern of disease is in keeping with the distribution of the Kir6.2 subunit of the K_{ATP} channel: as well as being present in the beta cells it is also in the brain, peripheral axons and skeletal muscle. Altered action at these sites is likely to be responsible for the neurological features.

Fortunately, the full DEND syndrome is relatively rare, but there is a more common, intermediate subgroup of patients with less severe developmental delay and neonatal diabetes but who do not have epilepsy.

Other mutations

Activating mutations do not always cause permanent neonatal diabetes. A minority of patients with mutations in the Kir6.2 gene have transient neonatal diabetes which resolves around the age of two years. Finally, a common polymorphism, E23K, present in approximately 40% of the population, predisposes to type 2 diabetes, increasing the risk by approximately 20%.

☐ FROM GENOTYPE TO FUNCTIONAL ABNORMALITY TO PHENOTYPE IN NEONATAL DIABETES

A striking feature is a strong genotype/phenotype relationship in Kir6.2: the vast majority of patients with mutations at R201 have isolated neonatal diabetes, whilst most patients with mutations at V59 have neurological features. Structural models show mutations at the R201 residue directly interfere with ATP binding to the Kir6.2 channel. The mutations that result in a more severe phenotype are in regions of the molecule involved in changing the conformation of the channel: the slide helix and the pore of the K_{ATP} channel. Functional studies show that the severity of the clinical phenotype is reflected in the functional changes seen in the mutated channel.[12] Therefore, the current remaining in the presence of ATP is reduced in all the disease associated mutations, but the severity of the reduction is less in TNDM than in PNDM which, in turn, is less than in DEND syndrome.[12,13] The clinical severity associated with most patients in Kir6.2 therefore directly reflects the functional severity of these mutations (Fig 6).

☐ FROM GENE TO TREATMENT IN NEONATAL DIABETES

Defining the genetic aetiology has the greatest impact if it improves treatment for patients. As soon as activating Kir6.2 mutations were found to cause PNDM, knowledge of the K_{ATP} channel suggested that sulphonylurea tablets might offer an alternative to insulin injections. Although mutations in the Kir6.2 subunit prevent an increase in ATP closing the K_{ATP} channel, sulphonylureas are known to be able to bind to the sulphonylurea receptor 1 (SUR1) subunit and close the K_{ATP} channel through

Type 2 diabetes	TNDM	PNDM alone	Intermediate DEND	DEND syndrome
			Clinical severity	
E23K	G53S G53R I182V	R201H Y330C Y330S R50Q R50P	V59M R201C	Q52R V59G C166Y C166F I296V
			Functional severity	

Fig 6 Clinical spectrum associated with specific Kir6.2 mutations and the polymorphisms (E23K) reflects the functional severity of the mutations *in vitro* (DEND syndrome = developmental delay, epilepsy and neonatal diabetes; PNDM = permanent neonatal diabetes mellitus; TNDM = transient neonatal diabetes mellitus).

an ATP independent route (Fig 7). Although patients with Kir6.2 mutations secrete no insulin in response to intravenous (iv) glucose, physiological tests show that they have good insulin secretion in response to iv tolbutamide.[10] This led to testing whether patients could transfer from insulin to sulphonylurea tablets. High doses of glibenclamide or other sulphonylureas enabled most patients to discontinue insulin completely and to show improved glycaemic control (Fig 8).[11,13] This is the first time that insulin-dependent patients have been able to be effectively treated with tablets.

Do the neurological features resulting from K_{ATP} channel activation also improve with sulphonylureas? Glibenclamide binds to both SUR1 and SUR2, so it should act

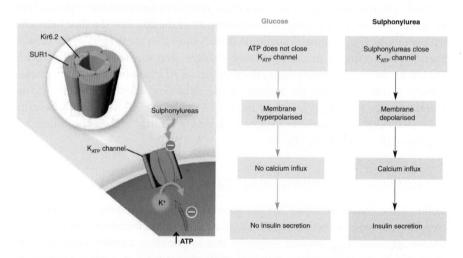

Fig 7 Diagram showing that patients with a mutation in Kir6.2 cannot close the K_{ATP} channel and hence secrete insulin in the presence of increased ATP, but can secrete insulin when the channel is closed independently of ATP by sulphonylureas (adapted from Ref 10).

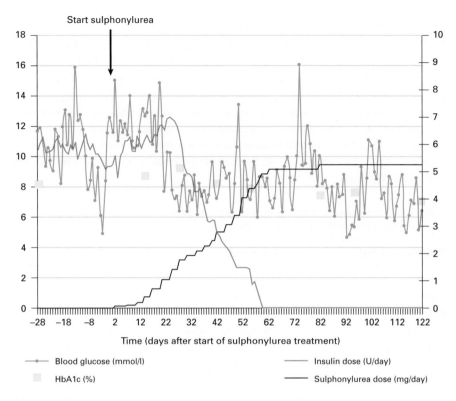

Fig 8 Sulphonylurea treatment in an apparently insulin-dependent infant with permanent neonatal diabetes mellitus (PNDM) caused by a mutation in Kir6.2, showing measurements of capillary blood glucose (mean of 4–6 daily measurements) (blue), glycosylated haemoglobin (HbA$_{1c}$) (green), administered dose of sulphonylurea (red) and insulin requirement (orange). The arrow indicates initiation of oral sulphonylurea (glibenclamide). The dose was increased every three days, with a parallel reduction in the insulin dose according to capillary glucose measurements made at home. As revealed by HbA$_{1c}$ measurements, the metabolic control did not deteriorate after insulin was discontinued. Reproduced from Ref 11 with permission of the American Diabetes Association.

in nerve, muscle and brain, but to act in most of the brain it would need to cross the blood–brain barrier which is uncertain in man. *In vitro* tests suggest that mutations associated with DEND syndrome respond poorly to sulphonylureas compared with mutations associated with isolated diabetes.[12] In keeping with this, three patients with the full set of DEND syndrome features were unable to discontinue insulin. However, most patients with mild developmental delay and diabetes associated with the V59M mutation not only discontinued insulin with glibenclamide but also showed improved muscle strength, concentration and speech. In some cases the change was dramatic: a two-year old patient, who was unable to stand unaided, was able to walk without help within days of starting sulphonylurea treatment. It is hard to prove causality in these cases, especially as the children and their parents were reluctant to return to insulin, but the timing certainly suggests that neurological features improve with sulphonylureas.

☐ CONCLUSIONS

We have shown that making a diagnosis of monogenic diabetes is important as it can have a dramatic effect on the treatment a patient should receive (Table 1). These patients are seen not infrequently: although they represent only 1–2% of all diabetic patients, 20–40,000 people have monogenic diabetes in the UK. The recognition of these patients will remain a clinical skill, with molecular genetic testing confirming the diagnosis. As technological advances continue in molecular genetics, the price of testing is likely to fall and it will become more widely used. It is important that, while numbers of patients are limited, we learn the appropriate use of molecular genetics in the diabetic clinic.

Table 1 Making a diagnosis of genetic diabetes alters treatment in diabetes: the initial pharmacological treatment in the different subgroups.

Diabetes aetiology	Treatment
Type 1	Insulin
Type 2	Metformin
MODY GCK	None
MODY HNF1α	Low-dose silphonylurea
Neonatal Kir6.2	High-dose sulphonylurea

GCK = glucokinase; HNF = hepatic nuclear factor; SU = sulphonylurea.

☐ ACKNOWLEDGEMENTS

I would like to thank all my colleagues in the Peninsula Medical School, Exeter, who have contributed to the work and ideas in this article, and to Diabetes UK and the Wellcome Trust, the principal funders of our work.

REFERENCES

1 Tattersall RB. Mild familial diabetes with dominant inheritance. *Q J Med* 1974;**43**:339–57.

2 Stride A, Hattersley AT. Different genes, different diabetes: lessons from maturity-onset diabetes of the young. Review. *Ann Med* 2002;**34**:207–16.

3 Fajans SS, Bell GI, Polonsky KS. Molecular mechanisms and clinical pathophysiology of maturity-onset diabetes of the young. Review. *N Engl J Med* 2001;**345**:971–80.

4 Stride A, Vaxillaire M, Tuomi T, Barbetti F *et al.* The genetic abnormality in the beta cell determines the response to an oral glucose load. *Diabetologia* 2002;**45**:427–35.

5 Page RC, Hattersley AT, Levy JC, Barrow B *et al.* Clinical characteristics of subjects with a missense mutation in glucokinase. *Diabet Med* 1995;**12**:209–17.

6 Pearson ER, Liddell WG, Shepherd M, Corrall RJ, Hattersley AT. Sensitivity to sulphonylureas in patients with hepatocyte nuclear factor-1 alpha gene mutations: evidence for pharmacogenetics in diabetes. *Diabet Med* 2000;**17**:543–5.

7 Pearson ER, Starkey BJ, Powell RJ, Gribble FM *et al.* Genetic cause of hyperglycaemia and response to treatment in diabetes. *Lancet* 2003;**362**:1275–81.

8 Shepherd M, Pearson ER, Houghton J, Salt G *et al.* No deterioration in glycemic control in HNF-1alpha maturity-onset diabetes of the young following transfer from long-term insulin to sulphonylureas. *Diabetes Care* 2003;**26**:3191–2.

9   Shepherd M, Hattersley AT. 'I don't feel like a diabetic any more': the impact of stopping insulin in patients with maturity onset diabetes of the young following genetic testing. *Clin Med* 2004;**4**:144–7.

10 Gloyn AL, Pearson ER, Antcliff JF, Proks P *et al.* Activating mutations in the gene encoding the ATP-sensitive potassium-channel subunit Kir6.2 and permanent neonatal diabetes. *N Engl J Med* 2004;**350**:1838–49.

11 Sagen JV, Raeder H, Hathout E, Shehadeh N *et al.* Permanent neonatal diabetes due to mutations in KCNJ11 encoding Kir6.2: patient characteristics and initial response to sulfonylurea therapy. *Diabetes* 2004;**53**:2713–8.

12 Proks P, Antcliff JF, Lippiat J, Gloyn AL *et al.* Molecular basis of Kir6.2 mutations associated with neonatal diabetes or neonatal diabetes plus neurological features. *Proc Natl Acad Sci USA* 2004;**101**:17539–44.

13 Hattersley AT, Ashcroft FM. Activating mutations in Kir6.2 and neonated diabetes: new clinical syndromes, new scientific insights, and new therapy. *Diabetes* 2005;**54**:2503–13.

☐ ENDOCRINOLOGY SELF ASSESSMENT QUESTIONS

Vitamin D deficiency

1 In the regulation of calcium and phosphate balance:
   (a) Vitamin D increases intestinal calcium and phosphate absorption
   (b) Vitamin D decreases calcium and phosphate absorption from bone
   (c) Vitamin D inhibits synthesis and secretion of parathyroid hormone
   (d) Parathyroid hormone decreases renal phosphate excretion
   (e) Parathyroid hormone reduces conversion of 25(OH)-vitamin D to
       1α,25-dihydroxyvitamin D

2 In the synthesis of vitamin D, the 1α-hydroxylation step:
   (a) Occurs in the liver
   (b) Is performed by a member of the cytochrome P450 enzyme pathway
   (c) Can occur in bone and cartilage
   (d) Results in the biologically inactive form of vitamin D
   (e) Is inhibited by calcium

3 Vitamin D deficiency:
   (a) Is more common in countries in southern latitudes
   (b) Is more common in housebound people because of their lack of
       absorption of ultraviolet A light
   (c) Is a risk factor for hip fracture in older people
   (d) Is rare in people with dark skin pigmentation
   (e) May result from inadequate dietary intake

4 Measurement of 25-hydroxy vitamin D (25(OH)D):
   (a) May be performed with radioimmunoassays
   (b) Is highly complicated, requiring specific handling
   (c) May display seasonal variations in results
   (d) Is well standardised between laboratories
   (e) May differ between ethnic groups

5 When considering interactions between vitamin D and parathyroid hormone:
   (a) Vitamin D deficiency may result in secondary hyperparathyroidism.
   (b) In primary hyperparathyroidism, coexistent vitamin D deficiency may
       worsen bone disease.
   (c) It is useful to measure parathyroid hormone in the context of a low
       normal level of vitamin D
   (d) In primary hyperparathyroidism, coexistent vitamin D deficiency is an
       indication for early surgical intervention.
   (e) In patients with coexistent vitamin D deficiency and primary
       hyperparathyroidism, treatment with long-acting vitamin D analogues is
       indicated

Genetics of endocrine cancer syndromes

1   A patient with multiple endocrine neoplasia type 1 is at a higher risk of
developing tumours of the:
   (a) Adrenal medulla
   (b) Pancreatic exocrine cells
   (c) Parathyroid glands
   (d) Posterior pituitary gland
   (e) Thyroid C cells

2   Regarding multiple endocrine neoplasia type 2:
   (a) Thyroid papillary tumours are found commonly
   (b) The three variants are caused by three different genes
   (c) Total thyroidectomy at the earliest opportunity is the treatment of choice
       for multiple endocrine neoplasia type 2b
   (d) Megacolon is a feature of multiple endocrine neoplasia type 2b
   (e) Genetic tests should be offered only to patients older than 20 years

3   Phaeochromocytomas are a recognised feature of:
   (a) Multiple endocrine neoplasia type 1
   (b) Multiple endocrine neoplasia type 2a
   (c) Von Hippel-Lindau disease
   (d) Neurofibromatosis type 1
   (e) Carney syndrome

Molecular genetics goes to the diabetic clinic

1   Patients with maturity-onset diabetes of the young (MODY) due to a mutation
in the transcription factor hepatic nuclear factor (HNF)–1α:
   (a) Usually have a parent diagnosed as having diabetes
   (b) Show mild lifelong hyperglycaemia which rarely requires pharmacological
       treatment
   (c) Show evidence of pharmacogenetics by being very sensitive to the
       hypoglycaemic effect of Metformin
   (d) Should not be treated with sulphonylureas due to their reduced hepatic
       function which means this drug may accumulate due to reduced hepatic
       metabolism.
   (e) Are frequently misdiagnosed as having type 1 diabetes

2   Patients who present with diabetes in the neonatal period:
   (a) May have normal glucose tolerance by the age of 12 weeks
   (b) May have epilepsy as a result of a mutation affecting the K_{ATP} channel in
       the brain
   (c) Can always discontinue insulin and be managed by diet within the first
       year of diagnosis
   (d) Will, in most cases have at least one diabetic parent
   (e) Are frequently diabetic as a result of exposure to maternal hyperglycaemia
       in utero

3   Insulin in treatment in patients with diabetes:
  (a) Indicates that the patient is insulin dependent and therefore will develop ketoacidosis if insulin is withdrawn
  (b) Is always needed for patients with glucokinase mutations
  (c) Can be replaced with sulphonylurea therapy in most patients with neonatal diabetes due to a Kir6.2 mutation
  (d) Is the treatment of choice for patients with type 1 diabetes
  (e) Can be replaced with sulphonylurea therapy for many patients with mutations in the MODY gene HNF1α

Transplantation

Update on organ donation

Michael Wilks

Although some success can be claimed in the creation of a significant but small increase in organ transplantation rates, the picture is far from good. Overall, the gap between the supply of organs from all sources and the demand, as measured by the size of the waiting list for donation, continues to increase. As at 31 December 2003, the combined active and suspended waiting list topped 7,000 patients, while the supply of organs from deceased donors decreased to below 700 – continuing a steady fall over the past few years. When the fact that a potential donor can provide life-saving or life-enhancing surgery for up to five recipients is remembered, this fall is alarming.

The single silver lining to this dark cloud is the increase in rates of live donation, which almost exclusively comprises live donations of kidneys. As a result, total transplantation rates remained static through the 1990s but recently showed a small rise. That this rise is almost entirely the result of increases in live donations – the rate of which has tripled in the past 10 years – suggests two main facts:

☐ The current reliance on heart-beating donors (from intensive care units) will, for reasons set out below, prove, in the medium term at least, to be misplaced.

☐ Dramatic increases in the rates of live donation will be the sole means of achieving a significant increase in overall transplant figures – although non-heart beating donors also should receive more attention as a source of organs.

What are the reasons behind such a dismal performance in relation to heart-beating donors? As most of these come from intensive care units, we need to examine the situation there first. The problems at the level of the intensive care unit are primarily the lack of adequate beds (particularly beds dedicated to continuing, as a priority, the ventilation of a potential donor) and also a very variable commitment on the part of teams in intensive care units to the principle of organ donation. Such variability is understandable in the face of the pressures of the work and the shortages of beds, but some of this is attitudinal and can be addressed.

More seriously, the level of refusal by relatives asked to sanction organ retrieval is a cause for major concern. An audit of 256 hospitals between April and June 2003 showed a 48% refusal rate among relatives who were asked specifically about organ donation. The reason for this is not clear – although it is tempting to blame the organ retention 'scandals' at Alder Hey and elsewhere, it is far from certain whether people, in fact, are confused about the difference between organ retention and organ donation. The answer may be more subtle – that the 'Alder Hey' effect makes families more respectful of their loved one's wishes. As most of us have neither obtained an organ donor card nor joined the organ donor register and as we are poor at discussing our wishes with people close to us, most families approached by doctors will simply not know what their now dead or dying relative wanted. In such a position, the default position will be to refuse.

This situation argues strongly for a change in the law in favour of a presumption of consent or willingness to donate. Although a change to presumed consent would not, and should not, take away the need to approach relatives, the character and content of an approach would change from one that asked permission to one that confirmed that there was no dissent. Obviously, in some circumstances it would not be appropriate to continue with a request in the face of hostility or distress, but these occasions should be relatively infrequent, as a national debate about the change in the law would have taken place. The British Medical Association and other bodies strongly support such a change, and it is disappointing that the government has failed to use the new Human Tissue Bill to enact it.

In the face of a seemingly intractable problem, what can be done to create a lasting and confident increase in the number of donors and the resulting transplant rate? A number of issues exist, and these cannot be separated out but need addressing as a 'package'. For instance, a presumed consent law would do little to improve organ donation without an increase in the number of transplant units in which the increased number of operations could be performed.

The first issue is a rights-based approach and a consideration of the rights of the sick. While not denying the mistakes that led to Alder Hey, and the anguish suffered by relatives, it is time to redress the balance in favour of the rights of those on the waiting list for an organ, while remaining sensitive to the views and feelings of families who lose relatives in traumatic ways. A presumed consent law recognises that balance and is well overdue.

Secondly, as the variable rates of donation from broadly similar intensive care units shows, communication and consent at the bedside can be improved greatly in the interests of family agreement. A wider issue of communication exists, as the spectacular success of the transplant programme in Spain shows. There, a crucial factor is the linking of potential donors and recipients through transplant coordinators who facilitate communication between intensive care units and transplants teams.

Thirdly, a major campaign of public information to increase the number of people who carry an organ donor card and are registered on the organ donor register is essential. This can be done more creatively, linking donation to driving licence renewals, the electoral register, reward cards and the like.

Fourthly, a stronger argument can be made for investment in the transplant programme on economic grounds. The current annual cost for haemodialysis is £35,000 and for peritoneal dialysis £20,000. A transplant operation costs £20,000, and the annual costs of immunosuppressant therapy would be around £6,500. Surgery therefore produces a small net economic benefit in the first year, followed by substantial benefits year on year. Enthusiasm for this superficially overwhelming case must be tempered by the fact that improving transplant activity will simply allow more people to be treated more quickly, but the case in humanitarian terms is unanswerable.

Fifthly, the case for a substantial investment, combined with a publicity programme to highlight its relatively low risk, should be made in relation to an intensive live donor programme for renal transplantation. From the evidence of the last few years, this would seem to be the only effective medium-term initiative that will narrow the gap between supply and demand. The Human Tissue Bill contains welcome provisions to help this process; it also paves the way for creating fewer barriers to non-heart beating donation, but the impact this element will have on overall rates remains less easy to predict.

The final issue is payment for organs. This is portrayed as a way in which sick but wealthy first-world citizens can buy organs from healthy but poor donors from the developing world. This is ethically unacceptable and exploitative. Whatever the arguments for or against this practice, as a solution it is unnecessary. What can, and what I suggest should, be considered is a controlled market in organs – within the National Health Service and with effective controls against abuse. Such a system currently is illegal and remains unaddressed in any serious way by the profession and by politicians. The well-rehearsed arguments against this practice melt away in the context of a controlled market, and the rights of those who are sick, as already highlighted, deserve more consideration.

It is quite correct to say, in this case, that desperate situations do not justify desperate remedies, but the situation is desperate – with one person on the waiting list for an organ dying every day for the lack of it. We should not rule out any effective and ethically robust method in the face of this level of mortality.

Use of adult stem cells to mitigate the effects of diabetes

Paul G Shiels

☐ INTRODUCTION

Worldwide, 150 million people have diabetes. Despite insulin therapy, late complications such as retinopathy, nephropathy and neuropathy are not uncommon. Transplantation of cadaveric islets offers one means of treating the problem of type 1 diabetes, although this is compromised through lack of available organs. Stem-cell therapies, however, offer a potential means to address this problem.[1,2] Although much published literature documents success in converting stem cells into insulin secreting, glucose-responsive cells, these need to be re-evaluated after reports that cells can adsorb insulin present in growth media.[3]

☐ STEM CELLS

Stem cells are unspecialised cells that have the capacity to proliferate for long periods in culture and that can be induced to become specialised cell types. They can be isolated primarily from embryos or adults, although stem cells from adults seem to have distinct characters and functions.

Stem cells have three general properties that distinguish them from other cells in the body; they are:

☐ unspecialised and do not have an apparent specific developmental function

☐ capable of self-proliferation for long periods in culture; unlike other primary cell types, which senesce, stem cells are able to renew themselves

☐ able to give rise to specialised cell types with specific functions (eg neurones, beta cells and cardiomyocytes).

☐ EMBRYONIC STEM CELLS

These cells typically are derived from the inner cell mass of the blastocyst of fertilised embryos. Their use has led to major moral and ethical debate about stem cells derived from human embryos.

No defined standard test exists to characterise cells unambiguously as embryonic stem cells (ESCs). The typical characterisation relies on a prolonged period of undifferentiated growth in culture and the expression of a marker called Oct 4 (a factor required for maintenance of self-renewal characteristics) in combination with a variety of cell-surface markers. This is correlated with karyotype analysis to ensure the gross genetic integrity of the cells and determination of whether the cells can be recultured after freeze/thaw cycling. Further correlates are the determination of pluripotency in vitro and the capacity to form teratomas after injection into an immunosuppressed mouse.

Directed differentiation of ESCs, grown in specific-culture media, can enrich for particular types of cells. Pure cell populations derived from this procedure are potential therapies for diabetes and Parkinson's disease; however, this has proved difficult to achieve in practice. Typically, such cell populations are heterogeneous but enriched for a particular cell type.

□ ADULT STEM CELLS

Adult stem cells (ASCs) are undifferentiated cells found among the differentiated cells of an adult tissue or organ. These are unspecialised and can renew themselves while maintaining a capacity to differentiate into the major cell types of the tissue or organ. The numbers of ASCs in any tissue seems limited, but they are believed to maintain and affect tissue repair. The origin of adult stem cells in mature tissues is unknown, and their degree of plasticity remains to be determined. Their use in transplantation is recognised widely: adult stem cells from bone marrow have been used in transplants for 30 years. The use of adult non-haematopoietic stem cells and their efficacy, plasticity and safety in long-term follow up remains unproven. Reports of non-stromal ASCs remain debated in the field, although neural stem cells now are established and accepted as a bone fide type of ASC.

Although the proven pluripotent character of ESCs and the ability to grow them in large numbers makes them attractive candidates for cell-based therapies, this is also a double-edged sword. Their potency and our inability to obtain pure cell populations for transplantation run the risk of neoplasias being generated. Adult stem cells thus are an attractive alternative. They can be derived from 'self', so any patient would receive their own cells and not have to suffer the deleterious side effects of immunosuppression to prevent rejection, including a significantly enhanced risk of cancer. Limited potency/plasticity also is considered to be an enhanced safety factor, in that aberrant cell differentiation would be limited and the risk of neoplasia reduced.

□ MAKING INSULIN-PRODUCING CELLS WITH STEM CELLS

One approach to facilitate the generation of beta cells has involved expansion and differentiation of adult human pancreatic progenitor cells, which are related closely with the beta cell lineage; this would avoid the controversy and technical problems associated with the use of pluripotent stem cells.[4] Evidence that such stem cells reside in the pancreatic ducts has been provided by rodent models of pancreas regeneration.[5]

In vitro, mouse ductal cells have been shown to provide a source of pancreatic progenitors.[6] Endocrine differentiation also has been reported in cultures enriched for human pancreatic duct cells. The exact nature of any pancreatic progenitor/stem cells still is controversial. In addition to the duct epithelial cell, a further candidate islet progenitor cell has been described on the basis of expression of the neural stem cell marker nestin and lack of known islet and duct cell markers.[7]

Such nestin-positive cells have been reported to differentiate in vitro into pancreatic endocrine, exocrine and hepatic phenotypes.[8] Differentiation of insulin-producing cells from murine ESCs also has been described as involving a nestin-expressing intermediate cell type.[9] This is contrary to established descriptive analyses of the developing mouse and human pancreas, which would preclude a role for any nestin-expressing cells in islet differentiation.

A more traditionally accepted view is that pancreatic endocrine progenitor/stem cells express PDX-1, a known marker for insulin-producing cells.[3] Such a cell type has been shown to be amenable to in-vitro manipulation and, when grown in the presence of fibroblast growth factor-7 (FGF-7), to stimulate proliferation of ductal cells. Furthermore, growth on Matrigel™ supplemented with nicotinamide has been reported to initiate and stimulate endocrine differentiation.[9] These data have been supported by the identification of a similar human cell population. These cells have been reported to require serum-free growth conditions and the use of Matrigel™ as absolute essentials. They have been induced in vitro to produce islet-like structures that produce insulin in response to glucose stimulation. Critically, no evidence was found for the development of endocrine cells from nestin-positive stem cells.[10]

☐ ISOLATION AND CHARACTERISATION OF PANCREATIC-DERIVED PATHFINDER CELLS

I have sought to tackle the problems associated with stem-cell derivation through an approach that focuses on damage repair rather than development. This has involved an adaptation of pre-existing methods to isolate nestin-positive cells (termed pancreatic-derived pathfinder cells (PDPCs)), from the pancreatic ducts of adult rats. These cells can be induced, when grown in an appropriate medium, to form islet-like clusters that express PDX-1, insulin somatostatin, pancreatic polypeptide and glucagon. Importantly, they also can give rise to neurones (Fig 1).

The islet cell clusters, when examined by transmission electron microscopy, show the presence of dense core vesicles typical of islets in vivo. Although these cells

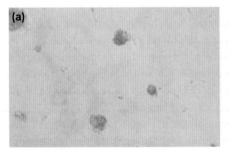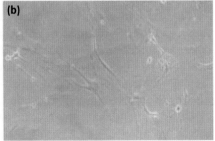

Fig 1 Cells derived from pancreatic-derived pathfinder cells: (a) light micrograph of islet cells and (b) neuronal-like cells.

express insulin, the time needed to isolate and differentiate the nestin-positive PDPCs is considerable. This places the cells under conditions of elevated oxidant stress while in culture. Cellular damage acquired during this period may manifest only after transplant. This is neither readily, nor easily, addressed at a practical level. The most basic solutions to mitigate this damage might involve growing the cells in the presence of antioxidants and limiting the period for expansion/differentiation.

To avoid these issues associated with cellular damage when growing and differentiating cells in culture, which in turn may lead to post-transplant complications including carcinogenesis, we have used PDPCs directly to treat disease. This allows us to address whether the PDPCs differentiate in vivo to repair damage, whether they might stimulate the host tissue to do so, or whether a combination of host and donor cell actions is involved.

We have used a streptozotocin-induced model of diabetes (STZ model)[3] with a concordant xenotransplant of rat cells, specifically to track the fate of the PDPCs and to provide a functional assay. Rat cells were put into a diabetic mouse to determine just what the PDPCs would do with respect to generating insulin-producing cells. Treatment involved tail-vein injections of PDPCs into the mice, with no complex surgery. This is in contrast to the transplantation of fully formed islets under the kidney capsule of NOD (non-obese diabetic) or NOD–STZ diabetic mice and the injection of islets into the hepatic portal vein of transplant recipients.

Control groups for our PDPC experiment received saline or rat bone marrow three days after the animals were rendered diabetic by treatment with streptozotocin. Blood glucose was monitored every three days for the duration of the experiment (33 days). Figure 2 shows the results. The choice of rat bone marrow as an extra control allowed us to evaluate previous observations that indicated that bone marrow-derived cells could, on transplantation, give rise to insulin-producing cells in streptozotocin-treated animals.

Animals treated with PDPCs survived treatment with streptozotocin, unlike the control animals (Fig 2). After administration of streptozotocin, blood glucose in all groups rose from a mean of 7 mM/l to 45 mM/l. This situation persisted, with the saline-treated controls proving non-viable by day 19, when blood glucose levels peaked at 50 mM/l. The bone-marrow control group survived until day 21, when the animals had to be sacrificed in accordance with animal licence conditions. Animals treated with PDPC survived throughout this period and beyond – to day 33, when the animals were sacrificed.

The survival of the PDPC-treated animals was highly significant (Table 1). Although normolglycaemia was not achieved, the blood glucose levels stabilised by day 6, at a mean value of 20 mM/l. Bone marrow-treated animals did show a significant survival advantage over saline controls (Table 1). This observation is in keeping with reports that indicate that cells derived from bone marrow have the capacity to engender insulin production after transplantation.

To establish whether the lack of normoglycaemia was the result of cell loss because of immune attack or insufficient numbers delivered by the intravenous route, replicate transplant experiments were performed in the presence and absence of ciclosporin and with 1,500,000 cells or a repeat injection of 1,500,000 PDPCs at

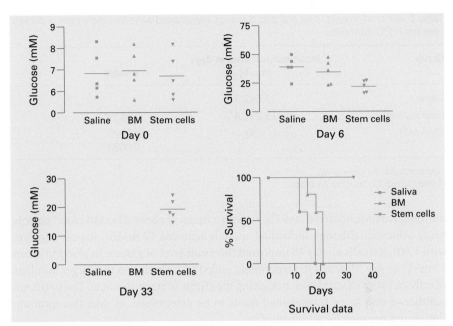

Fig 2 Blood glucose measurement (mM/l) in STZ diabetic mice given saline, bone marrow (BM) or pancreatic-derived pathfinder cells (stem cells).

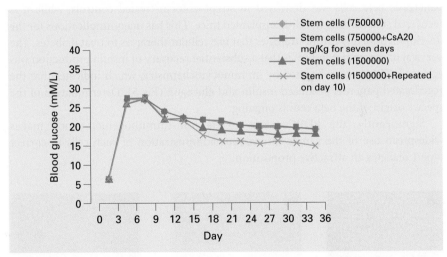

Fig 3 Blood glucose measurements (mM/l) after administration of pancreatic-derived pathfinder cells with immunosuppression.

day 10 after treatment with streptozotocin. Figure 3 shows the results of this particular protocol.

Treatment with ciclosporin seemed to have no effect on blood glucose levels, which suggests that the PDPCs are non-immunogenic; this is in keeping with observations with human nestin islet precursor (NIP) cells. When the number of PDPCs was doubled, no significant improvement in blood glucose levels to near

Table 1 Statistical analysis of survival data in animals transplanted with saline, bone-marrow derived cells and PDPC stem cells.

Group	Mean survival time in days (n = 6)	p value
Saline	15.0±2.7	
Bone marrow	19.2±2.4	0.0439*
Stem cells	>30	0.0025*
		0.0034†

*Compared with the saline group.
†Compared with the bone-marrow group.

normolglycaemia occurred (see Fig 3), with a mean of about 20 mM/l blood glucose being achieved (although individual animals achieved 12 mM/l). Repeat injection with 1,500,000 cells on day 10 improved the mean level of glucose in blood to about 15 mM/l by day 33 (when the experiment ended). This indicates that larger numbers of cells are more efficacious in mitigating the effects of streptozotocin. The optimum number of cells to be transplanted needs to be determined, as does the optimum timing and regimen for administration.

Post-mortem analysis of the treated animals and control groups showed that treatment with PDPCs regenerated the pancreatic beta cells (Fig 4). The structure of pancreatic beta cells was destroyed in streptozotocin-treated controls, while it is recovered substantially in cell-transplanted mice. This has major implications for the development of any future strategies that use cellular therapies to treat diabetes. The survival of these mice indicates that a substantial recovery of insulin production was achieved. This is corroborated by immunocytochemistry, which indicates that the regenerated pancreas produced insulin and glucagon (Fig 5). Determination of the species origin of the beta cells is ongoing.

Significantly, the PDPCs seem to be non-immunogenic, which makes widespread use of the simple intravenous administration of such cells to correct type 1 diabetes an attractive proposition.

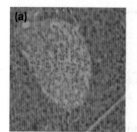 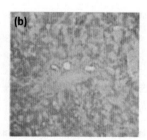 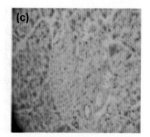

Fig 4 Post-mortem analysis of STZ diabetic mice treated with pancreatic-derived pathfinder cells: (a) light photomicrograph of a haematoxylin-and-eosin (H/E)-stained section of untreated murine pancreas, (b) light photomicrograph of an H/E-stained section of an STZ-treated murine pancreas showing loss of beta-cell mass in an islet and (c) light photomicrograph of an H/E-stained section of an STZ-treated murine pancreas after 30 days after intravenous injection of pancreatic-derived pathfinder cells.

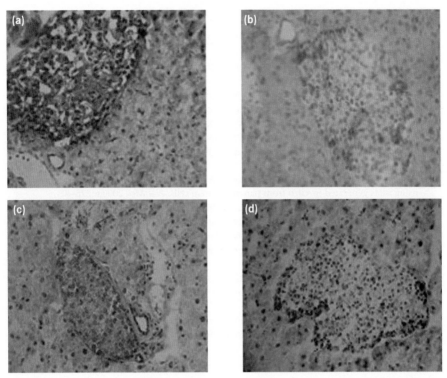

Fig 5 Immunohistochemical staining for insulin and glucagon in STZ diabetic mice treated with pancreatic-derived pathfinder cells: mouse pancreatic section stained for (a) insulin and (b) glucagon and pancreatic section from STZ treated mouse given pancreatic-derived pathfinder cells stained for (c) insulin and (d) glucagon.

☐ CONCLUSIONS

The use of adult cell types to affect recovery from streptozotocin-induced diabetes is exciting. Should these observations translate into a human clinical setting, a successful cellular therapeutic for diabetes may emerge. This, of course, is not without precedent, given the successful history of bone-marrow transplantation. The advantages of using an adult cell type should allow the development of patient-specific therapies free from immunosuppression. This, I would argue, would negate – the future use of islet transplants, and the associated problems. Much more work on defining the character and action of PDPCs in vivo is still needed, although the simple approach to therapy described in this article yet might be applicable to the treatment of degenerative disorders such as Parkinson's disease, especially in light of the observations that PDPCs can give rise to neurones.

☐ ACKNOWLEDGEMENTS

I would like to acknowledge the generous support of Darlinda's Charitable Trust and all of my collaborators, especially Dr Anthony Dorling and Dr Daxin Chen (Imperial College School of Medicine, London).

REFERENCES

1   Mummery C. Stem cell research: immortality or a healthy old age? *Eur J Endocrinol* 2004;**151** (Suppl. 3):U7–12.

2   Landry DW, Zucker HA. Embryonic death and the creation of human embryonic stem cells. *J Clin Invest* 2004;**114**:1184–6.

3   Colman A. Making new beta cells from stem cells. *Semin Cell Dev Biol* 2004;**15**:337–45.

4   Vinik A, Pittenger G, Rafaeloff R, Rosenberg L *et al.* Determinants of pancreatic islet cell mass: a balance between neogenesis and senescence/apoptosis. *Diabet Rev* 1996;**4**:235–63.

5   Bonner-Weir S, Baxter LA, Schuppin GT, Smith FE. A second pathway for regeneration of adult exocrine and endocrine pancreas. A possible recapitulation of embryonic development. *Diabetes* 1993;**42**:1715–20.

6   Ramiya VK, Maraist M, Arfors KE, Schatz DA *et al.* Reversal of insulin-dependent diabetes using islets generated in vitro from pancreatic stem cells. *Nat Med* 2000;**6**:278–82.

7   Zulewski H, Abraham EJ, Gerlach MJ, Daniel PB *et al.* Multipotential nestin-positive stem cells isolated from adult pancreatic islets differentiate ex vivo into pancreatic endocrine, exocrine, and hepatic phenotypes. *Diabetes* 2001;**50**:521–33.

8   Hunziker E, Stein M. Nestin-expressing cells in the pancreatic islets of Langerhans. *Biochem Biophys Res Commun* 2000;**271**:116–9.

9   Otonkoski T, Beattie GM, Mally MI, Ricordi C *et al.* Nicotinamide is a potent inducer of endocrine differentiation in cultured human fetal pancreatic cells. *J Clin Invest* 1993;**92**: 1459–66.

10 Gao R, Ustinov J, Pulkkinen MA, Lundin K *et al.* Characterization of endocrine progenitor cells and critical factors for their differentiation in adult pancreatic cell culture. *Diabetes* 2003;**52**:2007–15.

☐ TRANSPLANTATION SELF ASSESSMENT QUESTIONS

Stem cells

1   Stem cells:
  (a) Are specialised cells with defined developmental functions
  (b) Are unspecialised cells with no apparent developmental functions
  (c) Are short lived cells only found in embryos
  (d) Cannot give rise to specialised cell types
  (e) Are found only in the bone marrow

2   Pancreatic stem cells:
  (a) Are found only in pancreatic ductal epithelium
  (b) Are found in pancreatic ducts and express nestin
  (c) Are found in pancreatic ducts and do not express nestin
  (d) Are not found in the pancreas
  (e) Express pyruvate dehydrogenase complex protein X (PDX-1)

3   STZ diabetic mice:
  (a) Have no pancreatic endocrine cells
  (b) Have no pancreatic exocrine cells
  (c) Lose pancreatic alpha cells
  (d) Lose pancreatic beta cells
  (e) Are non-obese diabetic mice

Renal

Management of chronic kidney disease: population-based approach

Rachel J Middleton and Donal J O'Donoghue

☐ INTRODUCTION

Chronic kidney disease (CKD) is defined as the presence of kidney damage or decreased level of kidney function for three months or more, irrespective of the underlying renal diagnosis.[1] Glomerular filtration rate (GFR), which provides a measure of the solute excretory capacity of the kidney, is used to define the level of kidney function. This definition has been central to the development of a staging classification of CKD, produced by the National Kidney Foundation Kidney Dialysis Outcomes Quality Initiative (K/DOQI) (Table 1). The classification has been adopted widely in clinical practice and is used as the basis for the recommendations in the recently published National Service Framework for Renal Services.[2] The five stages of CKD are highly predictive of prognosis. This classification enables comparative epidemiological studies to be performed across the globe in an effort to gain a better understanding of the risk factors, associations and impact of CKD.

Table 1 Stages of chronic kidney disease according to glomerular filtration rate.

Stage*	GFR (ml/min)
1†	≥90
2†	60–89
3	30–59
4	15–29
5	<15

*All stages require the abnormality to be present for at least three months.
†Require further evidence of kidney damage such as proteinuria, haematuria or abnormal renal imaging for CKD to be present.

Glomerular filtration rate can be estimated from serum creatinine with a formula derived from empiric observations. Estimated GFR (eGFR) has been well validated in populations with CKD and can be reported automatically by clinical biochemistry laboratories.[3,4] At all stages, CKD is a risk factor for cardiovascular disease, conferring an increased risk of ischaemic heart disease, congestive heart failure and cerebrovascular disease and an increased mortality from acute cardiovascular events. A patient aged 25 years on dialysis has a similar risk of death from a cardiovascular event as a 75-year-old person in the general population. Even an 80-year-old patient on dialysis has a cardiovascular risk five times greater than their peers without CKD. This increased cardiovascular risk begins early in the course of CKD. Early detection and a systematic approach to management of CKD are essential to reduce cardiovascular comorbidity and reduce the risk of renal progression (Fig 1).

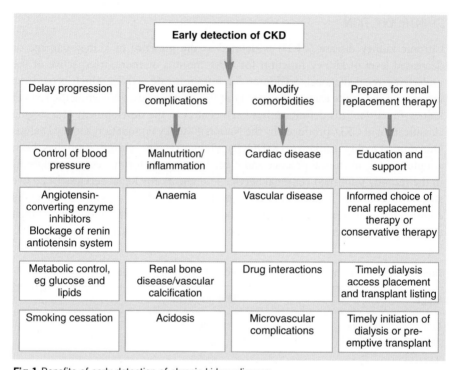

Fig 1 Benefits of early detection of chronic kidney disease.

☐ IDENTIFICATION OF CKD

The kidney not only has a solute excretory function but also has other major roles in, for example, regulation of blood pressure, bone homeostasis, regulation of haemoglobin concentration, drug clearance and volume control. The kidneys' excretory capacity is used to measure kidney function in clinical practice.

Serum creatinine is the most commonly recognised measure of renal excretory function, being readily available and inexpensive to measure. Creatinine is produced by skeletal muscle, and its plasma concentration therefore is proportional to muscle mass. Factors that affect muscle mass, such as age, body size, sex and race, must be taken into consideration to interpret serum creatinine accurately. A 78-year-old Caucasian woman with a serum creatinine of 105 µmol/l (a level considered to be in the normal range for many laboratories) would have a GFR of <50 ml/min. The creatinine value would give a GFR of approximately 70 ml/min in a 44-year-old Caucasian man. If the same man were of black ethnicity, the GFR would be even greater, at around 85 ml/min.

Creatinine is filtered freely in the kidney by the glomerulus, but it also is secreted by the proximal tubule, so formulae based on the urinary excretion of creatinine, such as 24-hour creatinine clearance (CrCl), will overestimate GFR. Imprecise 24-hour urine volume collection also contributes to inaccuracies in CrCl.

Inulin is filtered freely across the glomerulus and is the gold standard marker of renal function. Inulin clearance and clearance of radioisotopes such as iothalamate are time consuming and costly, so they are impractical in routine practice and are used more often as a research tool. Isotope GFR has the additional risk of exposure to radiation.

Measurement of serum creatinine is not harmonised between laboratories – even the same analyser may be calibrated differently in individual laboratories. This variation in serum creatinine measurements makes inter-laboratory comparison difficult. Future development of standardised serum creatinine assays, eg with isotope dilution mass spectrometry, could eliminate calibration errors.

Several equations to produce an estimation of GFR have been developed with serum creatinine in addition to factors such as age, sex, weight and race. The most widely used of these are the Cockcroft-Gault equation and the four-variable modification of diet in renal disease (MDRD) equation. The Schwartz formula can be used to estimate GFR in children. The Cockcroft-Gault formula first was validated in 236 Caucasian adults; it is modelled on creatinine clearance and, in the same way, may overestimate GFR. Knowledge of a patient's weight is necessary for the Cockcroft-Gault formula, which can mean it is an inconvenient method for determining renal function in practice. The four-variable MDRD formula was derived from isotope GFR measurements in 1,628 patients with CKD. It requires age, sex, race and serum creatinine only (see below) and therefore is quick and easy to calculate in all patients:

Four-variable MDRD GFR: $eGFR = 186(sCr/88.4)^{-1.154} \times age^{-0.203}$

 – $\times 0.742$ if female
 – $\times 1.21$ if black (but no adjustment is recommended currently for the Asian population)

Both the Cockcroft-Gault and MDRD equations have been validated in patients with CKD. In people with normal kidney function, both may underestimate renal function compared with isotope GFR. In patients with CKD with GFR <60 ml/min, 90% have a MDRD-GFR accurate to within 30% of an isotope GFR; this represents an improvement compared with serum creatinine alone. Glomerular filtration rate can be interpreted as a percentage of kidney function, which is a concept easily grasped by patients and healthcare practitioners.

☐ STAGES AND PREVALENCE OF CHRONIC KIDNEY DISEASE.

The K/DOQI classification encompasses the spectrum of CKD from normal renal function to end-stage renal failure (Table 1). A GFR ≥60 ml/min for at least three months, with other evidence of kidney damage such as proteinuria on urine dipstick, abnormal renal imaging or a known histological lesion, confirms a diagnosis of CKD stages 1 and 2. A GFR <60 ml/min for at least three months establishes the diagnosis of CKD stage 3–5.

The K/DOQI staging classification is highly predictive of prognosis. The stage of CKD influences an individual's risk of progression to end-stage renal failure, the development of complications and comorbidity secondary to CKD and the risk of death.

The staging classification and the MDRD formula for calculating GFR have enabled population estimates of the prevalence of CKD. The Third National Health and Nutrition Examination Survey (NHANES III) found the prevalence of CKD in adults in the United States to be 11% (19.2 million) of the population, with 4.6% (8.3 million) having moderate to severe CKD (stage 3–5).[5] The prevalence of CKD increases with age and presence of diabetes or hypertension. The same American data found the prevalence of CKD stage 3–5 to be 20.6% in those ≥65 years. Data from the United Kingdom are comparable: the New Opportunities for Early Renal Intervention by Computerised Assessment study (NeoErica), which interrogated general practitioners' databases from 12 practices in east Kent, west Surrey and Salford, found the prevalence of CKD stage 3–5 to be 5.1% of the population.

The forthcoming CKD guidelines, jointly produced by the Royal College of Physicians and Renal Association, as well as the recently published renal National Service Framework, recommend that clinical biochemistry laboratories automatically report formulae-based estimates of kidney function, together with creatinine measurements.[2,6] Routine reporting of eGFR will identify a considerable number of the population with previously unrecognised CKD, which will have major implications for the individual and the healthcare system. The healthcare system will need to develop new strategies and collaboration between primary care teams and secondary care to appropriately manage the potential 2.5 million individuals with CKD in the United Kingdom today.

From an individual perspective, early identification of impaired renal function will allow implementation of cardio–renal protective strategies, treatment of related complications and avoidance of nephrotoxic drugs to prevent or delay progression of CKD and reduce cardiovascular risk. A label of CKD may have adverse psychosocial consequences for an individual, as although usually asymptomatic, CKD augments the risk of cardiovascular morbidity and mortality.

☐ GENERIC APPROACH TO MANAGEMENT

Clinical history, examination or investigation may establish an underlying renal diagnosis or uncover a multi-system disorder that warrants specific treatment. In addition, general management principles can be applied to all patients with CKD to retard renal progression, decrease cardiovascular risk, manage renal complications and prepare for end-stage renal failure. The renal National Service Framework and the United Kingdom's CKD draft guidelines focus attention on these key areas.[2,6]

Delay progression of chronic kidney disease

The rate of progression of CKD is determined by the underlying cause of CKD and the presence of risk factors such as hypertension and proteinuria. A primary renal diagnosis of diabetic nephropathy, for example, is associated with more rapid progression of CKD than obstructive uropathy. A diagnosis of glomerulonephritis, vasculitis or myeloma may require specific immunosuppressive therapy to treat the disease and induce remission, and will often be apparent from clinical examination, urinalysis, or biochemical or immunological findings. It is not always necessary or possible, however, to obtain a definitive histological renal diagnosis, and treatment can focus on modifying risk factors that are known to adversely affect cardiovascular risk and rate of renal progression.

Meticulous attention to blood pressure control and proteinuria excretion, particularly blockade of the renin–angiotensin system with angiotensin-converting enzyme (ACE) inhibitors or angiotensin II receptor blockers alone or as dual therapy, was clearly shown to delay progression of CKD in a recent meta-analysis.[7] Systolic blood pressure between 110 mmHg and 129 mmHg was associated with the lowest risk of progression of CKD. The risk of progressive renal disease was significantly greater in those with proteinuria >1 g/day than in those with proteinuria <1 g/day. Guidelines recommend blood pressure control to less than 130/80 mmHg in the presence of CKD, and tighter blood pressure control (to less than 120/75 mmHg) in patients with CKD and proteinuria >1 g/day.[6]

Despite the recommendations for ACE inhibitors as first-line management for hypertension and proteinuria in CKD, the number of people being prescribed ACE inhibitors for such indications is suboptimal. Up to a 30% increase in serum creatinine is acceptable after introduction of ACE inhibition or angiotensin II receptor blockers.[8] Patients with CKD, who are at the highest risk of mortality after a cardiovascular event, are less likely to receive appropriate reperfusion therapy or cardioprotective drugs.[9] Medicines management in CKD also includes modification of drug dosage in line with estimated renal drug clearance and avoidance of nephrotoxic drugs. Use of metformin may cause lactic acidosis in patients with CKD and non-steroidal anti-inflammatory drugs reduce renal blood flow, so both should be used with caution. The risks and benefits of nephrotoxic drugs need to be weighed up on an individual basis, and close renal monitoring is needed if they are started.

Prevent uraemic complications

Complications secondary to uraemia, such as anaemia, renal bone disease, acidosis, malnutrition and inflammation, can occur early in the continuum of CKD. Their presence is determined largely by the stage of CKD rather than the underlying cause of CKD.

Renal-related anaemia may occur as early as stage 2 CKD, when the serum creatinine level is likely to be normal. Active management of uraemic complications therefore requires prior acknowledgement of the presence of CKD to enable appropriate surveillance and treatment. Uraemic complications have an adverse impact on morbidity and mortality if left uncorrected. Anaemia is associated with left ventricular hypertrophy, hospitalisation and increased mortality in CKD; partial correction of anaemia with erythropoietin and iron can lead to improvement in clinical outcomes.[10]

Low levels of calcium and high levels of phosphate and parathyroid hormone are the biochemical hallmarks of renal bone disease and are evident in stage 3 CKD. Clinically, the abnormal bone profile may present as bone pain; fractures; and extraosseous calcification in cardiac muscle, valves and vasculature, which leads to cardiovascular disease or calciphylaxis necrotic lesions of the skin secondary to small vessel calcification. Modification of the abnormal bone profile with vitamin D and phosphate binders, or acidosis with bicarbonate replacement, frequently is necessary long before a patient needs dialysis or transplantation.

Modify comorbidity

Only a very small proportion of the population with CKD progresses to end-stage renal failure. One explanation for this is the excessive mortality seen in CKD.

Chronic kidney disease is a potent risk factor for cardiovascular disease and mortality. The risk of death, cardiovascular events and hospitalisation increases with worsening stages of CKD, such that patients with stage 4 CKD have a three times greater risk of death than those with GFR ≥60 ml/min, and those with stage 5 CKD have a risk of death almost six times greater. Patients with stage 4 and 5 CKD also have greater risks of cardiovascular events compared with patients with GFR ≥60 ml/min (hazards ratios 2.8 and 3.4, respectively).[11] Even in severe renal failure, the risk of death or cardiovascular event is greater than the risk of end-stage renal failure. The pathogenesis of the excess cardiovascular risk in CKD is multifactorial: risk factors for CKD, such as hypertension and diabetes, also are traditional risk factors for cardiovascular disease. The uraemic environment is associated with an increase in non-traditional cardiovascular risk factors, such as hyperhomocysteinaemia, inflammation and anaemia. Cardiovascular disease itself is also a risk factor for CKD via atherosclerosis or low-output cardiac failure.

The Asian population has a higher incidence of CKD, in part because of an increase in prevalence of diabetes and hypertension in the Asian population.

A key aim of the management plan for a patient with CKD should be appropriate modification of associated comorbidities such as cardiovascular disease and diabetic neuropathy and retinopathy.

Preparation for renal replacement therapy

Most people with early CKD can be managed in an integrated fashion, with the majority of care being delivered in a primary care setting. Education of patients, practice nurses and general practitioners, in conjunction with opportunities to discuss patients with complex disease with the renal specialist team, is key to the success of this approach. Patients with rapidly progressing CKD (decline in GFR >5 ml/min/year) and most of those with stage 4 and 5 CKD should be referred for specialist nephrology evaluation. A patient who 'crash-lands' into renal services as a uraemic emergency can experience serious consequences, with greater use of temporary dialysis catheters, increased hospitalisation, increased mortality and reduced access to transplantation waiting lists.[12]

The multi-skilled renal team has a central role in the delivery of care to patients who are approaching end-stage renal failure. Such patients benefit from education and information about dialysis and transplantation that enables an informed choice about the mode of renal replacement therapy or the option of conservative therapy. The renal National Service Framework's core standards recommend that patient care be delivered in a multidisciplinary team environment one year before renal replacement therapy and that vascular access should be created successfully six months before.[2] Both interventions are associated with improved long-term survival. Renal transplantation also is recognised by the renal National Service Framework as the most cost-effective form of renal replacement therapy, providing the best quality of life and independence for patients, and suitable patients should be listed for transplantation once GFR reaches <15 ml/min or within six months of dialysis being started. Pre-emptive transplantation – that is, before renal replacement therapy is started – is the optimum, with superior long-term graft outcomes compared with transplantation after two years on dialysis (graft survival at 10 years: 69% *v* 39%).

☐ SUMMARY

Chronic kidney disease is common, and 5% of the population in the United Kingdom is likely to have moderate-to-severe renal failure (CKD stages 3–5). Effective management of this population requires a coordinated approach across the healthcare system, analogous to the well-established models of care used in diabetes and cardiovascular disease. Management of an individual with CKD in the early stages should focus on comorbid risk factors, in common with diabetes and cardiovascular disease, such as smoking cessation, blood pressure control and primary and secondary prevention of cardiovascular disease. Medicines management, minimisation of proteinuria and treatment of uraemic complications require specific attention in CKD, and as the disease progresses, preparation for renal replacement therapy should be provided in a multi-skilled renal environment.

REFERENCES

1   National Kidney Foundation Kidney Disease Outcomes Quality Initiative. Part 4. Definition and classification of stages of chronic kidney disease. *Am J Kidney Dis* 2002;**39** (Suppl 1):S46–75.

2   Department of Health. *The national service framework for renal services.* London: Stationery Office, 2004.

3   Levey AS, Bosch JP, Lewis JB, Greene T *et al.* A more accurate method to estimate glomerular filtration rate from serum creatinine: a new prediction equation. Modification of Diet in Renal Disease Study Group. *Ann Intern Med* 1999;**130**:461–70.

4   Poggio ED, Wang X, Greene T, Van Lente F *et al.* Performance of the modification of diet in renal disease and Cockroft-Gault equations in the estimation of GFR in health and in chronic kidney disease. *J Am Soc Nephrol* 2005;**16**:459–66.

5 Coresh J, Astor BC, Greene T, Eknoyan G *et al.* Prevalence of chronic kidney disease and decreased kidney function in the adult US population: third national health and nutrition examination survey. *Am J Kid Dis* 2003;**41**:1–12.

6 Joint Specialty Committee of the Royal College of Physicians and Renal Association. *UK guidelines for the management of chronic kidney disease.* London: Royal College of Physicians, Renal Association, 2005.

7 Jafar TH, Stark PC, Schmid CH, Landa M *et al.* Progression of chronic kidney disease: the role of blood pressure control, proteinuria, and angiotensin-converting enzyme inhibition: a patient-level meta-analysis. *Ann Intern Med* 2003;**139**:244–52.

8 Bakris GL, Weir MR. Angiotensin-converting enzyme inhibitor-associated elevations in serum creatinine: is this a cause for concern? *Arch Intern Med* 2000;**160**:685–93.

9 Wright RS, Reeder GS, Herzog CA, Albright RC *et al.* Acute myocardial infarction and renal dysfunction: a high-risk combination. *Ann Intern Med* 2002;**137**:563–70.

10 Levin A, Thompson CR, Ethier J, Carlisle EJ *et al.* Left ventricular mass index increase in early renal disease: impact of decline in hemoglobin. *Am J Kid Dis* 1999;**34**:125–34.

11 Go AS, Chertow GM, Fan D, McCulloch CE *et al.* Chronic kidney disease and the risk of death, cardiovascular events, and hospitalization. *N Engl J Med* 2004;**351**:1296–305.

12 Roderick P, Jones C, Drey N, Blakeley S *et al.* Late referral for end-stage renal disease: a region-wide survey in the south west of England. *Nephrol Dial Transplant* 2002;**17**:1252–9.

Inherited renal diseases

Anand Saggar

☐ INTRODUCTION

Inherited kidney disorders are many and varied, and it is not possible to discuss even those conditions with a proven inheritable component in this brief article. As they may become apparent at any time in life, however, their correct diagnosis is essential and, for some conditions, an early diagnosis may influence outcome. Accurate and timely genetic counselling requires knowledge about the natural history of the disorder and understanding of the genetic factors and correct mode of inheritance. Importantly, early diagnosis allows the risk of the disorder in other family members to be defined and opens up options for prenatal diagnosis.

Clinical geneticists play an important role in the diagnosis of paediatric and late-onset genetic conditions. Contrary to the popular image of a 'geneticist' who pours over detailed genetic maps, we actually see patients all the time, endeavouring to deliver information sensitively and accurately. We are interested, of course, in moving from the gene to the actual organ and so to the disease itself, but in the end, genetics is about the disease process.

Diagnoses are made in traditional ways, particularly by taking a family history – an important take-home message. We are taught to do this as medical students, but sadly this skill often is neglected. Clinical information to aid the diagnosis also can be obtained from drawing a family pedigree, physical examination, clinical and laboratory investigations and family photographs.

☐ CLASSIFICATION

Inherited renal disorders can be classified broadly into seven categories (Table 1). As with the spectrum of non-renal diseases (Fig 1), many multifactorial, non-Mendelian disorders widely thought to have environmental determinants now have significant genetic elements to their presentation or penetrance. For example, susceptibility to malarial parasites is determined by sickle-cell status, and, similarly, genetic determinants of diabetes are being identified and a gene for resistance to HIV seroconversion is known. The underlying causative gene mutations for many cancer syndromes also now have been identified. Within the kidney disorders, genes now have been found for many of the cystic diseases, renal cancers, renal malformations and monogenic forms of hypertension, and loci are being sought for many other conditions – for example, vesicoureteric reflux.

Table 1 Categorisation of renal disease.

Category	Example
Congenital malformations	Agenesis Dysplasia (see also Table 2)

Chromosomal disorders
  Urinary tract defects associated with Dysmorphic
  syndromes associated with renal involvement
	Trisomy 13, 18, 21
	Brancio-oculo-facial syndrome
	Beckwith-Wiedeman syndrome
	Vater syndrome

Primary hereditary nephropathies	Congenital nephrotic syndrome Alport syndrome Cystic renal diseases (see also Table 3) Immunoglobulin A nephropathy
Primary inherited metabolic diseases of kidney	Cystinosis X-linked hypercalciuric nephrolithiasis
Genetic syndromes with a renal component	Sickle cell disease Haemophilia Acute intermittent porphyria Nail Patella syndrome Alpha-1 antitrypsin deficiency Wilson's disease
Inherited renal cancer syndromes	Birt Hogg Dube syndrome Familial renal carcinoma

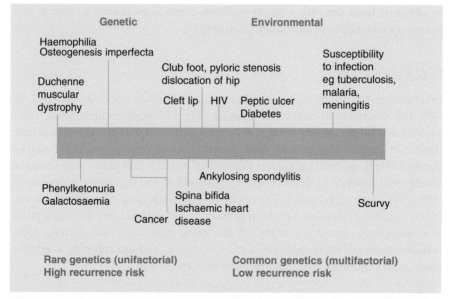

Fig 1 Human diseases as a spectrum ranging from those which are largely environmental in causation to those which are entirely genetic, illustrating the increasing recognition of genetic component(s) within multifactorial disorders.

The mammalian kidney derives from two tissue compartments in the embryo:

☐ the ureteric bud epithelium, which branches to form the collecting duct system

☐ the renal mesenchyme, which transforms to make the components of the nephron, including the glomerular and proximal tubular epithelia.

The increasing use of fetal ultrasound scanning has led to many more people with congenital malformations of the urinary tract being diagnosed. These disorders now account for about 30% for all prenatally diagnosed anomalies. Many may have minimal clinical significance, and others may be more serious, such as bilateral renal agenesis or dysplasia. The frequency of prenatally diagnosed anomalies makes it unsurprising that congenital malformations of the kidney and lower urinary tract are common causes of chronic renal failure in infants and young children. Table 2 gives the spectrum of congenital malformations of the kidney and lower urinary tract.

Table 2 Spectrum of abnormalities of the kidney and lower urinary tract.

Upper urinary tract	Lower urinary tract
Renal agenesis	Agenesis
Renal dysplasia	Hydronephrosis
Renal hypoplasia	Duplication of the ureters
Duplex kidney	Vesicoureteric reflux
Horseshoe kidney	Posterior urethral valves

☐ AUTOSOMAL DOMINANT POLCYSTIC KIDNEY DISEASE (ADPKD)

Space does not permit a full discussion of all the inherited renal disorders, so I will concentrate on autosomal dominant polycystic kidney disease (ADPKD) – one of the hepato–renal fibrocystic diseases (Table 3). It is the most common inherited renal disorder and one to which most doctors inevitably will be exposed. It is worth observing, however, that autosomal dominant polycystic liver disease (PLD) without renal cysts is now considered a genetic separate entity from the massive cystic liver disease seen in ADPKD (Fig 2). Thus, if a patient has massive cystic liver disease, it should not necessarily be assumed to be associated with cystic kidney disease.

Table 3 The hepato–renal fibrocystic diseases.

Autosomal dominant polycystic kidney disease
Autosomal recessive polycystic kidney disease
Autosomal dominant polycystic liver disease (without kidney cysts)
Nephronopthesis
Bardet-Biedl syndrome

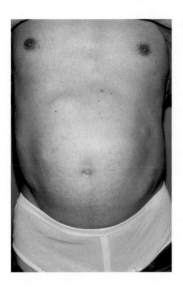

Fig 2 Clinical appearance of a patient with massive polycystic kidneys and liver.

Autosomal dominant polycystic kidney disease remains the silent disease despite being twice as common as multiple sclerosis and affecting more people than cystic fibrosis, muscular dystrophy, haemophilia, Down syndrome and sickle cell anaemia combined. It is characterised by the progressive development and enlargement of bilateral renal cysts and often leads to end-stage renal disease (ESRD) by late middle age. Patients typically present with haematuria, loin pain and/or hypertension in the third or fourth decade of life. It is, however, a multi-system disorder, with many renal and extra-renal complications. These include hepatic cysts, cerebral intracranial aneurysms (ICA), cardiac valvular anomalies, left ventricular hypertrophy and abdominal hernias.[1] About 4–6% of the population who undergo dialysis have this diagnosis. Autosomal dominant polycystic kidney disease has an overall symptomatic prevalence of one in 800, but it is extremely variable clinically – a phenomenon called variable penetrance. It affects all races, although little is known about non-white Caucasian populations. The condition also has been described in many animal models, including mice, rats, antelopes, cats, pigeons and even goldfish!

□ MAKING THE DIAGNOSIS

Although ADPKD presents mainly in adult life, 2% of people may present in infancy, which is why the term adult polycystic kidney disease has been abandoned. Clinical expression ranges from incidental findings at autopsy to ESRD by the age of 30 years. Detection of renal cysts is possible before the onset of symptoms, and ultrasonography is the most reliable diagnostic method. Recently, the criteria for ultrasound diagnosis have been revised to allow for the chance findings in older people of cysts that occur as a consequence of ageing and independent of ADPKD.[2] As renal cysts are extremely unusual before the age of 30 years, the presence of two cysts in one or both kidneys in a person younger than 30 years without a family history of ADPKD is considered diagnostic. From the ages of 30–59 years, observation of two cysts in each kidney may be needed, and for people older than 60 years, in whom isolated kidney cysts are common, at least four cysts may be needed in each kidney to establish a reliable positive diagnosis. In people younger than 30 years, isolated kidney cysts are very rare, so the finding of even one cyst raises a strong suspicion of ADPKD, particularly in a person with a 50% *a priori* risk because of a positive family history. The use of modern-day scanners means that the risk of a false-negative scan in a first-degree relative of someone affected with ADPKD approximates to less than 10% at the age of 20 years and less than 1% at the age of 30 years.[2] These figures can be reduced further by the use of fine-cut renal computed tomography scanning.

☐ CLINICAL PRESENTATION AND COMPLICATIONS

The common presenting symptoms and signs in patients with autosomal dominant polycystic kidney disease are:

- ☐ renal pain
- ☐ hypertension
- ☐ haematuria
- ☐ urinary tract infection
- ☐ cyst infection
- ☐ nephrolithiasis
- ☐ renal failure.

Haematuria occurs in 30–50% of patients and may be the first presenting sign at around 30 years of age. More rarely, bleeding may occur into a renal cyst. Urinary tract infection also occurs commonly in the bladder, the kidney tissue or cyst fluid and ideally requires a non-ionised, lipid-soluble antibiotic that has good cyst penetration. No good data exists on length of treatment for cyst infections, but patients often need several weeks of therapy. The treatment of such infections can be protracted and difficult and therefore is best done under the supervision of specialist units. Nephrolithiasis occurs in about 25% of patients with ADPKD and is an important consideration in patients who present with pain or haematuria. More rarely, patients may present with massive hepatic liver disease, which is most commonly seen in women and is associated with intake of oestrogen. The liver usually remains functionally unaffected, but considerable pressure effects, increased feelings of satiety and rarely, extrinsic compression problems associated with thrombosis of the hepatic or portal veins may be present. In such rare symptomatic cases, hepatic transplantation or partial hepatectomy has been required (see review by Torres[3]).

The most important functional abnormality is renal failure. The family history cannot be used to determine when or which patients will progress to dialysis. About

50% of patients will have ESRD by the age of 53 years, but this is highly variable, with a range of 2–80 years, even within families. This variation is presumed to be the result of the stochastic nature of pathogenic second mutational hits and other genetic modifiers within and between families.

Hypertension occurs in 60% of polycystic patients before renal impairment and in almost all patients once significant renal dysfunction is present. Hypertension remains poorly controlled in patients with ADPKD. There seems to be some consensus emerging that blood pressure should be kept lower than 130/70 mmHg. Detection and early treatment of hypertension on the assumption that it will delay progression of renal disease and other types of target organ damage represents one of the best justifications for early diagnosis of ADPKD. The crucial and yet still unanswered question, however, is the extent to which lower blood pressure alters renal function and at what level of blood pressure the rate of decline in renal function is altered significantly. The choice of hypertensive agent is at present guided mostly by effectiveness and patient compliance. Theoretical advantages exist to using angiotensin-converting enzyme (ACE) inhibitors early in the course of the disease. They are well tolerated and also have been shown to be renoprotective in patients with other renal diseases independent of blood pressure control and to reduce proteinuria significantly in patients with ADPKD. In the later stages of decline in renal function, however, ACE inhibitors may in some patients significantly exacerbate renal failure or induce hyperkalaemia, or both. The factors associated with a worse renal prognosis in ADPKD are:

☐   history of hypertension

☐   repeated haematuria

☐   proteinuria

☐   urine infection (in males)

☐   massive polycystic kidney disease

☐   male sex

☐   black race

☐   concurrence of a sickle cell trait

☐   more than two children (in women).

The association of intracranial aneurysms in patients with ADPKD has been established for many years. Overall, the prevalence is about 4–10% in the population of patients with ADPKD. Subarachnoid haemorrhage (SAH) as a cause of death is recorded in about 0.7% of the general population but in about 6% of patients with ADPKD. Aneurysm rupture is life threatening and has a worse prognosis in patients with ADPKD than the 30–50% mortality seen in the general population. Nonetheless, a substantial proportion of intracranial aneurysms in patients with ADPKD do not rupture, remain asymptomatic and can be multiple. This makes it very difficult to know which patients should have surgery or indeed even be screened. The only characteristic clearly associated with intracranial aneurysms in patients with ADPKD is a family history of the same. Intracranial aneurysms in patients with ADPKD seem to be almost three times more frequent in patients with a definite family history of intracranial aneurysms or SAH than in those without. Interestingly, 30% of patients with ruptured intracranial aneurysms had had normal blood pressure (reviewed by Saggar-Malik[1]).

Screening now is offered only to families with a history of aneurysm, unruptured or otherwise, or where there is a clear-cut history of SAH. Before magnetic resonance imaging became available, risk–benefit analysis did not justify screening by carotid angiography, but the advent of magnetic resonance angiography has changed things. At-risk patients now are screened for silent intracranial aneurysms and aneurysm ablation can, in selected cases, be done by the endovascular route. Magnetic resonance angiography can identify intracranial aneurysms >2 mm diameter and has an 80% sensitivity with approximately 90% specificity.[4] When screening is offered and no intracranial aneurysms are found, scans are repeated after five years, When an intracranial aneurysm is identified, rescreening should be offered in one year, depending on the size of the aneurysm, its stability and related symptoms. The problem question remains: at what aneurysm size should there be intervention? No good or clear data exist on this, but if the aneurysm is bigger than 10 mm, surgery always would be recommended. If aneurysms are smaller than 5 mm, we tend not to do anything but observe; for aneurysms between 5 mm and 10 mm in size, the most appropriate action is to perhaps monitor symptoms and the rate of growth by regular review.

☐ GENETICS OF ADKPD

The notion that polycystic kidney disease was inheritable was suggested first in 1925; however, it took almost another 60 or 70 years before the actual genes were identified. In 1994, the PKD-1 gene on chromosome 16 was identified, and the second gene (PKD-2) was found on chromosome 4 in 1996.[5,6] Present estimates indicate that about 80% of cases of ADPKD are the result of the PKD-1 gene in white European populations. The prevalence of PKD-2 among older patients with ADPKD is about 40%.

A large multicentre study looked at survival in 333 patients with PKD-1 and 291 patients with PKD-2.[7] A 16-year difference was seen in median survival to ESRF or death between patients with PKD-1 and those with PKD-2. Mutations at the PKD-1 locus resulted in a clinically more severe form of the disease (median age of ESRD of about 53 years) than mutations in the PKD-2 gene (median age of ESRD of about 69 years) (Fig 3). Clearly, PKD-2 has a better outlook and prognosis, but genotyping cannot be offered routinely on a clinical level. Importantly, very little difference was seen in phenotypic presentation.[7]

It long has been recognised that polycystic kidney disease not only has intrafamilial variability but that the cysts are very focal and affect only about 4% of nephrons. This variability is suggested to be the result of the somatic acquisition of second hits – the classical Knudson two-hit model. Wild-type inactivation of PKD-1 and PKD-2 has been reported, and almost a quarter of cysts show loss of

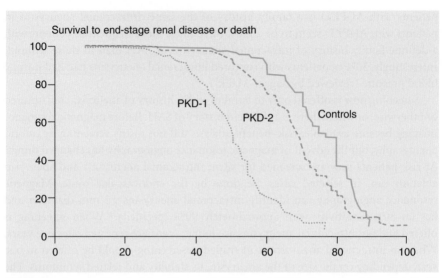

Fig 3. Renal survival in years in patients with PKD-1 and PKD-2. Reproduced from Ref 7 with permission from Elsevier.

heterozygosity.[8] Similar findings have been reported for liver cyst cells.[8] The proposed functions of the polycystins are signal regulation of intracellular calcium, cell-cycle, G-protein coupled receptors, cell adhesion and Wnt pathways. The probable cell locations of the polycystins are at the cell matrix, cell–cell surface and on the cilial mechanosensors.[9]

The cilia form complexes with the cellular centrosome, which is part of the cell cytoskeleton. Dysfunction of this complex has an impact on cell polarity and organelle transportation. This can lead to cellular disorganisation of microtubules and disruption in cell signalling, cell cycling and cellular differentiation. Recently, it has become increasingly apparent that the ciliated cells of the renal tubules respond to flow and that this flow-activated cilial movement in turn activates calcium signalling through cyclic adenosine monophosphate, which initiates downstream cell signalling and activity.[10]

Considerable lessons have been learned from other cystic disorders, such as nephronopthesis, Jouberts syndrome and Bardet-Beidl syndrome, which have considerable extra-renal features (Table 4). The common factor seems to be the role of primary or modified cilia. For example, motile and non-motile cilia regulate laterality and lead to activation of left-sided determining genes within the nodal cilia of embryonic cells.[11] An understanding of the genes implicated in ADPKD undoubtedly will lead to better understanding of cellular organisation and cell differentiation.

Mutation screening in patients with ADPKD has been difficult – not least of all because of the genomic reiteration of the more proximal part of the PKD-1 transcript on chromosome 16. The genetic heterogeneity at the PKD-1 and PKD-2 loci (with most mutations being unique within only a single family) has complicated things further. Many different mutations in PKD-1/PKD-2 have been described, and

Table 4 Extra-renal features of other cilia-related renal cystic diseases.

Disease	Feature
Nephronopthesis (NPHP)	Situs inversus (NPHP2)
	Retinitis pigmentosa (Senior-Loken syndrome)
	Oculomotor apraxia (Cogan syndrome)
Joubert	Cerebellar vermis agenesis
	Ocular coloboma
	Retinal dystrophy
	Hyperpnea/psychomotor retardation
Bardet-Biedl	Retinal dystrophy
	Obesity
	Polydactyly
	Mental retardation
	Genital anomalies; hypogonadism
	Diabetes mellitus
	Congenital hepatic fibrosis
	Congenital heart defects

no clear hotspot exists. Semi-automatic methods of mutational analysis that use denaturing high-performance liquid chromatography (DHPLC) have been developed; consequently, costs for gene screening for polycystic kidney disease are decreasing. Mutation screening with DHPLC reported that, overall, 70% of all mutations (across both PKD-1 and PKD-2) were detected.[12]

Treatment prospects for the future remain promising, although human and animal studies previously have not always shown consistent results. Careful control of blood pressure, prompt treatment of infection, reduction in microalbuminuria and the early treatment of complications undoubtedly will reduce morbidity and mortality. More recently, a lot of work has looked at the use of novel agents to specifically reduce cyst formation, and phase III human trials with vasopressin 2 receptor antagonists, which show great potential, are due to begin in 2005.[13]

☐ NON-ADPKD CYSTIC RENAL DISEASES

Simple or degenerative cysts commonly occur in the kidneys and have no sinister portent; however, many other important renal disorders are associated with renal cysts.

Medullary cystic kidney disease is a group of inherited cystic nephropathies characterised by juvenile-onset recessive (nephronopthesis) or adult-onset dominant (medullary cystic disease) inheritance. The main features are renal cyst formation in the medulla or corticomedullary junction. Genes have been identified for both forms and testing is available nationally. (For a more detailed description of this group of disorders, see Saggar-Malik.[1])

Tuberous sclerosis complex (TSC) affects one in 10,000 people and is a dominantly inherited multi-system disorder associated with severe developmental delay, epilepsy, characteristic skin lesions, renal angiomyolipomas and renal cysts.

Reports also have been made of associated focal segmental glomerular sclerosis. Renal complications include:

- [ ] renal cysts

- [ ] renal angiomyolipomas

- [ ] renal cell carcinoma

- [ ] focal segmented glomerular sclerosis

- [ ] perirenal lymphangiomatous cysts

- [ ] end-stage renal failure.

Two genes have been identified for TSC – one is on chromosome 9 (TSC1) and the other on chromosome 16 (TSC2), which is head to head with the PKD-1 gene. The more severe forms of TSC associated with renal cysts, hypertension and end-stage renal failure almost certainly are the result of contiguous gene deletions that span the PKD-1 and TSC-2 genes. In TSC, the renal angiomyolipomas, which affect 60–80% of patients, can haemorrhage intratumorally or retoperitoneally. The association with hypertension and progressive slow growth increases the risk of haemorrhage. Very rarely (in 1–2% of people), angiomyolipomas may disclose an underlying renal cell carcinoma.

A further cystic condition with autosomal dominant inheritance is Von-Hippel Lindau disease, which maps to chromosome 3p25.5. This condition is a multi-system disorder associated with renal cell carcinoma, retinal angiomas, cerebellar haemangioblastoma, phaeochromocytomas, pancreatic cysts and islet cell tumours. Patients with this disease require lifelong screening and the early treatment of complications in specialised units that have access to genetic and renal advice.

Oral-facial-digital syndrome is a X-linked condition in which clefting, polydactyly or syndactyly (fusion of the fingers) occurs, together with dental abnormalities and cystic kidneys.

☐ FAMILIAL RENAL CANCER SYNDROMES

Recently, much work has been done to examine inherited renal cancer syndromes, particularly those of a syndromic nature.

Birt Hogg Dube syndrome is a dominant condition associated with fibrofolliculomas (little fleshy lumps on the skin and the face), lung cysts (which may lead to pneumothoraces, recurrent colonic polyps and tumours) and kidney cancer in 15% of patients. The renal tumours usually are chromophobe carcinoma or renal oncocytoma. The inheritance is autosomal dominant (gene locus 17p11.2). The presentation usually is late onset after the age of 30 years, and the patients require bowel and renal screening. A family history from a person who presents with kidney cancer or has colonic polyps, together with a good physical examination, often will lead to the correct diagnosis of an inheritable condition.

A new condition of hereditary leiomyomatosis renal call carcinoma (HLRCC), in which there are cutaneous leiomyomas (small, pea-sized, fleshy cutaneous lumps), uterine leiomyomas (fibroids) and renal cell carcinoma (usually papillary type II) has been described. Interestingly, the gene mutation has been identified to be the HLRCC gene, which is in the mitochondrial fumarase hydratase pathway. Why mutations in this Krebs's cycle pathway should cause cancer is unknown.

☐ CONCLUSIONS

Greater understanding of the clinical presentation, complications and underlying genetic components of renal diseases has done much to improve the management of inherited renal disorders, as well as reducing the rate of disease progression in some conditions. Molecular biological intervention therapy recently came of age and is generating tremendous excitement. Although gene therapy for renal disease is still too immature for general clinical application, perhaps the greatest benefit to date has been in the treatment of renal malignancies, with some protocols against renal cancer showing possible inhibition of growth in certain cancer types.

Not all inheritable renal diseases are treatable or complications preventable. Furthermore, early diagnosis of some conditions may not have value, as patients become uninsurable. With all potential deteriorating renal conditions, however, patients must be offered the best advice and accurate facts. Morbidity and mortality clearly need to be reduced where possible – through screening or adequate treatment of complications.

REFERENCES

1   Saggar-Malik AK, Somlo S. Autosomal dominant polycystic kidney disease. In: Flinter F, Maher E, Saggar-Malik AK (eds), *The genetics of renal disease.* Oxford: Oxford University Press, 2003.

2   Ravine D, Gibson RN, Walker RG, Sheffield LJ *et al.* Evaluation of ultrasonographic diagnostic criteria for autosomal dominant polycystic kidney disease 1. *Lancet* 1994;**343**:824–7.

3   Torres VE. Polycystic liver disease. In: Watson ML, Torres VE (eds), *Polycystic kidney disease.* Oxford: Oxford University Press, 1996:500–29.

4   Huston J III, Nichols DA, Luetmer PH, Goodwin JT *et al.* Blinded prospective evaluation of sensitivity of MR angiography to known intracranial aneurysms: importance of aneurysm size. *Am J Neuroradiol* 1994;**15**:1607–14.

5   The European Polycystic Kidney Disease Consortium. The polycystic kidney disease 1 gene encodes a 14 kb transcript and lies within a duplicated region on chromosome 16. *Cell* 1994;**77**:881–94.

6   Mochizuki T, Wu G, Hayashi T, Xenophontos SL *et al.* PKD2, a gene for polycystic kidney disease that encodes an integral membrane protein. *Science* 1996;**272**:1339–42.

7   Hateboer N, v Dijk MA, Bogdanova N, Coto E *et al.* Comparison of phenotypes of polycystic kidney disease types 1 and 2. *Lancet* 1999;**353**:103–7.

8   Pei Y, Watnick T, He N, Wang K *et al.* Somatic PKD2 mutations in individual kidney and liver cysts support a 'two-hit' model of cystogenesis in type 2 autosomal dominant polycystic kidney disease. *J Am Soc Nephrol* 1999;**10**:1524–9.

9   Boletta A, Germino GG. Role of polycystins in renal tubulogenesis. *Trends Cell Biol* 2003; **13**:484–92.

10 Nauli SM, Alenghat FJ, Luo Y, Williams E *et al.* Polycystins 1 and 2 mediate mechanosensation in the primary cilium of kidney cells. *Nat Genet* 2003;**33**:129–37.

11 Tabin CJ, Vogan KJ. A two-cilia model for vertebrate left-right axis specification. *Genes Dev* 2003;**17**:1–6.

12   Rossetti S, Chauveau D, Walker D, Saggar-Malik A *et al.* A complete mutation screen of the ADPKD genes by DHPLC. *Kidney Int* 2002;**61**:1588–99.

13   Wang X, Gattone V 2nd, Harris PC, Torres VE. Effectiveness of vasopressin V2 receptor antagonists OPC-31260 and OPC-41061 on polycystic kidney disease development in the PCK rat. *J Am Soc Nephrol* 2005;**16**:846–51.

Other resources

For more information see **www.pkdcharity.org.uk**

☐ RENAL SELF ASSESSMENT QUESTIONS

Management of chronic kidney disease: population-based approach

1   Assessment of renal function:
    (a) Glomerular filtration rate measures the solute excretory function of the kidney
    (b) Measurement of creatinine clearance is the best method of determining renal function
    (c) Creatinine is the ideal marker of renal function, as it is filtered freely by the glomerulus without tubular reabsorption or secretion
    (d) Abnormal urine dipstick is an essential requirement when making a diagnosis of chronic kidney disease
    (e) Formulae that correct creatinine for muscle mass improve the accuracy of renal function assessment compared with serum creatinine

2   Complications of chronic kidney disease:
    (a) Anaemia is a late complication of chronic kidney disease
    (b) The stage of chronic kidney disease can determine the risk of developing complications of chronic kidney disease
    (c) Chronic kidney disease is a risk factor for cardiovascular disease
    (d) Cardiovascular disease is a risk factor for chronic kidney disease
    (e) High levels of calcium and low levels of phosphate are key features of renal bone disease

3   Medicines management in chronic kidney disease:
    (a) Dual therapy with angiotensin-converting enzyme inhibitors and angiotensin II receptor blockers are contraindicated
    (b) Metformin may cause lactic acidosis
    (c) Angiotensin-converting enzyme inhibitors should be discontinued if serum creatinine rises after their introduction by 15%
    (d) Target blood pressure is 130/80 mmHg in all patients
    (e) Treatment of anaemia with iron and erythropoietin improves long-term outcomes

Inherited renal diseases

1   The following features are characteristics of autosomal dominant polycystic kidney disease:
    (a) Arachnoid cysts
    (b) Cerebral aneurysms
    (c) Nephrolithiasis
    (d) Learning difficulties
    (e) Branchial cysts

2   With respect to tuberous sclerosis, the following statements are true:
   (a) Most patients have normal intelligence
   (b) Hypertension occurs frequently
   (c) Patients may present with myoclonic jerks
   (d) Renal angiomyolipomas eventually become malignant
   (e) Focal segmental glomerulosclerosis is more common

3   Cystic kidney disease can be associated with:
   (a) Polydactyly
   (b) Cerebellar haemangiomas
   (c) Developmental delay
   (d) Cleft lip
   (e) X-linked inheritance

4   With respect to dominant polycystic kidney disease:
   (a) It can present *in utero*
   (b) Renal tumours occur more frequently
   (c) Mutations on chromosome 4 are not associated with berry aneurysms
   (d) Renal transplantation has a higher rate of failure because of infection
   (e) Cerebral aneurysms may be single or multiple

5   Renal tumours:
   (a) Can be familial
   (b) Can be associated with bowel polyps
   (c) Can be associated with uterine polyps
   (d) May be caused by fumarase hydratase gene mutations
   (e) May present as a pneumothorax with lung cysts

Neurology

Update in multiple sclerosis

David Miller

☐ INTRODUCTION

Multiple sclerosis (MS) is the most common chronic neurological disorder to produce locomotor disability in young adults living in the United Kingdom. It has a population prevalence of one in 600 to one in 800 and usually presents between the ages of 20 and 40 years. Although 50% of cases will have severe neurological impairments after 15 years from onset – including paraplegia, ataxia, tremor, sphincter disturbance and cognitive impairment – significant numbers of patients experience a benign long-term course, with 30% having minimal or no disability after 15 years.

Considerable progress has been made in recent years in both our understanding and management of MS. This update reviews key aspects of recent developments in: aetiology, pathogenesis, diagnosis and management.

☐ AETIOLOGY

Genetic factors

The main genetic association is with major histocompatibility complex (MHC) loci on chromosome 6, which are involved in immune regulation. In northern European populations, the principal association is with human leucocyte antigen (HLA)-DR15, while in Sardinia (where MS is very common) the association is with HLA-DR3. Full genome screenings have confirmed the association with MHC alleles but also identified several additional loci, albeit with a weaker effect and less consistent across different populations. Multiple sclerosis has been recognised to have an increased familial risk, and a series of elegant studies have shown that this excess risk is explained by the extent of genetic sharing. The rate of concordance is highest for monozygotic twins (30%) and is significantly higher in full biological non-twin siblings (3.1%) than in half siblings (1.9%) or adopted siblings (0.1%), which is the general risk for the population.[1]

Environmental factors

The striking geographical distribution of the disease indicates a predilection for cooler temperate latitudes in the northern and southern hemispheres. Although some latitudinal risk can be attributed to differences in the population frequency of susceptibility genes (eg more genetic susceptibility in Scottish than English populations), such an explanation does not account for the striking gradient of prevalence between southern and northern Australia: here, the influence of environmental factors seems clear. Migration studies from the United Kingdom (a high-risk region) to South Africa and Australia (both regions with lower risk) also suggest a role for environmental factors. Such factors seem to operate from early life. A serological association with infection with Epstein-Barr virus has been reported in childhood MS,[2] and a higher risk for MS has been described in those who develop infectious mononucleosis as adolescents. The nature of the link between Epstein-Barr virus infection and MS is uncertain but perhaps most likely reflects an immunopathogenic response, possibly as a result of molecular mimicry between viral and myelin epitopes. Recently, the risk for MS has been shown to be modified by month of birth, with a 10% higher prevalence reported in those born in May in the northern hemisphere and a 10% lower prevalence for those born in November.[3]

☐ PATHOGENESIS

Recent insights have developed in the pathogenesis of acute and chronic lesions and – by implication – in our understanding of the early relapsing–remitting and later progressive phase of the disease.[4]

Acute lesions

The 'classic' acute lesion is one in which breakdown of the blood–brain barrier occurs, with trafficking of activated lymphocytes into the perivenous white matter, where – through immune-mediated mechanisms – they trigger breakdown of myelin. Macrophages are prominent in acute lesions and have a role in antigen presentation as well as myelin phagocytosis. Such lesions, when they occur in clinically eloquent locations, are liable to cause relapse. Remission occurs as a result of several factors, including resolution of inflammation, restoration of conduction in demyelinated fibres by sodium channel insertion along the internodal membrane, remyelination (which is common in early MS) and cortical adaptation.

Recent work suggests immunopathogenic heterogeneity, with several distinct subtypes of acute lesions described in different patients:[5] cell-mediated breakdown of myelin and primary destruction or loss of oligodendrocytes, associated with macrophage activation. Some investigators have suggested that individual patients have a unique pathogenic mechanism, but concordance between pathogenic and clinical subtypes has not emerged. The apparent occurrence of oligodendrocyte apoptosis in the absence of an obvious immunopathogenic process challenges the dogma that MS is an autoimmune disease – at least in some instances.[6]

Chronic lesions

A striking observation from the last decade of research is that profound axonal loss occurs in chronic lesions: this is shown directly at post mortem and indirectly with putative magnetic resonance markers of axonal loss such as low N-acetyl aspartate on magnetic resonance spectroscopy or atrophy of the brain or spinal cord – all of which are more pronounced in progressive forms of MS.[7] Loss of axons likely accounts for irreversible and progressive disability. Although some loss of axons occurs directly as a result of the acute inflammatory processes described above, an unresolved question is what causes apparent continuing loss of axons when evidence for persistent inflammation is minimal. A possible explanation is failure of remyelination, because demyelinated fibres with an increased number of internodal sodium channels may be more susceptible to death as a result of unstable ion fluxes, which result in an intracellular increase in calcium. Other explanations may well exist, and a better understanding is needed of the mechanisms that underpin the evolution from milder relapsing remitting to secondary progressive MS with a poorer prognosis.

Normal appearing white matter

A variety of neuropathological abnormalities occur in macroscopically normal appearing white matter in MS. These include astrocyte hyperplasia, microglial activation, small areas of perivascular inflammation or demyelination and loss of axons. Quantitative magnetic resonance imaging techniques show abnormalities, even at the earliest clinical stages of the disease,[8] and some evidence suggests that the evolution of the changes on magnetic resonance images is related to clinical progression of disease. The possibility that changes that occur in normal appearing white matter are of primary pathogenic and prognostic importance warrants further investigation.

Cortical lesions

Recent neuropathological studies have shown that demyelinating lesions occur frequently in the cortex.[9] These are hard to see macroscopically, but careful microscopic examination shows their presence isolated to the cortex or in contiguity with demyelination of subjacent white matter. The cortical lesions show less inflammation than those found in white matter, and conventional magnetic resonance imaging fails to visualise them; however, progressive atrophy of grey matter occurs even in early MS. As for the pathology of normal appearing white matter, further investigation of abnormalities of the cortical grey matter is needed to determine their role in pathogenesis and prognosis.

☐ DIAGNOSIS

An early and accurate diagnosis of a chronic disease is desirable to enable counselling for individual patients and decisions on managing the disease. Nowadays openness with patients in whom the disease is suspected is much greater, and this is appropriate given the implications that a diagnosis of MS may have for lifestyle, work, insurance and treatment decisions. Diagnosis must be correct: considerable harm can be done if MS is diagnosed wrongly. The diagnosis should be made by an experienced neurologist and requires integration of complex information from history, examination and investigative findings, usually magnetic resonance imaging and sometimes cerebrospinal fluid and evoked potentials. Traditional criteria required clinical evidence for dissemination in space and time, but, since 2001, MS can be diagnosed within three months of onset with a single typical clinical episode (eg optic neuritis), with evidence from magnetic resonance imaging for dissemination in space and time.[10] The criteria for imaging are complex and require neurological and neuroradiological expertise to be applied properly. They also lack sensitivity in making an early diagnosis, and modifications may be needed to improve their accuracy and practicality. Revisions to the existing diagnostic criteria are expected in late 2005.

□ MANAGEMENT

The last decade has seen a major change in the patterns of care provided for patients with MS. This has involved many aspects of general and symptomatic management, in addition to the emergence of partially effective disease-modifying treatments.[11]

General aspects and symptomatic management

Optimal care for patients with MS requires multidisciplinary input. Those frequently involved are neurologists, rehabilitation physicians, general practitioners, psychiatrists, specialist nurses, physiotherapists, occupational therapists and speech therapists. Multiple sclerosis has become a subspecialty interest for an increasing number of neurologists in the UK, and the delivery of licensed disease-modifying treatments is provided through more than 60 regional neuroscience centres, each of which has designated neurologists responsible for prescribing. Ten years ago, the concept of a MS specialist nurse was almost unheard of, but now ~175 such nurses practice nationwide. Their role in providing a broad range of readily accessible advice and care to patients with MS has been a welcome and major step forward in achieving better care. In some centres, clinics are available for treating specific aspects of the disease, eg relapses and spasticity. Neurorehabilitation is useful, especially as patients develop moderate or increasing disabilities, and may be delivered through outpatient or inpatients services.

In 2003, the National Institute for Clinical Excellence (NICE) published comprehensive guidelines for the care of people with MS; these cover all aspects of diagnosis and ongoing management. Recent years have witnessed a steady increase in the range of symptomatic pharmacotherapies used in MS – for example, tolterodine for urinary urgency, gabapentin for neuropathic pain, sildenafil for erectile dysfunction and modafinil for MS-related fatigue.

Disease-modifying treatments

Immunosuppression

As evidence indicates that immune-mediated mechanisms of tissue damage are relevant in MS, numerous efforts have been made to treat the disease with global immunosuppressive strategies. By and large, these have been disappointing. Azathioprine reduces the rate of relapse, but only marginally, and it increases the long-term risk of neoplasia. No therapy has been shown to modify the progressive non-relapsing phase of MS, but strong immunosuppression in active relapsing disease associated with inflammatory lesions on magnetic resonance imaging can substantially reduce the frequency of relapse and inflammatory disease activity seen on magnetic resonance images. This has been shown most convincingly with mitoxantrone, and this drug is used to treat rapidly deteriorating MS because of relapses or MS with active magnetic resonance images, or both. Its use is limited by potential serious side effects, including a small risk of acute leukaemia (one in 500 cases) and dose-related cardiotoxicity.

Beta interferon

Beta interferon is a naturally occurring molecule that probably has several immunomodulatory actions, including downregulation of class II expression of MHC. Three licensed preparations are available; all have been prepared by recombinant DNA technology and are administered parenterally (subcutaneously or intramuscularly). All three have been shown to reduce relapse rate by about 30% in placebo-controlled trials of patients with relapsing–remitting MS of two years' duration. Some but not all studies have shown a modest reduction in the accumulation of disability, which is not surprising given that some relapses fail to recover completely. The positive effect on relapses is accompanied by a reduction in the number of new lesions on magnetic resonance imaging, which ranges from 50% to 80%. Beta interferon is not effective in progressive forms of MS, however, and – of critical importance – it is still not known whether treating early relapsing–remitting MS delays the development of secondary progression. Long-term follow up is needed to address the latter question, and, in the UK, this is being conducted as part of a risk-sharing scheme, in which more than 5,000 patients are being monitored through an annual disability assessment. This scheme was established by the Department of Health after NICE concluded that the licensed treatments are not cost effective but also recommended that they are provided to patients with active relapsing disease in a manner that ensures they are made cost effective. Under this scheme, cost effectiveness will be evaluated periodically on the basis of data derived from treated patients being compared with data from historical controls.

Head-to-head studies of the two beta interferon preparations given three or four times a week and the preparation given once weekly indicate that the former have a slightly greater effect in reducing the rate of relapse, although they also are more likely to produce neutralising antibodies, which may reduce efficacy. No data indicate whether any of the three drugs confer a longer term advantage, for example after five years of treatment. Side effects encountered with β interferon are flu-like symptoms (which normally resolve after a few weeks), myalgia, headache, injection site reactions (with subcutaneous preparations), lymphopaenia, altered liver function, menstrual disturbance, alopecia (rare) and (possibly) depression.

Glatiramer acetate

This licensed therapy is given by daily subcutaneous injections and, like β interferon, also reduces the rate of relapse by 30% in patients with relapsing–remitting MS. Whether it affects the evolution of disability in relapsing disease is unknown, and it is ineffective in primary progressive MS. Glatiramer acetate is thought to induce T-regulatory cells that dampen down immune responses against myelin. It can cause injection site reactions including lipoatrophy, and some patients develop an acute sense of panic, with dyspnoea or chest tightness, that is self limiting. Few reports of allergic reactions have been made.

Immunomodulatory therapies under investigation

A novel recent therapeutic approach has been to use anti-adhesion molecule therapies to block the trafficking of white cells across the blood–brain barrier. Such an approach is supported by the observation that gadolinium enhancement, which indicates breakdown of the blood–brain barrier, is often the earliest feature of the formation of new lesions on magnetic resonance imaging in patients with relapse onset MS and by evidence that acute lesions often are perivenular with cuffs of T-lymphocytes, which suggests that blood-borne white cells may trigger immune-mediated demyelination. A monoclonal anti-α4 integrin antibody called natalizumab has shown promising effects in placebo-controlled trials, resulting in a 90% reduction in the number of new enhancing lesions and a decrease of two thirds in the rate of relapse over two years. The drug was licensed for the treatment of relapsing MS by the Food and Drug Administration in the United States in November 2004; however, three cases of progressive multifocal leucoencephalopathy (a serious and frequently fatal CNS infection that usually occurs in immunocompromised individuals) have been reported recently in patients who received natalizumab. As a result, the treatment was discontinued in all patients in February 2005; at the time of going to press, its future role in MS remains to be determined.

A considerable number of other immunomodulatory therapies are undergoing investigation in MS. These include daclizumab (an anti-interleukin 2 antibody shown to reduce new enhancing lesions by 80%), campath-1H (a pan-lymphocyte-depleting monoclonal antibody shown to reduce enhancing lesions by 90%) and several other types of cytokine and chemokine blockade.

Neuroprotection

Where the existing licensed disease-modifying treatments are thought to be immunomodulatory and anti-inflammatory, thus diminishing the rate of relapse, progressively increasing disability in MS is widely believed to be the result of increasing neuroaxonal loss that is not necessarily related to inflammation. Proposed mechanisms of axonal loss include a lack of trophic support from oligodendrocytes and myelin, unstable ion current in axons because of an excess of sodium channels in demyelinated axons (which, however, may have the beneficial effect of enabling conduction in the presence of demyelination) or low-grade damage mediated by microglia or other inflammatory molecules. Interest thus exists in applying neuroprotective strategies in progressive MS. A trial of lamotrigine (a sodium-channel blocker) funded by the MS Society of Great Britain and Northern Ireland is due to start later in 2005. In addition to assessing disability, magnetic resonance imaging is being used to measure atrophy to evaluate potential neuroprotective agents.

Remyelination

Much current interest is in remyelination as a means to restore function but also to protect axons and enhance their long-term survival. Current neuroscience research is investigating several strategies, including neurotrophic factors, remyelinating immunoglobulins and stem cells. Along with developing therapeutic strategies, tools are needed to detect remyelination when it occurs: measurement of the magnetisation transfer ratio on magnetic resonance images may be useful.

□ CONCLUSION

The perception and understanding of MS has undergone enormous change in the last decade. Diagnosis is made earlier and more confidently, and a culture of openness exists with patients throughout all stages of the illness – from prediagnosis onwards. Diagnosis is more reliable, and magnetic resonance imaging is a sensitive tool for monitoring and understanding the course of MS. Much has been learnt about the underlying pathogenic mechanisms, and partially effective treatments have become available for relapsing–remitting MS. Trial designs have improved, as have the tools for therapeutic monitoring. We are still a long way short of preventing disease progression and reversing disabilities, but the prospects for continued progress in meeting these challenges seem better than ever.

REFERENCES

1   Ebers GC, Sadovnick AD, Dyment DA, Yee IM *et al.* Parent-of-origin effect in multiple sclerosis: observations in half-siblings. *Lancet* 2004;**363**:1773–4.

2   Alotaibi S, Kennedy J, Tellier R, Stephens D *et al.* Epstein-Barr virus in pediatric multiple sclerosis. *JAMA* 2004;**291**:1875–9.

3   Willer CJ, Dyment DA, Sadovnick AD, Rothwell PM *et al.* Timing of birth and risk of multiple sclerosis: population based study. *BMJ* 2005;**330**:120.

4   Compston A, Coles A. Multiple sclerosis. *Lancet* 2002;**359**:1221–31.

5   Lucchinetti C, Bruck W, Parisi J, Scheithauer B *et al.* Heterogeneity of multiple sclerosis lesions: implications for the pathogenesis of demyelination. *Ann Neurol* 2000;**47**:707–17.

6   Barnett MH, Prineas JW. Relapsing and remitting multiple sclerosis: pathology of the newly forming lesion. *Ann Neurol* 2004;**55**:458–68.

7   Miller DH, Barkhof F, Frank JA, Parker GJ *et al.* Measurement of atrophy in multiple sclerosis: pathological basis, methodological aspects and clinical relevance. *Brain* 2002;**125**:1676–95.

8   Fernando KT, McLean MA, Chard DT, MacManus DG *et al.* Elevated white matter myo-inositol in clinically isolated syndromes suggestive of multiple sclerosis. *Brain* 2004;**127**: 1361–9.

9   Peterson JW, Bo L, Mork S, Chang A *et al.* Transected neuritis, apoptotic neurons, and reduced inflammation in cortical multiple sclerosis lesions. *Ann Neurol* 2001;**50**:389–400.

10 McDonald WI, Compston A, Edan G, Goodkin D *et al.* Recommended diagnostic criteria for multiple sclerosis: guidelines from the International Panel on the Diagnosis of Multiple Sclerosis. *Ann Neurol* 2001;**50**:121–7.

11 Noseworthy JH. Management of multiple sclerosis: current trials and future options. *Curr Opin Neurol* 2003;**16**:289–97.

Advances in headache management

Peter J Goadsby

☐ INTRODUCTION

Headache dominates neurology outpatient appointments[1] and is one of the most common disorders that present to doctors. A day with severe migraine is considered by the World Health Organization to be as disabling as a day spent quadriplegic.[2] There is thus a need to know about headache disorders and a considerable opportunity to make many patients much better. Traditionally, headache has been consigned little time for teaching among the pressures of ever-increasing knowledge in the world of increasing patient expectations. Many developments in headache in recent times have particular relevance to clinical practice, and, as such, doctors need to follow these changes to optimise the care of their patients. I have highlighted here some developments that cut across the neurobiology of headache and its clinical management. Interested readers are referred to a recent monograph for a more detailed account of the broader management of headache disorders.[3]

☐ CLASSIFICATION OF HEADACHE

The development and promulgation of the International Headache Society's diagnostic criteria in 1988 was perhaps one of the great advances of the late twentieth century for headache. The criteria provided clear and homogenous populations that formed the basis of all the important studies in the 1990s. They did not suffer from the vagueness of the 1962 *Ad Hoc* classification, but in this research strength, the classification has its clinical Achilles' heel. Although it is essential to define clear populations for research, this can force artificial distinctions in clinical practice. Many things in biology exist with a continuous distribution. Presentation of some individual headache syndromes might be expected to be on some clinical continuum, and it thus can be difficult to make diagnoses and define appropriate management. In this light, it is not surprising that patients based in headache clinics sometimes have not fitted the system, although for most patients it does work very well.

The second edition of the classification has seen fine tuning of the migraine classification and the inclusion of some important headache types not previously dealt with at all.[4] The classification of migraine has been modified for paediatric populations by allowing less feature-full headaches. In addition, some further thought has been given to the childhood periodic syndromes – cyclical vomiting, abdominal migraine and benign paroxysmal vertigo of childhood – that so often portend migraine in adolescence and adulthood.

Section three on cluster and related headaches has been altered to accommodate the range of phenotypes of what have been termed the trigeminal autonomic cephalalgias (TACs).[5] These syndromes share the pathophysiological feature of pronounced activation of the cranial parasympathetic autonomic outflow in association with the pain.[6] The terminology in section three has been standardised, such that chronic implies the form of the disorder that does not have breaks of at least one month and episodic is the form that has breaks of a month or more. Both cluster headache and paroxysmal hemicrania have episodic forms, and this is now recognised. Short-lasting attacks of unilateral neuralgiform headache with conjunctival injection and tearing (SUNCT) has been included.

Other headaches not previously recognised in the 1988 classification include hemicrania continua, hypnic headache and primary thunderclap headache. These are important, as the first two respond well to therapy and the latter has important management implications. Hemicrania continua is very sensitive to indomethacin,[7] and hypnic headache usually responds to lithium.[8]

Chronic daily headache

The most controversial issue in headache classification, indeed in some respects in clinical practice, is how to deal with the problem of frequent, daily or near-daily headache. Some 5% of North American and Western European populations have headache on 15 days or more a month for, on average, four or more hours a day. If shorter lasting headaches are included, chronic daily headache is simply a syndrome defined by frequent headache[9] – not just tension-type headache. Chronic daily headache may be associated with medication overuse but it is not compulsory. It often is equated incorrectly with the concept of transformed migraine, which is a subset of chronic daily headache (Table 1). Similarly, although the International Headache Society has narrowly defined new daily persistent headache,[4] I use it in the syndromic sense, which helps me remember to look for the important secondary causes (Table 2). The concept that migraine sufferers may have a less severe daily headache is not new at all, being recognised by luminaries of the nineteenth century, including Gowers. The revised International Headache Society has adopted the term chronic migraine for patients who experience migraine without aura for 15 days or more a month. This seems a biologically implausible dichotomy. Moreover, the committee has not been explicit in its reasoning for excluding patients with probable migraine from the umbrella of chronic migraine. In my clinical practice, I take this as an omission, and I use transformed migraine, as Silberstein-Lipton have evolved the concept (Table 3), to indicate 15 days or more a month of migraine or probable migraine. It seems to make more biological sense, as we see similarities, for example, in functional brain imaging in episodic and chronic migraine.[10–13]

□ GENETICS OF HEADACHE

For the moment, the genetics of headache is the genetics of migraine. It seems logical to suppose all the primary headaches have a predisposition that is in some way

Table 1 Classification of chronic daily headache (headache on 15 days or more a month that may be due to a range of underlying mechanisms and may be complicated by *or* caused by medication overuse).

Primary		Secondary*
More than four hours a day	**Less than four hours a day**	

Chronic migraine
Transformed migraine†
	Chronic cluster headache‡	Post-traumatic:
		  Head injury
		  Iatrogenic
		  Post-infectious

Chronic tension-type headache	Chronic paroxysmal hemicrania	Inflammatory:
		  Giant cell arteritis
		  Sarcoidosis
		  Behçet's syndrome

Hemicrania continua	Short-lasting attacks of unilateral neuralgiform headache with conjunctival injection and tearing	Chronic infection of the central nervous system
New daily persistent headache**	Hypnic headache	Medication overuse headache

*List is illustrative rather than exhaustive.
†Chronic migraine is a term used by international classification of headache disorders (IHCD)-2 that is, in essence, migraine without aura for 15 days or more a month. Transformed migraine is a more useful term in clinical practice. A current working definition is included in Table 3.
‡Patients with chronic cluster headache may have more than fours a day of headache. The inclusion of the syndrome here is to emphasise that, by and large, the attacks themselves are less than four hours in duration.
**This term is used by ICHD-II,[4] but I find the more generic approach of Table 2 clinically practical.

Table 2 Differential diagnosis of new daily persistent headache.

Primary (phenotype)	Secondary (cause)
• Migrainous-type • Featureless (no sensory sensitivity*)	• Subarachnoid haemorrhage • Low-volume headache • Raised cerebral spinal fluid-pressure headache • Post-traumatic headache† • Chronic meningitis

*No sensitivity to light, sound, smells, head movement or throbbing component to the headache.
†Indicates trauma in the broad sense of insult to cranial structures, such as blunt trauma or post-infective triggers to headache.

activated by physiological means and other life events, such as puberty. Clinically, each of cluster headache, paroxysmal hemicrania and SUNCT can be seen to run in families. Overall, it seems a good way to understand primary headache. For migraine, the description of missense mutations in the $Ca_V2.1$ subunit of the P/Q voltage-gated Ca^{2+} channel gene on chromosome 19 in families with familial

Table 3 Transformed migraine – modified Silberstein-Lipton/American Headache Society criteria.

A	Headache frequency ≥15 days/month for three months
B	Average headache duration of ≥4 hours/day (if untreated)
C	Headache fulfilling International Headache Society's criteria for migraine without aura (1.1), migraine with aura (1.2) or probable migraine (1.6) on ≥50% of the headache days
D	Does not meet International Headache Society's criteria for chronic tension-type headache (2.3), hypnic headache (4.5), hemicrania continua (4.7) or new daily persistent headache (4.8)
E	Not attributed to another disorder

Comment:
- Headache may fulfil any combination of 1.1, 1.2, and 1.6 on 50% or more of total headache days per month.
- It is important to detect patients with medication overuse (use of an acute attack treatment for more than 10 days a month), as this problem needs to be addressed if treatment with a preventive is to be successful.

hemiplegic migraine (FHM) was a milestone in the field.[14] This effort was boosted further by the description of mutations in *ATP1A2*, which encodes the α_2 subunit of the Na^+/K^+ pump. Some families with more routine forms of migraine can be linked to chromosome 19 and some to the X chromosome, and migraine is part of the phenotype of mitochondrial cytopathies; however, the genotype–phenotype correlations remain disappointing. Clearly we will reach a point when the known syndromes can be checked by DNA analysis of apparently affected patients, and hopefully this will guide therapy.

☐ PATHOPHYSIOLOGY OF HEADACHE

Classic neurology as promulgated by Gowers sought to provide anatomical answers to clinical questions. In many ways, Sherington changed this and sought a physiological approach. The anatomical approach has been very successful, but the problems of primary headache will need a physiological approach to clinical neurology (after Lance JW[3]). To some extent, human functional imaging begins to do this. In the 1960s and 1970s, migraine was considered a vascular phenomenon, and it often still is referred to incorrectly as a vascular headache. Wolff summarised the referral patterns of intracranial pain-producing structures in his classic book; he took the view that migraine aura was the result of vasoconstriction and the subsequent headache the result of a reactive vasodilatation. Olesen debunked this link. The spreading depression theory points out that the flow changes after metabolic demand blood flow alterations in response to vasoneuronal coupling.[15] When the features of attack, such as nausea, photophobia and phonophobia (which do not occur in all cases), or of the premonitory phase, such as yawning or diuresis, are considered, the vascular hypothesis seems unattractive. The totality of the attack might suggest that the brain, brainstem or diencephalon indeed were likely to be the sites of the *lesion*.

Positive emission tomography (PET) scanning in acute migraine showed activations in the rostral brainstem that persisted after the successful treatment of the attack but were not present interictally.[16] These changes are not seen in experimentally induced ophthalmic division pain[17] or cluster headache.[18] We observed a patient in a bout of cluster headache who had a phenotypic migraine in the PET scanner and had brainstem changes consistent with migraine and not cluster headache.[10] From images of further spontaneous attacks, the dorsal rostral pons seems a crucial area activated consistently in migraine.[11] In chronic migraine, defined as migraine without aura on 15 days or more a month for more than six months,[4] the same area of the dorsolateral pons is activated on PET,[13] which suggests that infrequent and frequent migraine are the same problem. Use of blood oxygen level-dependent (BOLD) contrast, functional magnetic resonance imaging holds the promise of allowing study of single patients and determination of the site of abnormal activation.[19] Moreover, magnetic resonance angiography has allowed flow changes seen in migraine and cluster headache[10,18] to be shown as simply a result of ophthalmic division pain – not a cause of the syndrome.[20,21]

Another recent finding with neuroimaging that further supports the importance of the brainstem, particularly the dorsolateral pons, in migraine is that changes lateralise with the attack. Study of attacks of typical migraine triggered by nitroglycerin shows that patients with left-sided attacks have left-sided brain activation and patients with right-sided attacks have right-sided activation, while patients with bilateral pain have bilateral activation.[12] These data suggest that the dorsolateral pons is pivotal in the phenotypic expression of migraine as a lateralised syndrome. These changes persist after resolution of the pain with a triptan, are not present interictally and were not seen in a control group scanned with the same design but in whom migraine did not develop. Moreover, the pontine change is not seen during the dull bilateral nitroglycerin-induced headache phase in controls or patients with migraine.[12] An understanding of the candidate areas in the pons, such as the nucleus locus coeruleus (the major noradrenergic nucleus of the brain), may provide insights into the disorder and direction for preventive management.

☐ MIGRAINE – WHAT NEW TREATMENTS CAN WE EXPECT?

Triptans (serotonin 5-HT$_{1B/1D}$ receptor agonists) served as foot soldiers for the advances in migraine during the latter part of the twentieth century. Many patients with migraine were liberated in a way that they had not previously experienced, clinical trial guidelines were refined and revised and clinical studies were well organised and uniform. After sumatriptan came zolmitriptan, naratriptan, rizatriptan, almotriptan, eletriptan and frovatriptan;[22] donitriptan has just finished preclinical development. Ergotamine, the mainstay of specific acute treatment for most of the twentieth century after its initial description in the nineteenth century, is now treatment of choice in few indications.[23] Patients clearly want rapid, complete and consistent pain relief, but how they decide between the available treatments is not established entirely. That most patients do have preferences for individual triptans when asked is established. Table 4 sets out some situations in which the various triptans may be helpful.

Table 4 Clinical stratification of acute specific migraine treatments.

Clinical situation	Treatment options

Failed analgesics or non-steroidal anti-inflammatory drugs	First tier:
	  Sumatriptan 50 mg or 100 mg orally
	  Rizatriptan 10 mg orally
	  Almotriptan 12.5 mg
	  Eletriptan 40 mg orally
	  Zolmitriptan 2.5 mg orally
	Slower effect or better tolerability:
	  Naratriptan 2.5 mg
	  Frovatriptan 2.5 mg
	Infrequent headache:
	  Ergotamine 1–2 mg orally
	  Dihydroergotamine nasal spray 2 mg

Early nausea or problems taking tablets	Sumatriptan 20 mg nasal spray Zolmitriptan 5 mg nasal spray Rizatriptan 10 mg orally disintegrating wafer Zolmitriptan 2.5 mg dispersible
Headache recurrence	Ergotamine 2 mg (perhaps most effective as needed and usually with caffeine) Naratriptan 2.5 mg orally Eletriptan 80 mg
Tolerating acute treatments poorly	Naratriptan 2.5 mg Frovatriptan 2.5 mg
Early vomiting	Sumatriptan 25 mg as needed Sumatriptan suppositories

Menstrual-related headache	Prevention:
	  Ergotamine orally at night
	  Oestrogen patches
	Treatment:
	  Triptans
	  Dihydroergotamine nasal spray

Very rapidly developing symptoms	Sumatriptan 6 mg subcutaneously Dihydroergotamine 1 mg intramuscularly

New treatments

Of the unmet needs, three readily come to mind.

First, a considerable need exists for the development of preventive medications. On average, two-thirds of patients will have a 50% reduction in headache frequency with most preventive drugs. They can then choose between the potential for sleepiness, exercise intolerance, erectile impotence, nightmares, dry mouth, weight gain, tremor, hair loss and fetal deformities as possible side effects. That patients with migraine do make such choices is an important statement about the level of disability they experience. The recent reporting of positive clinical trials with topiramate established its use in migraine.

Second, treatments for non-vascular acute attacks are needed for patients who cannot be given triptans or ergot derivatives. Publication of a clinical trial in which

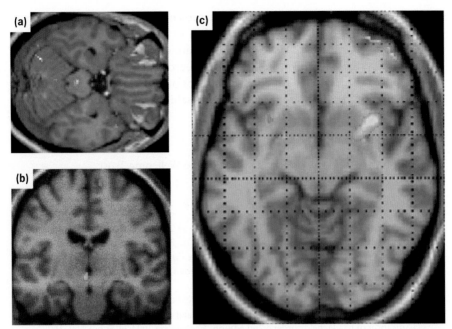

Figure 1 Positron emission tomography findings in **(a)** migraine[10] **(b)** cluster headache[18] and **(c)** experimental head pain[17]. Activation of rostral brainstem structures in migraine and posterior hypothalamic grey matter in cluster headache seem relatively specific for the syndromes, as neither are seen in experimental ophthalmic (first) division head pain. The findings support the view that primary neurovascular headaches, migraine and cluster headache fundamentally are disorders of the nervous system. Figures 1a and 1b reprinted from Refs 10 and 18 respectively with permission from Elsevier; Fig 1c reprinted from Ref 17 with permission from the International Association for the Study of Pain.

BIBN4096BS – a potent, specific, calcitonin gene-related peptide antagonist – was effective compared with placebo in acute migraine[24] at once answers the pressing pathophysiological issue of the primacy of the nerves and vessels and provides the beginning of a crucial advance in therapy. It is useful to observe that the advance was predicted by laboratory work more than a decade ago,[25,26] and the translation of the basic experimental work to clinical practice illustrates the importance of basic neurobiology to advancing clinical practice. Vasoconstriction is clearly not now needed to abort acute migraine. Indeed, a recent demonstration that sildenafil, a phosphodiesterase inhibitor, will induce migraine without changes in cerebral vessel diameter provides perhaps the last nail in the coffin for the vascular theory. From a therapeutic viewpoint, the development of non-vasoconstrictor treatments for migraine offers an important development in terms of safety, which will be welcomed by doctors and patients alike.

□ CONCLUSION

To say that the future of headache is bright is no exaggeration. A better classification and new understanding of the basic cause in terms of genetics, the pathophysiology from functional brain imaging and the management in terms of new therapies is very promising. Headache is the most common of human maladies, which is its greatest limitation. Familiarity is a horrible limitation to interrogation of a subject, and so it is with headache. For the established neurologist, headache is a necessity, for our patients a major cause of disability and for our community a major burden of cost. Advances in medicine can alleviate the disability and the burden.

□ ACKNOWLEDGEMENTS

The work of the author has been supported by the Wellcome Trust.

REFERENCES

1   Carson AJ, Ringbauer B, MacKenzie L, Warlow C *et al.* Neurological disease, emotional disorder, and disability: they are related: a study of 300 consecutive new referrals to a neurology outpatient department. *J Neurol Neurosurg Psychiatry* 2000;**68**:202–6.

2   Menken M, Munsat TL, Toole JF. The global burden of disease study: implications for neurology. *Arch Neurol* 2000;**57**:418–20.

3   Lance JW, Goadsby PJ. *Mechanism and management of headache.* New York: Elsevier, 2005.

4   Headache Classification Committee of the International Headache Society. The international classification of headache disorders: 2nd edition. *Cephalalgia* 2004;**24**(Suppl 1):9–160.

5   Goadsby PJ, Lipton RB. A review of paroxysmal hemicranias, SUNCT syndrome and other short-lasting headaches with autonomic features, including new cases. *Brain* 1997;**120**: 193–209.

6   May A, Goadsby PJ. The trigeminovascular system in humans: pathophysiological implications for primary headache syndromes of the neural influences on the cerebral circulation. *J Cereb Blood Flow Metab* 1999;**19**:115–27.

7   Matharu MS, Boes CJ, Goadsby PJ. Management of trigeminal autonomic cephalalgias and hemicrania continua. *Drugs* 2003;**63**:1637–77.

8   Dodick DW, Mosek AC, Campbell JK. The hypnic ('alarm clock') headache syndrome. *Cephalalgia* 1998;**18**:152–6.

9   Welch KM, Goadsby PJ. Chronic daily headache: nosology and pathophysiology. *Curr Opin Neurol* 2002;**15**:287–95.

10 Bahra A, Matharu MS, Buchel C, Frackowiak RS *et al.* Brainstem activation specific to migraine headache. *Lancet* 2001;**357**:1016–7.

11 Afridi S, Giffin NJ, Kaube H, Friston KJ *et al.* A PET study in spontaneous migraine. *Arch Neurol* 2005;**62**:1270–75.

12 Afridi S, Matharu MS, Lee L, Kaube H *et al.* A PET study exploring the laterality of brainstem activation in migraine using glyceryl trinitrate. *Brain* 2005;**128**:932–9.

13 Matharu MS, Bartsch T, Ward N, Frackowiak RS *et al.* Central neuromodulation in chronic migraine patients with suboccipital stimulators: a PET study. *Brain* 2004;**127**:220–30.

14 Ferrari MD, Haan J, Palotie A. Genetics of migraine. In: Olesen J, Tfelt-Hansen P, Welch KMA (eds), *The headaches.* Philadelphia: Lippincott Williams & Wilkins, 2003.

15 Lauritzen M. Pathophysiology of the migraine aura. The spreading depression theory. *Brain* 1994;**117**:199–210.

16 Weiller C, May A, Limmroth V, Juptner M *et al.* Brain stem activation in spontaneous human migraine attacks. *Nat Med* 1995;**1**:658–60.

17 May A, Kaube H, Buchel C, Eichten C *et al.* Experimental cranial pain elicited by capsaicin: a PET study. *Pain* 1998;**74**:61–6.

18 May A, Bahra A, Buchel C, Frackowiak RS *et al.* Hypothalamic activation in cluster headache attacks. *Lancet* 1998;**352**:275–8.

19 May A, Bahra A, Buchel C, Turner R *et al.* Functional magnetic resonance imaging in spontaneous attacks of SUNCT: short-lasting neuralgiform headache with conjunctival injection and tearing. *Ann Neurol* 1999;46:791–4.

20 May A, Buchel C, Turner R, Frackowiak RSJ *et al.* Neurovascular dilatation of intracranial vessels in experimental headache. *Cephalalgia* 1999;19:464–5.

21 May A, Buchel C, Turner R, Goadsby PJ. Magnetic resonance angiography in facial and other pain: neurovascular mechanisms of trigeminal sensation. *J Cereb Blood Flow Metab* 2001;21: 1171–6.

22 Goadsby PJ. The pharmacology of headache. *Prog Neurobiol* 2000;62:509–25.

23 Tfelt-Hansen P, Saxena PR, Dahlof C, Pascual J *et al.* Ergotamine in the acute treatment of migraine: a review and European consensus. *Brain* 2000;123:9–18.

24 Olesen J, Diener HC, Husstedt IW, Goadsby PJ *et al.* Calcitonin gene-related peptide (CGRP) receptor antagonist BIBN 4096 BS for the acute treatment of migraine. *N Engl J Med* 2004; 350:1104–10.

25 Goadsby PJ, Edvinsson L, Ekman R. Release of vasoactive peptides in the extracerebral circulation of humans and the cat during activation of the trigeminovascular system. *Ann Neurol* 1988;23:193–6.

26 Goadsby PJ, Edvinsson L, Ekman R. Vasoactive peptide release in the extracerebral circulation of humans during migraine headache. *Ann Neurol* 1990;28:183–7.

□ NEUROLOGY SELF ASSESSMENT QUESTIONS

Update in multiple sclerosis

1 The following are implicated in the aetio-pathogenesis of multiple sclerosis:
   (a) Human leucocyte antigen genes
   (b) Neurotoxins
   (c) Trauma
   (d) Environmental triggers, probably including viral infections
   (e) T lymphocytes

2 Regarding the pathophysiology of multiple sclerosis:
   (a) Relapses are the result of acute inflammatory lesions and an abnormal blood–brain barrier
   (b) Remyelination is uncommon in early multiple sclerosis
   (c) Most permanent disability is the result of demyelination with conduction block
   (d) Most permanent disability is the result of axonal loss
   (e) Cortical lesions are common but hard to detect on magnetic resonance imaging

3 By current criteria, the diagnosis of multiple sclerosis can be made:
   (a) With no clinical symptoms but typical magnetic resonance imaging and cerebrospinal fluid abnormalities
   (b) After one typical clinical episode plus magnetic resonance imaging evidence for dissemination in space and time
   (c) After one clinical episode plus a single abnormal magnetic resonance imaging scan at symptom onset
   (d) In people with normal magnetic resonance images
   (e) After two typical clinical episodes disseminated in space and time

4 Beta interferon has proved efficacy in the following types of multiple sclerosis:
   (a) Relapsing–remitting multiple sclerosis with frequent relapses
   (b) Relapsing–remitting multiple sclerosis with no relapses for 10 years
   (c) Secondary progressive multiple sclerosis without relapses
   (d) Primary progressive multiple sclerosis
   (e) Acute relapses of multiple sclerosis (shortens relapse duration)

Advances in headache management

1 Referring to chronic daily headache:
   (a) This is an uncommon disorder that affects fewer than 0.1% of the population
   (b) Means the same thing as chronic tension-type headache
   (c) Always is associated with overuse of prescribed drugs
   (d) Has primary and secondary forms

2   Migraine:
   (a) Is a disorder of the cranial vessels
   (b) Requires each of nausea, photophobia and phonophobia to make the
        diagnosis
   (c) Can occur daily
   (d) Generally lacks a significant family history

3   Migraine is associated with:
   (a) Activations in functional brain imaging in the dorsolateral pons
   (b) Activations in functional brain imaging in the frontal cortex cingulate
        cortex not seen in other headache types
   (c) Almost no significant incidence in childhood
   (d) May require a combination of preventive and acute attack treatments

Hepatology

Advances in viral hepatitis

Nikolai Naoumov

Chronic infections with the hepatitis B virus (HBV) or hepatitis C virus (HCV) are the principal causes of hepatitis, cirrhosis and hepatocellular carcinoma worldwide. Infection with HBV is one of the most common viral infections in humans. More than 2 billion people worldwide are estimated to have been exposed to the virus and 400 million are chronic carriers of HBV.[1,2] About 170 million people worldwide have chronic HCV infection, and a proportion of them will develop cirrhosis and liver cancer.[3] Chronic HCV infection can be associated with several extrahepatic manifestations, including essential mixed cryoglobulinaemia, B-cell non-Hodgkin's lymphoma, glomerulonephritis, seronegative arthritis and neurological conditions.

During the last few years, major advances in viral hepatitis have occurred in several directions.

☐ Advances in the standardisation of nomenclature and definitions of different stages of infection and treatment response.

☐ New insights into the molecular biology of HBV and HCV as well as the mechanisms of antiviral immune response in the host.

☐ Increasing range of treatment options, particularly with potent antiviral agents for patients with hepatitis B.

☐ Clinical evidence of the major impact of antiviral treatment in controlling progression of liver disease and reducing the rate of complications.

☐ CHRONIC HEPATITIS B

Standardisation of nomenclature and definitions

Chronic infection with the hepatitis B virus is defined as persistence of hepatitis B surface antigen (HBsAg) in the serum for more than six months.[1] Patients with chronic hepatitis B are characterised with virological and biochemical parameters, as well as liver histology (Table 1). Quantification of serum HBV DNA is essential to define the level of viral replication in a patient with chronic HBV infection. Currently, the value of 10^5 viral DNA copies/ml is considered to be a level of replication below which no significant necroinflammatory changes occur in the liver.[1] This is not an absolute cut-off value, however, and should be interpreted in conjunction with the results of other investigations performed on more than one

Table 1 Standardisation of terminology in chronic HBV infection.

Terms		Diagnostic criteria
Chronic hepatitis B	1	Serum HBsAg positivity longer than six months
	2	Persistent or intermittent elevation of ALT/AST levels
	3	Serum HBV DNA >10^5 copies/ml
	4	Liver biopsy with a necroinflammatory score ≥4
Inactive HBsAg carrier	1	Serum HBsAg positivity greater than six months
	2	HBeAg negative; anti-HBe positive
	3	Serum HBV DNA <10^5 copies/ml
	4	Persistently normal serum ALT/AST levels
	5	Liver biopsy* showing absence of significant inflammation (necroinflammatory score <4)
Resolved hepatitis B	1	Serum HBsAg negative; anti-HBc positive
	2	Normal serum ALT levels
	3	History of known acute or chronic hepatitis B
	4	Undetectable serum HBV DNA (hybridisation assays)†

*Liver biopsy in these circumstances is optional.
†HBV DNA may de detectable using sensitive PCR assays.

occasion. One of the current limitations is that the diagnostic assays for HBV DNA quantification are not standardised: they have different sensitivities and units to measure viraemia levels. Thus, results may differ between laboratories, and this needs to be borne in mind in clinical practice.

Molecular characteristics of HBV

One of the new developments over the last few years has been the recognition of different genotypes of HBV. At present, eight HBV genotypes have been identified, designated genotypes A–H. These naturally occurring variants of the virus differ in approximately 10% of the nucleotide sequences over the entire HBV genome. The distribution of HBV genotypes worldwide has a distinct geographical pattern: genotype A is prevalent in northern Europe and the United States, genotypes B and C are found exclusively in the Far East, while genotype D is predominant in southern Europe and the Middle East. Genotype E almost entirely is restricted to West Africa, while HBV genotype F was found in Central and South America.[4] The other two genotypes have been reported in individual cases in France and the United States (genotype G) and patients from Central America (genotype H). With the accumulating knowledge on the impact of different HBV genotypes, determination of the HBV genotype is likely to become part of routine diagnosis for patients with chronic hepatitis B over the next few years. The data so far indicate that certain HBV genotypes (genotype A and B in particular) respond better to treatment with interferon than genotypes C and D. The impact of different HBV genotypes on the severity of chronic hepatitis B is under investigation.

Immunopathogenesis of chronic HBV infection

The diversity of clinical manifestations and the outcome of HBV infection depend primarily on the host's immune response to the virus. The dominant cause of viral persistence in patients with chronic HBV infection is weak T-cell reactivity to viral antigens. The validity of this concept was shown directly in patients with haematological malignancies who also had chronic infection with HBV. In such patients, bone-marrow transplantation with marrow from human leucocyte antigen (HLA)-matched donors with natural immunity to HBV led to resolution of chronic HBV infection and clearance of HBsAg.[5] Resolution of HBV infection, however, is now known not to mean viral eradication, as HBV DNA usually persists in the liver and mononuclear cells – even in patients with natural immunity to HBV. Sensitive poly-merase chain reaction-based assays can detect HBV DNA in these patients. As long as they have strong T-cell reactivity to the virus, however, no significant level of replica-tion or liver inflammation is seen. Thus, the concept emerging over the last few years is that after exposure to hepatitis B virus, sterilising immunity does not occur. Instead, the infection is similar to that with the herpes simplex or Epstein-Barr viruses, where the viral genome persists in the host. This maintains the T-cell memory, and, if the person has adequate antiviral T-cell reactivity from both CD4+ and CD8+ T-lymphocytes, HBV replication is kept under control and there is no hepatic inflammation.

In patients with chronic hepatitis B, two different forms now are recognised: hepatitis Be Ag (HBeAg) positive and anti-hepatitis Be (anti-HBe) positive.[1] Patients with anti-HBe-positive chronic hepatitis B usually are infected with a mutant strain of HBV that is unable to produce HBeAg as a result of mutations in the precore region. The presence of precore mutant HBV does not imply a more severe hepatitis B. This form of chronic hepatitis B is increasingly common in areas in which the HBV genotypes B, C or D are prevalent, and the clinical course is characterised by fluctuating levels of HBV DNA, which are mirrored by fluctuating levels of alanine aminotransferase and progressive liver disease.

New treatments for chronic hepatitis B

The ultimate goal of therapy in patients with chronic hepatitis B is to reduce progression of liver disease and reverse fibrosis (Fig 1). Accumulating evidence indicates that long-term suppression of HBV replication ($<10^5$ copies/ml) is the key to achieving this goal. In a proportion of patients, antiviral treatment can achieve sustained control of HBV replication – that is, suppression of HBV replication continues after antiviral treatment stops. This is achieved in one third of patients with HBeAg-positive chronic hepatitis B after seroconversion to anti-HBe and in 15–20% of patients with anti-HBe positive chronic hepatitis B. In the remaining patients with chronic hepatitis B, suppression of HBV replication requires maintained inhibition – that is, continuous antiviral therapy for years.

Currently, three drugs are licensed for the treatment of chronic hepatitis B: interferon alpha, which is given parenterally, and two oral drugs – lamivudine and adefovir dipivoxil. Treatment with interferon is of finite duration, durability of response is good and no drug-resistant mutations have been reported. Recent data

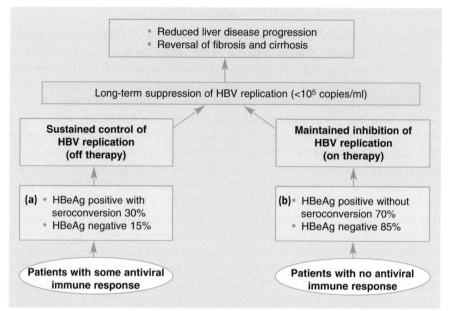

Fig 1 Achieving the goals of therapy in chronic hepatitis B. (a) Antiviral treatment with a finite duration can achieve sustained suppression of hepatitis B virus replication in a proportion of patients – amongst HBeAg positive chronic hepatitis B these are patients with seroconversion to anti-HBe (20–30% after 12 months of treatment) and approximately 15% of HBeAg negative chronic hepatitis B. These patients usually have some antiviral immune reactivity. (b) Patients who remain HBeAg positive on treatment (after 12 months approximately 70%), and the majority of HBeAg negative chronic hepatitis B would require long-term therapy to maintain the inhibition of HBV replication, in order to achieve the goals of therapy.

with pegylated interferon show that 12 months of treatment is associated with HBeAg seroconversion in one third of patients. The limitations of interferon treatment are the parenteral application, cost and considerable side effects. Lamivudine offers the advantage of having minimal side effects; however, long-term treatment leads to emergence of drug-resistant HBV mutants. Adefovir dipivoxil has a moderate antiviral effect; its main advantage is that it is effective against lamivudine-resistant HBV. Long-term treatment with adefovir is associated with a much lower rate of drug resistance. Renal toxicity is a possible concern with long-term use of adefovir.

Several new antiviral agents are in phase III clinical trials and are expected to be licensed for clinical use in the next few years. These include entecavir, telbivudine, tenofovir, and clevudine (L-FMAU). The new pegylated interferon has shown improved efficacy compared with standard interferon, in addition to convenience (administration is by once-weekly injections).

The success of antiviral treatment for chronic hepatitis B in the last few years is illustrated by three recent studies. In a prospective, double-blind, placebo-controlled trial, more than 600 patients with compensated cirrhosis or very advanced liver fibrosis were randomised to receive lamivudine or placebo.[6] Disease progression during the study was defined as an increase in the Child-Pugh score of at least two points or development of hepatocellular carcinoma, renal insufficiency or bleeding varices. The study was terminated after 32 months by the Study Review Board because of a significant difference between the lamivudine-treated patients and placebo group in terms of disease progression. Only 7.8% of patients treated with lamivudine experienced disease progression compared with 18% of the placebo group.[6]

The second example is the use of lamivudine to prevent reactivation of HBV in patients who need chemotherapy for the treatment of solid tumours or haematological malignancies.[7] The use of lamivudine to suppress HBV replication in parallel with chemotherapy is now established as an effective treatment that, given in parallel with chemotherapy for all patients positive for HBsAg, is effective in preventing post-chemotherapy flares with hepatitis and liver failure.

Prolonged treatment with lamivudine is associated with development of treatment-resistant HBV mutants. One of the major benefits of adefovir dipivoxil is that it is effective against lamivudine-resistant HBV.[8] Treatment with adefovir dipivoxil added to lamivudine in patients with chronic hepatitis B with compensated or decompensated liver disease is associated with effective virus suppression and marked improvement in liver function tests.

☐ CHRONIC HEPATITIS C

Hepatitis C virus is a small, enveloped RNA virus. The viral genome comprises 9,600 nucleotides and encodes a single polyprotein that is cleaved into 10 polypeptides, including structural and non-structural proteins.[4] The virus replicates predominantly in the cytoplasm of hepatocytes, where it has no cytopathic effect. Six major genotypes (1–6) and more than 50 subtypes of HCV have been identified. Different genotypes of HCV have distinct geographical distributions in their prevalence. Genotype 1a is the prototype and is most common in the United States and northern Europe. Genotype 1b has a worldwide distribution. Genotype 2 represents 10–30% of all genotypes of HCV and particularly is common in Japan and Northern Italy. Genotype 4 is the most common genotype in Africa and the Middle East. The HCV genotypes differ little in clinical expression, and no difference is seen in clinical outcomes or severity of liver disease. Infection with any genotype can lead to cirrhosis, end-stage liver disease or hepatocellular carcinoma. Two features of different HCV genotype infections deserve special attention. Firstly, genotype 3 has been associated with a propensity to steatosis on liver biopsy, which resolves after disappearance of HCV infection. Secondly, the HCV genotype is most important in determining the duration and likelihood of response to current antiviral treatments.

Natural course of HCV infection

In acute infection, HCV RNA can be detected in the serum of almost all patients within 1–2 weeks of exposure. Levels of alanine aminotransferase in serum, which are indicative of hepatocyte necrosis, start to increase between two and eight weeks after exposure. About one third of adults with acute HCV infection will develop clinical symptoms with jaundice. The average onset of symptoms is one week (range 3–12 weeks) after exposure.[3]

Chronic HCV infection is defined as persistence of HCV RNA in the serum for at least six months. Patients who develop chronic infection are less likely to have symptoms or jaundice than those with acute resolving hepatitis C. Once chronic infection is established, levels of HCV RNA in serum tend to stabilise, and spontaneous resolution of chronic HCV infection is very rare – in prospective studies, this has been observed in <2% of patients with chronic HCV infection.

Liver histology shows chronic mononuclear cell infiltrate and a variable degree of fibrosis. The degree of necroinflammatory activity and the pattern of fibrosis are considered the best prognostic features for predicting future worsening of fibrosis and development of cirrhosis. These factors make liver biopsy the gold standard for grading and staging of chronic hepatitis C.

Long-term complications of chronic hepatitis C

The major long-term complications of chronic hepatitis C are cirrhosis, end-stage liver disease and hepatocellular carcinoma.[3] Progression to cirrhosis often is clinically silent, and some patients are not known to have HCV infection until they present with signs of end-stage liver disease. Infection with HCV has a variable course and outcome. During chronic HCV infection, progressive worsening of fibrosis can occur in a proportion of patients. Hepatocellular carcinoma appears typically after decades of infection, usually in a patient with underlying cirrhosis. Between 55% and 85% of patients with acute HCV infection develop chronic infection. Successful antiviral treatment leads to resolution of chronic HCV infection, which is associated with marked improvement in clinical symptoms and liver histology, including resolution of hepatic inflammation and reversal of fibrosis.

After the discovery of HCV and the subsequent introduction of diagnostic assays, the incidence of acute HCV infection declined markedly; however, this has little impact on the existing pool of patients with chronic hepatitis C and related liver and extrahepatic complications. Analysis of the burden of HCV-related liver diseases in the United States projected that the proportion of patients with cirrhosis will

Table 2 Definitions of response to antiviral treatment in patients with chronic hepatitis C.

Response	Definition
Biochemical	Normalisation of serum ALT
Virological	Serum HCV RNA (qualitative and quantitative testing)
Early virological response	HCV RNA not detectable or $>2 \log_{10}$ decrease in viraemia
End-of-treatment response	HCV RNA not detectable
Sustained virological response	HCV RNA not detectable six months after end of treatment
Histological	Liver biopsy – score of inflammation grade and stage of fibrosis

increase from 16% to 32% by 2020 in the untreated population.[9] Complications of cirrhosis also are projected to increase over the next 20 years, with hepatic decompensation up 106%, hepatocellular carcinoma up 81% and liver-related deaths up 180%. Many more patients would need to be treated to alter this trend in liver complications.

Treatment of chronic hepatitis C

During the last decade, remarkable improvements have been achieved in the results of treatment in patients with chronic hepatitis C (Fig 2). Interferon alpha emerged as the early treatment option, but only a very small proportion of patients achieved a sustained virological response. The addition of ribavirin to standard interferon treatment significantly improved the long-term virological response. More recently, the development of pegylated interferon plus ribavirin has shown a further improvement in outcomes in patients with genotypes 2 and 3, achieving sustained virological response in up to 80% after six months; in patients with genotype 1, the rate of sustained virological response is 50% after 12 months of treatment.[10]

Long-term follow up of patients with a sustained virological response clearly shows the benefit of clearance of HCV, as it leads to regression of fibrosis in a substantial proportion of patients. Pooled individual data from 3,010 treatment-naïve patients with pre-treatment and post-treatment liver biopsies shows that all treatment regimens significantly reduce the progression of fibrosis, with reversal of cirrhosis in 49% of patients with baseline cirrhosis in the liver biopsy.[11] Although the issue of possible sampling error is frequently mentioned, there is no doubt that a sustained virological response is associated with regression of fibrosis and improved prognosis in patients with chronic HCV infection. Meta-analysis of 14 clinical trials with interferon also favours the treatment option in prevention of

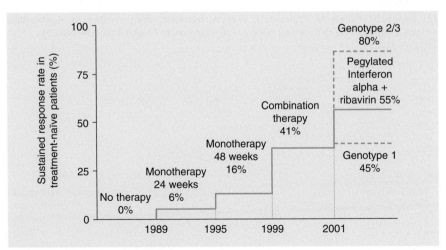

Fig 2 Improvement in sustained response rates with evolution of treatment regimens in chronic hepatitis C.

hepatocellular carcinoma in patients with HCV cirrhosis.[12] The preventative effect is more evident in patients with a sustained virological response, and as this has steadily increased with the use of pegylated interferon plus ribavirin, the beneficial effect in preventing hepatocellular carcinoma would be more apparent in future analyses.

REFERENCES

1   EASL Jury. EASL International Consensus Conference on Hepatitis B. 13-14 September, 2002: Geneva, Switzerland. Consensus statement (short version). *J Hepatol* 2003;**38**:533–40.

2   Ganem D, Prince AM. Hepatitis B virus infection – natural history and clinical consequences. *N Engl J Med* 2004;**350**:1118–29.

3   Lauer GM, Walker BD. Hepatitis C virus infection. *N Engl J Med* 2001;**345**:41–52.

4   Naoumov NV. Hepatitis viruses, including TTV. In: Warrell D, Cox T, Firth J, Benz E. *Oxford textbook of medicine. Volume 1*. Oxford: Oxford University Press, 2003: 414–9.

5   Lau GK, Suri D, Liang R, Rigopoulou EI *et al.* Resolution of chronic hepatitis B and anti-HBs seroconversion in humans by adoptive transfer of immunity to hepatitis B core antigen. *Gastroenterology* 2002;**122**:614–24.

6   Liaw YF, Sung JJ, Chow WC, Farrell G *et al.* Lamivudine for patients with chronic hepatitis B and advanced liver disease. *N Engl J Med* 2004;**351**:1521–31.

7   Lau GK, Yiu HH, Fong DY, Cheng HC *et al.* Early is superior to deferred preemptive lamivudine therapy for hepatitis B patients undergoing chemotherapy. *Gastroenterology* 2003;**125**:1742–9.

8   Perrillo R, Hann HW, Mutimer D, Willems B *et al.* Adefovir dipivoxil added to ongoing lamivudine in chronic hepatitis B with YMDD mutant hepatitis B virus. *Gastroenterology* 2004;**126**:81–90.

9   Davis GL, Albright JE, Cook SF, Rosenberg DM. Projecting future complications of chronic hepatitis C in the United States. *Liver Transpl* 2003;**9**:331–8.

10   Poynard T. Treatment of hepatitis C virus: the first decade. *Semin Liver Dis* 2004;**24** (Suppl 2):19–24.

11   Poynard T, McHutchison J, Manns M, Trepo C *et al.* Impact of pegylated interferon alfa-2b and ribavirin on liver fibrosis in patients with chronic hepatitis C. *Gastroenterology* 2002;**122**: 1303–13.

12   Camma C, Giunta M, Andreone P, Craxi A. Interferon and prevention of hepatocellular carcinoma in viral cirrhosis: an evidence-based approach. *J Hepatol* 2001;**34**:593–602.

Primary biliary cirrhosis

David EJ Jones, Julia L Newton

☐ INTRODUCTION

Primary biliary cirrhosis (PBC) was first described in the 1850s. The first detailed descriptions, made a century later, were of a rare, rapidly progressive and uniformly fatal form of chronic liver disease. Over the next 50 years, it has become clear, however, that the disease is significantly more common, and the spectrum of disease severity significantly broader, than previously thought. The explanation for this evolution in the clinical picture is increased efficiency of diagnosis of less clinically overt and milder forms of the disease. The pitfall associated with this evolution, however, is that some aspects of the older literature that relates to PBC has lost its relevance to the typical modern patient, who has a relatively low risk of death from liver disease but is much more likely to experience prolonged impairment of their health-related quality of life. Current estimates suggest disease prevalence rates of up to 35 per 100,000, with a significant (10:1) female predominance. The highest rates of incidence are seen in middle age. The cumulative effect of these demographic effects is that PBC affects up to one in 700 women older than 45 years in high-prevalence geographical areas such as northeastern England.[1]

This review aims to give a modern perspective on the pathogenesis, clinical features and treatment of PBC.

☐ PATHOGENESIS

Primary biliary cirrhosis is characterised by damage to, and ultimately loss of, the biliary epithelial cells (BEC) that line the small intrahepatic bile ducts (Fig 1). Loss of bile ducts results in progressive cholestasis, with characteristic biochemical and symptomatic sequelae outlined below. Retention of hydrophobic bile salts in particular results in a cycle of secondary BEC and hepatocyte damage that amplifies tissue damage and contributes to the progressive development of portal tract fibrosis and cirrhosis. The rate of progression to cirrhosis varies significantly among patients, for reasons that at present are unclear. Hepatocellular function typically is maintained well until late in the disease process, although decompensation, when it occurs, can be rapid, creating practical problems in terms of the optimum timing of liver transplantation.

Damage to the BEC typically is accompanied by the formulation of granulomas and a significant, T-cell rich, portal tract, mononuclear cell infiltrate.[2] The T-cell infiltrate is mixed in phenotype, although CD8+ effector T-cells predominate in the

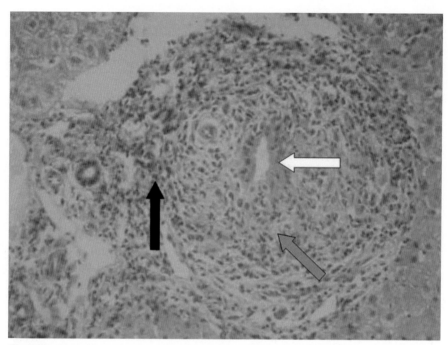

Fig 1 Bile duct lesion in classic early primary biliary cirrhosis. The damaged bile duct (white arrow) is accompanied by a T-cell rich mononuclear cell infiltrate (grey arrow) and granuloma formation (black arrow). Immunohistochemical studies confirm that the T-cell phenotype is mixed, with CD8+ cells typically predominating around the bile duct.

areas directly adjacent to damaged ducts. The BEC in effected ducts have been shown to express markers indicative of apoptosis, which leads to the view that apoptosis, triggered by infiltrating T-cells, is a key effector process for target cell damage.[3] It should be borne in mind, however, that apoptosis of BEC could represent, in part at least, a secondary phenomenon that results from the effects of retained hydrophobic bile salts. Indeed, studies of very early disease (which are difficult to perform because patients rarely undergo liver biopsy at this most informative stage) have suggested the presence of little apoptosis of BEC. An alternative mechanism for early 'loss' of BEC – epithelial to mesenchymal transition (EMT) driven by TGF-β-expressing T-cells – has been proposed. If applicable, this mechanism may hold important implications for the development of future treatments given its potential reversibility.

Broad consensus is that the pathogenesis of PBC has a significant autoimmune component, with the implication that the effector responses that mediate BEC apoptosis and/or EMT themselves are autoreactive. Primary biliary cirrhosis certainly is characterised by the almost universal presence of autoantibody and autoreactive T-cell responses. The predominant of these responses in PBC are directed at members of the 2-oxoacid dehydrogenase family of multienzyme complexes present in the M2 fraction on the inner mitochondrial membrane, particularly pyruvate dehydrogenase complex (PDC) (Fig 2). The descriptive term

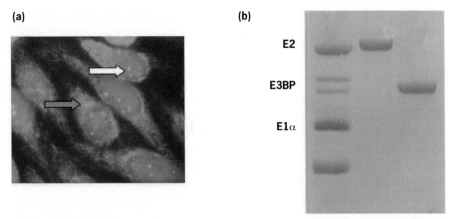

Fig 2 Autoantibodies in primary biliary cirrhosis. Autoantibodies in pooled sera from patients with primary biliary cirrhosis shown by immunofluorescence on HepG2 cells (a) mitochondrial (anti-mitochondrial antibodies) and multiple nuclear dot (antinuclear antibodies) staining patterns are shown (grey and white arrows, respectively). Immunoblot of the same sera against human pyruvate dehydrogenase complex (PDC) (b) reactivity with PDC-E2, PDC-E3BP and, in this serum aliquot, PDC-E1α is seen (left hand lane). Antibody reactive with recombinant PDC-E2 (middle lane) also shows reactivity with recombinant PDC-E3BP following elution (right hand lane), demonstrating cross-reactivity between PDC-E2 and PDC-E3BP.

for these collective mitochondrial antigen-directed autoantibody responses (anti-mitochondrial antibodies (AMA)), which was coined before the identification of individual target antigens, remains in common use to this day. The dominant AMA responses, seen in more than 95% of patients, are directed at the dihydrolipoamide acetyltrasferase (E2) and E3 binding-protein components of PDC.[3] These responses are fully cross-reactive and are directed against a unique domain motif shared between PDC-E2 and PDC-E3BP, which binds a lipoic acid cofactor essential for complex enzymatic function. Indeed, covalent modification of lipoic acid, potentially by environmental xenobiotics, has been implicated in bypassing normal immune tolerance mechanisms, thereby predisposing to the development of autoreactive immune responses to lipoic acid-containing proteins in genetically susceptible individuals.[4,5]

Autoreactive T-cell responses reactive with epitopes that span the lipoic acid-binding residue in PDC-E2 also are specific for patients with PBC and enriched in liver.[2,6] Given the target cell changes seen in liver tissue in patients with PBC, these autoreactive T-cells, which have been shown to have antigen specific cytotoxic capacity in vitro,[6] represent a plausible effector system for damage to BEC. Although the humoral compartment of the immune response seems to play little role in direct target cell damage, it may play a key upstream role in priming autoreactive T-cell responses.

Autoantibodies reactive with nuclear autoantigens are seen in a minority of, typically AMA-negative, patients with PBC (see Fig 2).[7] These antibodies, which show characteristic immunofluorescence patterns (multiple nuclear dot and nuclear rim) have been studied less well than AMA, and the T-cell responses to the associated autoantigens (Sp100 and gp210) have not been studied at all. The disease phenotype seems to be identical between patients positive for AMA and those positive for antinuclear antibodies.

☐ CLINICAL FEATURES

Changes in patterns of diagnosis and our increasing perception of the true spectrum of the disease have led to a significant broadening of the range of clinical phenotypes recognised in patients with PBC. Most patients who present in the modern era do not now exhibit the 'classic' form of end-stage disease described by Sheila Sherlock. Instead, they present with what might be described conveniently as 'non-classic' forms of disease – a grouping that would include asymptomatic disease and disease associated with non-stage specific symptoms.

'Classic' clinical features

The classic view of PBC is one of disease progression culminating in the development of biliary cirrhosis. Hepatocellular function subsequently decompensates (initially episodically with patient recovery but in the final stages of disease in a sustained fashion), which resulted ultimately, in the days before liver transplantation, in the patient's death. The classic clinical features of PBC therefore are chronic cholestasis and biliary cirrhosis, exemplified by the development of jaundice and pruritus, followed by ascites and the clinical features of portal hypertension and, latterly, hepatic encephalopathy (Fig 3). Patients are characterised by cholestatic serum biochemical markers (disproportionately increased levels of alkaline phosphatase, with progressive increases in conjugated bilirubin) and, in the end stages of the disease, reduced levels of serum albumin and prolongation of the prothrombin time. Cholesterol levels (predominantly high-density lipoprotein) characteristically are increased (again a cholestatic rather than PBC-specific feature)

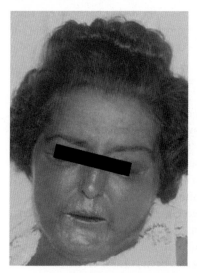

Fig 3 A patient with classic end-stage primary biliary cirrhosis. The patient has deep jaundice with skin pigmentation. The peri-orbital bruising is a consequence of coagulopathy and the imapirment of conscience level a consequence of encephalopathy. Note also the xanthelasmata and facial oedema.

and xanthelasma formation is common. This form of disease still is seen in the context of late-presenting patients and as an end stage of progression in patients who present with milder forms of the disease, although optimal clinical practice would be to transplant such patients long before the end stage of disease is reached.

'Non-classic' clinical features

The most common presentations of PBC in the modern era are asymptomatical after biochemical or serological screening (*vide infra*) or after development of symptoms that are not associated with progressive disease – most typically fatigue. Fatigue is well established now as a significant clinical problem in PBC, and one that can often reduce dramatically a patient's health-related quality of life.[8] It also is clear that no association exists between severity of fatigue and severity of underlying disease; indeed, fatigue often is at its most debilitating in patients with histologically and biochemically mild disease. An important corollary of this observation is that treatments that slow disease progression have no effect on fatigue and its impact on health-related quality of life. As the sole focus in development of treatment for PBC to date has been to slow progression of disease, the often very real clinical issues associated with fatigue have been neglected. This historical tendency towards a one-dimensional view of the disease is now being addressed widely.

As most patients now present with non-classic features, a key question arises as to the natural history of subsequent disease in such patients. Although the risk of disease progression remains, the disease course can be extremely prolonged, with a significant proportion of patients remaining in early stage disease throughout a normal lifespan.[9] In this respect, the prognosis associated with non-classic disease can be very good. However, two concerns are emerging. Firstly, even in patients who show little or no disease progression, health-related quality of life can remain significantly impaired over many years. This can lead to situations where doctors' perceptions about the management success (good because of little or no disease progression) and their patients' perceptions (bad because of little or no improvement in health-related quality of life) can diverge dramatically, damaging the therapeutic relationship. Secondly, emerging data from long-term follow-up studies suggest that, although liver-related mortality remains relatively low in patients with non-classic disease, their overall mortality is elevated significantly, with an excess of non-liver-related deaths.[1] One factor seems to be an increase in cardiac-related deaths (particularly sudden cardiac death). In this respect, it is worth noting that patients with PBC have a high (and stage-unrelated) prevalence of autonomic dysfunction; a finding that has, in other settings, been linked with an increased risk of sudden cardiac deaths. Further work in this area to delineate the non-liver risks faced by patients with PBC and determine the pathological processes underpinning these risks and potential interventions is needed badly.

Other clinical issues

In addition to specific features of the disease, issues of clinical importance relate to disease complications and associated disease processes.[10] Significant complicating processes typically are associated with advanced classic disease. These include increased risks of hepatocellular carcinoma (particularly increased in men) and osteoporosis. Given the condition's autoimmune aetiology, that the most significant disease associations in PBC are with other autoimmune conditions is unsurprising.[5] The most significant issue in terms of management is the potential for overlap with autoimmune hepatitis.

☐ DIAGNOSIS

Three parameters are important for the diagnosis of PBC (Fig 4):[1]

- ☐ the presence of cholestatic serum liver biochemistry

- ☐ the presence of compatible or diagnostic liver histology

- ☐ the presence of AMA or a PBC-associated ANA at a significant titre (conventionally >1:80).

Conventionally, the presence of all three features is regarded as indicative of 'definite PBC', two features as 'probable PBC' and one feature (typically AMA or ANA in the context of normal biochemistry) as 'possible PBC' (although follow-up studies suggest that these patients are at risk of developing more typical disease forms over time).[9] Many clinical centres (including the authors' own) are moving away from histological confirmation of uncomplicated disease. This has occurred as a result of concerns about the risks of biopsy and the potential for false negative results because of the patchy nature of disease. The 95% sensitivity and specificity of AMA detection for disease diagnosis make the combination of this finding with appropriate biochemistry sufficient in most situations.[7] The most commonly encountered situations in which biopsy still is highly useful are in:

- ☐ patients with possible overlap syndrome (significantly elevated immunoglobulin (Ig) G (rather than the increased IgM more typically seen in patients with PBC) or disproportional increases in transaminases)

- ☐ patients with potential AMA, ANA-negative disease

- ☐ patients in whom ascertainment of the stage of disease (ie the presence of stage IV or cirrhotic disease) is of clinical significance, such as in the context of transplant referral.

Monitoring of disease progression through repeat biopsy still has some value, although concerns about safety and the effects of disease non-homogeneity remain. Interest is emerging in non-invasive protocols for assessment of progression, including factors such as splenic size on ultrasound scanning and lowering of the platelet count as predictors of portal hypertension.

☐ TREATMENT

Therapy in PBC has two largely independent goals: prolongation of life and improvement of the quality of that life.

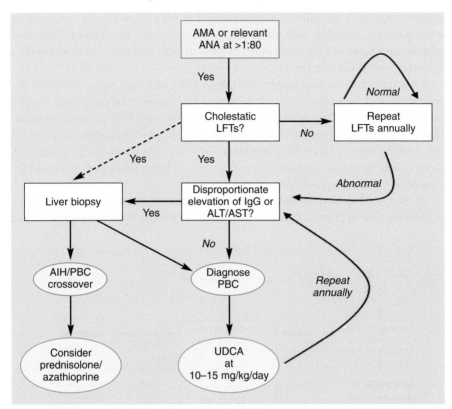

Fig 4 A suggested pathway for the diagnosis and treatment of primary biliary cirrhosis (PBC). This pathway reflects the authors' own clinical practice. The broken arrow represents an optional step (biopsy confirmation of otherwise uncomplicated disease). Immunoglobulin G (IgG) greater than 1.5 times the upper limit of normal (ULN) and/or aspartate aminotransferase (AST)/alanine aminotransferase (ALT) greater than four times the ULN, although lower thresholds should be applied in cases of particular concern. AIH = autoimmune hepatitis; AMA = antimitochondrial antibodies; ANA = antinuclear antibodies; LFTs = liver function tests; UDCA = ursodeoxycholic acid.

Mortality-directed treatment

The conventional goal of treatment in PBC has been to reduce mortality from development of end-stage disease. The only drug with evidence from randomised, placebo-controlled trials to support its generalised use is the hydrophilic bile acid ursodeoxycholic acid (UDCA); this probably has a (limited) beneficial effect through reduction of secondary damage in the liver that results from accumulation of toxic, hydrophobic bile acids (see Fig 4).[10] Even this agent is controversial, with a number of trials showing no benefit in terms of patient survival.[11] All trials agree that the drug itself is free of significant side effects. The consensus in the field is that UDCA probably is beneficial for patients if started before the development of cirrhosis. In light of our current understanding of the mechanisms of action, the contradictory findings of drug trials probably reflect suboptimal design (ie short-term use of the drug in patients with typically advanced disease). The use of prednisolone (with or without azathioprine) has been shown to be beneficial in some patients, although side-effect issues limit its use. In practice, immuno-suppressive treatment largely is limited to patients with PBC/autoimmune hepatitis crossover syndromes (see Fig 4).

Liver transplantation is highly effective in PBC, although concerns about the potential for disease recurrence are increasing.[12] A number of prognostic models (exemplified by the Mayo model) help with the optimum timing of transplantation, although the potential for rapid decline in the end stages of the disease and current and growing waiting times for transplantation should always be borne in mind. A useful rule of thumb is always to refer patients whose bilirubin exceeds 50 μmol/l for consideration of transplantation.

As the risk of death from end-stage liver disease has decreased, so the importance of reducing mortality from non-liver causes has increased. At present, however, the

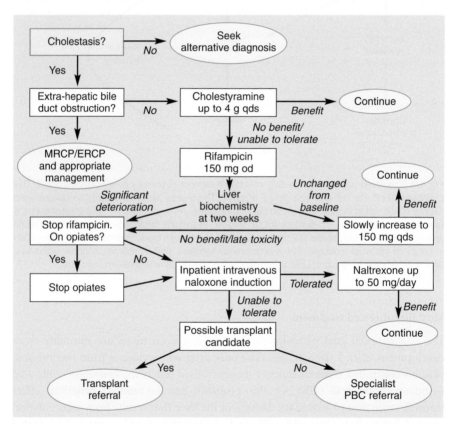

Fig 5 A suggested pathway for the management of pruritus in primary biliary cirrhosis. This pathway reflects the authors' own clinical practice. Some centres would advocate the use of opiate antagonist therapy before the use of rifampicin. The cautionary steps of checking liver function after the institution of rifampicin and the use of an intravenous naloxone induction step (where the dose is incrementally increased from 0.002 μg/kg/min to 0.2 μg/kg/min over 72 hours) reflect the potential clinical problems encountered with rifampicin and naltrexone (hepatotoxicity and opiate withdrawal reaction, respectively). ERCP = endoscopic retrograde cholangiopancreatography; MRCP = magnetic resonance cholangiopancreatography; od = once a day; qds = four times a day.

appropriate assessment and intervention is unclear, and further research is needed. The issue of cardiac risk in patients with non-classic disease is a particular concern at present.

Morbidity-directed treatment

The major factors in impairment of health-related quality of life in patients with PBC, other than the small subset with end-stage disease, are fatigue and pruritus. The mechanism that gives rise to fatigue remains unclear, although it is the subject of intensive ongoing research. At present, no evidence-supported treatments are available for fatigue in PBC. The possibility that associated disease processes such as hypothyroidism and anaemia secondary to B12 deficiency or coeliac disease (all of which are associated with PBC) and type II diabetes mellitus (which is common given the patient demographic) are giving rise to fatigue should be borne in mind. Pruritus, the most plausible mechanism for which is retention of endogenous opiates in cholestasis, is, in contrast to fatigue, relatively easily treated (Fig 5). Transplantation for symptom relief and improvement in health-related quality of life is controversial and should be avoided if possible.

REFERENCES

1   Prince M, Chetwynd A, Newman W, Metcalf JV *et al.* Survival and symptom progression in a geographically based cohort of patients with primary biliary cirrhosis: follow-up for up to 28 years. *Gastroenterology* 2002;**123**:1044–51.

2   Jones DE. Pathogenesis of primary biliary cirrhosis. *J Hepatol* 2003;**39**:639–48.

3   Yeaman SJ, Kirby JA, Jones DE. Autoreactive responses to pyruvate dehydrogenase complex in the pathogenesis of primary biliary cirrhosis. *Immunol Rev* 2000;**174**:238–49.

4   Palmer JM, Robe AJ, Burt AD, Kirby JA *et al.* Covalent modification as a mechanism for the breakdown of immune tolerance to pyruvate dehydrogenase complex in the mouse. *Hepatology* 2004;**39**:1583–92.

5   Jones DE, Donaldson PT. Genetic factors in the pathogenesis of primary biliary cirrhosis. *Clin Liver Dis* 2003;**7**:841–64.

6   Kita H, Matsumura S, He XS, Ansari AA *et al.* Quantitative and functional analysis of PDC-E2-specific autoreactive cytotoxic T lymphocytes in primary biliary cirrhosis. *J Clin Invest* 2002;**109**:1231–40.

7   Jones DE. Primary biliary cirrhosis. *Autoimmunity* 2004;**37**:325–8.

8   Goldblatt J, Taylor PJ, Lipman T, Prince MI *et al.* The true impact of fatigue in primary biliary cirrhosis: a population study. *Gastroenterology* 2002;**122**:1235–41.

9   Metcalf JV, Mitchison HC, Palmer JM, Jones DE *et al.* Natural history of early primary biliary cirrhosis. *Lancet* 1996;**348**:1399–402.

10 Heathcote EJ. Management of primary biliary cirrhosis. The American Association for the Study of Liver Diseases practice guidelines. *Hepatology* 2000;**31**:1005–13.

11 Goulis J, Leandro G, Burroughs AK. Randomised controlled trials of ursodeoxycholic-acid therapy for primary biliary cirrhosis: a meta-analysis. *Lancet* 1999;**354**:1053–60.

12 Liermann Garcia RF, Evangelista Garcia C, McMaster P, Neuberger J. Transplantation for primary biliary cirrhosis: retrospective analysis of 400 patients in a single center. *Hepatology* 2001;**33**:22–7.

☐ HEPATOLOGY SELF ASSESSMENT QUESTIONS

Advances in viral hepatitis

1   In patients with chronic hepatitis B, the level of hepatitis B virus replication is assessed by testing:
(a) HBeAg in serum
(b) Anti-HBe in serum
(c) Liver histology
(d) Levels of HBV DNA in serum
(e) Immunoglobulin M anti-HBc

2   Antiviral treatment in chronic hepatitis B is indicated:
(a) For all HBsAg-positive patients
(b) Only for HBeAg-positive patients
(c) For patients with levels of alanine aminotransferase greater than twice the upper level of normal and HBV DNA greater than 10^5 viral copies/ml
(d) Patients with raised levels of alanine aminotransferase, irrespective of levels of HBV DNA
(e) Patients with normal levels of alanine aminotransferase and levels of HBV DNA $<10^5$ viral copies/ml

3   In chronic hepatitis C, the presence of a sustained response to antiviral treatment is defined as HCV RNA not detectable at:
(a) End of treatment
(b) One month after stopping treatment
(c) Three months after stopping treatment
(d) Six months after stopping treatment
(e) One year after the end of treatment

4   The main side effect of ribavirin is:
(a) Headache
(b) Haemolytic anaemia
(c) Low platelets
(d) Flu-like symptoms
(e) Fever

Primary biliary cirrhosis

1   Primary biliary cirrhosis is:
(a) More common in women than men, in a ratio of 6:1
(b) Most common in women younger than 30 years
(c) More common in women than men, in a ratio of 10:1
(d) Increasing in prevalence in northern Europe
(e) Seen in one in 7,000 women older than 40 years in northern England

2   Primary biliary cirrhosis is characterised by:
  (a) Immune-mediated damage to hepatocytes
  (b) Immune-mediated damage to biliary epithelial cells
  (c) Apoptosis of biliary epithelial cells
  (d) Formation portal tract granulomas
  (e) A T-cell rich mononuclear cell infiltrate in which CD4+ cells predominate
      in the areas adjacent to bile ducts

3   Which of the following findings would be typical of a patient with early
     primary biliary cirrhosis?
  (a) Serum levels of anti-mitochondrial antibodies at a titre >1:80
  (b) Increased concentrations of serum bilirubin
  (c) Decreased concentrations of serum albumin
  (d) Prolonged prothrombin time
  (e) Increased concentrations of serum alkaline phosphatase

4   With respect to the treatment of primary biliary cirrhosis:
  (a) Most patients will benefit from high-dose prednisolone
  (b) Most patients will benefit from ursodeoxycholic acid
  (c) Rifampicin is effective at slowing disease progression
  (d) Naltrexone is effective at treating pruritus
  (e) Transplantation should be considered only once the level of bilirubin
      exceeds 200 µg/ml

Respiratory

Respiratory

Advances in therapy of asthma

Douglas Robinson

☐ INTRODUCTION

The publication of the British Thoracic Society/Scottish Intercollegiate Guideline Network's guidelines on management of asthma has provided, for the first time, an evidence-based framework for therapy.[1] This document highlights the good evidence base for anti-inflammatory treatment with inhaled steroids (ICS), the addition of long-acting β_2 agonists (LABA) if control is not achieved with moderate doses of ICS and the importance of self-management and education in the delivery of these highly effective drugs. The guidelines also focus, however, on the lack of evidence for treatment of more severe asthma at steps 4 and 5 and the continued morbidity from asthma despite current drugs. How then can we optimise treatment of asthma with existing therapies and what does the future hold for new treatments?

Optimal delivery of currently used drugs

One key message of the British guidelines for asthma management is the importance of written asthma management plans. These are underused despite excellent evidence that they can improve outcomes.[1] Current treatments include ICS combined with LABA. Recent developments suggest novel ways of using these drugs to achieve better asthma control, such as patient adjustment of therapy and increasing the dose in an aim to achieve control of asthma symptoms and lung function based on the guideline's definitions of control.[2,3]

New therapies for asthma

During the last 20 years, our understanding of the immunological basis of allergic asthma has increased and acceptance of the roles of immunoglobulin (Ig) E and T helper (Th) 2-type T cells in perpetuating airway inflammation and thus bronchial hyper-responsiveness and asthma symptoms has become widespread.[4] Perhaps the most exciting new development in asthma therapy has been the development of monoclonal antibodies that prevent IgE from binding to its high-affinity receptor (FcɛRI). The initiation of allergic reactions depends on cross-linking of allergen-specific IgE bound to high affinity receptors (FcɛRI) on mast cells and basophils: blocking such immediate hypersensitivity reactions thus clearly is an attractive target for allergic disease. A monoclonal antibody (termed E25) was developed that could bind to free IgE in the serum with very high affinity via the C3 portion that interacts with FcεRI. This antibody thus prevents binding of IgE to its receptor and does not cross-link any IgE already bound (an important feature, as this prevents any potential for severe allergic reactions or anaphylaxis to be triggered). This preparation, omalizumab, has been subject to a number of clinical studies in asthma and other allergic diseases.[5] Initial studies showed that anti-IgE could reduce not only the mast-cell dependent immediate response to inhaled allergen challenge (the early asthmatic reaction) but also the delayed late asthmatic reaction.[6] Although such activity could be the result of reduced activation of mast cells, it is also of note that high-affinity IgE receptors are found on dendritic cells – antigen-presenting cells that process allergen and activate Th2 cells – therefore, omalizumab may target both the IgE and T cell limbs of the allergic immune response.

A number of studies of omalizumab in moderate and severe allergic asthma in adults and children confirmed that the drug can reduce exacerbation rates. Most of these studies had a similar study design and included patients with continuing symptoms and/or impairment of lung function despite the use of ICS and sometimes oral corticosteroids (but not LABA). These studies were included recently in a systematic review for the Cochrane airways group's database.[7] One study gave two-weekly intravenous omalizumab to 317 patients. The initial 12-week, steroid-stable phase showed a reduction in asthma symptom score (primary endpoint) from 4.0 to 2.8 in the high- and low-dose active treatment groups and 3.1 in those treated with placebo. During the next eight weeks of steroid withdrawal, 78% of patients on active high-dose treatment could reduce their oral steroids by ≥50% compared with 57% in the low-dose group and 33% in the placebo group.[8] A significant increase also was seen in morning peak flow in the high-dose group compared with the placebo group at week 12, but no effect was noted on forced expiratory volume in one second (FEV_1) or dose of ICS (reviewed in Holgate[5]). Subsequent large studies used subcutaneous treatment and found that omalizumab reduced the rate of exacerbations (0.28 per patient for omalizumab versus 0.54 per patient for placebo in the steroid-stable phase of one study[9]) and modestly reduced the dose of ICS (this was maintained in a 24-week extension of the study). One study also showed a small but significant improvement in FEV_1 (reviewed in Holgate[5]). More recent studies in severe asthma confirm a reduction in rates of exacerbation but did not all show a reduction in the need for oral steroids or increase in lung function (reviewed in Holgate[5]). Overall, the systematic review concluded that omalizumab has activity in moderate and severe allergic asthma but that further comparative and paediatric data are required.[7] Studies in patients who already are taking LABA and other treatments in addition to ICS will be needed particularly, as this drug is likely to be expensive and perhaps most useful at steps 4 and 5 of the guidelines. The drug is licensed in the United States but not yet in Europe. It will be important to confirm whether this treatment can reduce exacerbation rates and the need for oral steroids: accurate targeting to those who may benefit will be important. It will be of interest to see if this approach also is useful in patients with non-allergic asthma, as evidence suggests local IgE synthesis in this condition.

☐ ANTI-TUMOUR NECROSIS FACTOR

Tumour necrosis factor-α is a proinflammatory cytokine that activates macrophages and increases adhesion molecule and chemokine expression in many inflammatory settings. Soluble-receptor therapy has shown dramatic benefit in patients with rheumatoid arthritis and inflammatory bowel disease, and expression of TNFα is increased in the airway in patients with asthma,[8] although other anti-inflammatory agents effective in arthritis have not always shown efficacy in asthma. Nonetheless, a recent open-label study reported only in abstract form suggested an ability to improve lung function and reduce symptoms of asthma in patients with severe asthma who are dependent on oral steroids.[9] Two recent double-blind, placebo-controlled studies, so far reported in abstract form only, suggest benefit in patients with severe asthma. The place of this treatment and the types of patients who might benefit await confirmation.

☐ OTHER ANTICYTOKINE AGENTS

Cytokines

Studies from animal models of airway allergen challenge allowed specific targeting of cytokines by gene disruption (knockouts), antibody treatment to block cytokine activity or the use of soluble receptors as blockers of cytokine activity. Such approaches suggested that interleukin (IL) 4, IL-5 and IL-13 would be valid targets for therapy, although it is of note that different models can give different results (reviewed in Robinson[10]). After initially promising data with an inhaled soluble IL-4 receptor in a model of provoked asthma after ICS treatment was withdrawn, however, follow-on studies in day-to-day use are thought not to have confirmed this early promise – although these have not been reported yet. The obvious reluctance of pharmaceutical companies to publish adverse data from trials has impacted on the publication of studies of anti-IL-4 and anti-IL-5, which is regrettable for patients with asthma who eagerly are awaiting effective new therapies.

Interleukin 13 has activities similar to those of IL-4, which is not surprising as it shares receptor components; blockade of IL-13, like that of IL-4, thus might be expected to impact on IgE switching and expression of adhesion molecules and chemokines. Murine experiments, however, suggest that IL-13, which also has its own unique receptor complex, may be an exciting target for asthma, since soluble IL-13Ralpha chain (which will bind IL-13) was able to block airway hyper-responsiveness in a model without affecting eosinophils or IgE. This approach has not been tested yet in humans.

Interleukin 5 emerged from the Th2/eosinophil hypothesis as perhaps the most attractive specific anti-asthma cytokine target: this cytokine is pivotal in eosinophil development, recruitment and survival, yet seems to have no other important function, and gene-deleted animals are healthy. Animal studies suggested that one dose of anti-IL-5 antibody could reduce airway hyper-responsiveness to allergen challenge for up to three months. An initial trial in 24 patients with mild asthma, however, showed that although anti-IL-5 could effectively reduce levels of eosinophils in blood and sputum, it had no effect on airway hyper-responsiveness or the late asthmatic reaction to inhaled allergen challenge.[11] A study with another anti-IL-5 monoclonal antibody in patients with more severe asthma similarly showed no clinical benefit.[12] This may be because anti-IL-5 antibody does not fully deplete levels of eosinophils in the airway – possibly because these cells have downregulated their IL-5 receptors so that they no longer are dependent on IL-5. Again, results of larger trials, apparently negative (from presentations in abstract form), have not been published yet.

Results of studies that looked at targeting IL-4 and IL-5 have led some to conclude that single cytokine targets are unrealistic.

Chemokines

Chemokines are small chemoattractant cytokines, initially described as acting to recruit specific cell types to sites of inflammation. They have cell specificity and also act in other ways, such as cell activation and degranulation. As they use 7-trans-membrane spanning receptors, similar to β adrenoreceptors, small molecule antagonists are being developed in work largely driven by the identification of chemokine receptors as co-receptors for HIV infection. In particular, chemokine receptor 3 (CCR3) is expressed by eosinophils, Th2 cells, mast cells and basophils and is another future target for asthma therapy.[13]

☐ IMMUNOTHERAPY FOR ASTHMA

Allergen immunotherapy was first described in 1911 and consists of injecting increasing doses of allergen extract subcutaneously into sensitised allergic patients. Allergen immunotherapy is effective for allergic asthma,[14] although current evidence is only for those with seasonal asthma to one pollen allergen or predominant house-dust related symptoms, and no comparative study with inhaled corticosteroids has been undertaken. The treatment is used widely in the United States but currently is contraindicated for asthma in the United Kingdom because surveys suggested that patients with asthma were most at risk of death associated with this therapy. Such risk results from the ability of the allergen extract given to sensitised patients to cross-link IgE, which leads to anaphylaxis or severe attacks of asthma: such risk is rare and controllable in a specialist hospital setting but greatly restricts the use of this treatment (it is licensed currently in the United Kingdom only for anaphylaxis related to bee and wasp venom – not for hayfever or other allergic diseases). Nonetheless, allergen immunotherapy offers the prospect of disease-modifying treatment for allergic disease: the current drugs suppress inflammation. A number of studies have suggested that allergen immunotherapy can reduce development of new allergen sensitivities in children with existing pollen or house-dust mite allergy, and the recent preventive allergy treatment (PAT) study suggested that allergen immunotherapy for grass or tree pollen in children with rhinitis could reduce the incidence of asthma over the three years of treatment. If allergen immunotherapy can be simplified and shown to be safe in the short and long term, such a preventive approach may become feasible.

A number of strategies are being explored to modify the regimen and thus reduce the anaphylactic potential: these include chemical modification of allergen molecules to reduce IgE binding, recombinant allergens with reduced IgE binding, use of allergen-derived peptides that do not bind IgE and use of adjuvants such as immunostimulatory DNA sequences to reduce the dose of allergen needed. In addition, it may be possible to combine anti-IgE therapy with allergen immunotherapy. Although some of these approaches have been used in initial trials, results are preliminary, and it will be some years before any such approach finds application in the clinic.[15]

□ WHO TO TREAT WITH NOVEL THERAPY: IS ALL ASTHMA THE SAME?

As novel biological approaches to treatment are used in asthma (and other chronic inflammatory diseases), it will be important to maximise therapeutic benefit from these expensive drugs. For example anti-IgE will cost £8,000–£10,000 per year per patient. Recent reviews have found that a systematic approach to characterise patients with severe asthma identifies a significant proportion of patients with poor treatment adherence or psychological input to symptoms, leaving only a proportion with true therapy-resistant asthma (TRA). To define whether subgroups exist within the group of patients with TRA and show that differential treatment responsiveness exists will be important.[16] Establishment of large national networks and collaborative groups will be an essential part of optimising treatment for the future in asthma.

REFERENCES

1 British Thoracic Society/Scottish Intercollegiate Guideline Network. British guideline on the management of asthma. *Thorax* 2003;**58**(Suppl 1):1–83.

2 Bateman ED, Boushey HA, Bousquet J, Busse WW *et al.* Can guideline-defined asthma control be achieved? The Gaining Optimal Asthma ControL study. *Am J Respir Crit Care Med* 2004;**170**:836–44.

3 O'Byrne PM, Bisgaard H, Godard PP, Pistolesi M *et al.* Budesonide/formoterol combination therapy as both maintenance and reliever medication in asthma. *Am J Respir Crit Care Med* 2005;**171**:129–36.

4 Busse WW, Lemanske RF. Asthma. *N Engl J Med* 2001;**344**:350–62.

5 Holgate ST, Djukanovic R, Casale T, Bousquet J. Anti-immunoglobulin E treatment with omalizumab in allergic diseases: an update on anti-inflammatory activity and clinical efficacy. *Clin Exp Allergy* 2005;**35**:408–16.

6 Fahy JV, Fleming HE, Wong HH, Liu JT *et al.* The effect of an anti-IgE monoclonal antibody on the early- and late-phase responses to allergen inhalation in asthmatic subjects. *Am J Respir Crit Care Med* 1997;**155**:1828–34.

7 Walker S, Monteil M, Phelan K, Lasserson TJ *et al.* Anti-IgE for chronic asthma in adults and children. *Cochrane Database Syst Rev* 2004:(2):CD003559

8 Ying S, Robinson DS, Varney V, Meng Q *et al.* TNF alpha mRNA expression in allergic inflammation. *Clin Exp Allergy* 1991;**21**:745–50.

9 Babu K, Arshad SH, Howarth PH, Chauhan AJ *et al.* Soluble tumor necrosis factor alpha (TNF-alpha) receptor (Enbrel) as effective therapeutic strategy in chronic severe asthma. *J Allergy Clin Immunol* 2003;**111**:Abstract 838.

10 Robinson-DS. Th-2 cytokines in allergic disease. *Br Med Bull* 2000;**56**:956–68.

11 Leckie MJ, ten Brinke A, Khan J, Diamant Z *et al.* Effects of an interleukin-5 blocking monoclonal antibody on eosinophils, airway hyper-responsiveness, and the late asthmatic response. *Lancet* 2000;**356**:2144–8.

12 Kips JC, Brian OJ, Langley SJ, Woodcock A *et al.* The effect of SCH55700, a humanized anti-hIL-5 antibody in severe persistent asthma: a pilot study. *Am J Respir Crit Care Med* 2003; **167**:1655–9.

13 Menzies-Gow A, Robinson DS. Eosinophil chemokines and their receptors: an attractive target in asthma? *Lancet* 2000;**355**:1741–3.

14 Durham SR, Walker SM, Varga EM, Jacobson MR *et al.* Long-term efficacy of grass pollen immunotherapy. *N Engl J Med* 1999;**341**:468–75.

15 Till SJ, Francis JN, Nouri-Aria K, Durham SR. Mechanisms of immunotherapy. *J Allergy Clin Immunol* 2004;**113**:1025–34.

16 Heaney LG, Robinson DS. Severe asthma treatment: need for characterising patients. *Lancet* 2005;**365**:974–6.

Respiratory tuberculosis

Peter Ormerod

The prevalence of tuberculosis is increasing worldwide, with a global estimated burden of more than nine million new clinical cases per annum (95% confidence interval (CI) 7.9–11.1), 1.87 million deaths (95% CI 1.5–2.4) and 34% of the world's population infected (nearly two billion people), as judged by a positive skin tuberculin test.[1] Tuberculosis has increased in England and Wales from a nadir of 5,000 cases in 1987 to nearly 7,000 cases per annum in 2005[2] – more than 40% of which are in Greater London. Very wide geographical and population group differences exist in the incidences of tuberculosis within England and Wales,[3] however – most cases are at respiratory sites.

These substantial variations in population rates for tuberculosis mean that clinical awareness needs to be maintained; this requires a working knowledge of the current epidemiology, risk groups and rates, as well as clinical patterns. The ethnic proportions of cases of tuberculosis have changed progressively over the last 15–20 years (Table 1), with a substantial majority of cases now in non-white ethnic groups and nearly 70% of cases in people who are not born in the United Kingdom. Within each population group, variations with age and time since first arrival in the United Kingdom exist. In the white ethnic group, an age gradient is seen: the rate in children and young adults (aged 16–25 years) is less than two in 100,000 per year but more than 15 in 100,000 per year in those older than 75 years.[5] Most cases in the white ethnic group now are in people older than 55 years, which represents reactivation of disease acquired earlier in life. The rate also increases with age in non-white ethnic groups. Duration of stay in the United Kingdom affects rates: rates are much higher in new arrivals to the United Kingdom than in British nationals and those resident in the country for some time: up to 800 in 100,000 per year for the first 1–3 years after first arrival but about eight-fold lower after 10 years of residence.[5] Within some populations, sub-groups can be at increased risk. The street homeless, who are predominantly white and male, have very high rates, with up to 1500 in 100,000 per year recorded in the 1990s.[6] An HIV-positive status increases the risk of clinical tuberculosis developing by between 60-fold and 150-fold. In sub-Saharan Africa, for example, nearly 80% of all patients with tuberculosis are co-infected with HIV. Table 2 gives other recognised risk factors for tuberculosis.

Some symptoms of respiratory tuberculosis, such as cough and haemoptysis, also are common in non-tuberculous chest diseases. Only fever, weight loss and night sweats are found more commonly in tuberculosis than other diseases. The chest X-ray often is very suggestive, but activity of disease is determined from sputum microscopy and culture. Certain patterns on X-ray are suggestive of

Table 1 Rates and proportions of tuberculosis cases in different ethnic groups in England and Wales.*

Ethnic group	1988[4]	1998[5]	2002[2]
Cases (%)			
White	53	38	27
Indian subcontinent	39	38	37
Black–African	1.7	15	21
Other ethnic groups	6	11	15
Population group tuberculosis rates per 100,000 per year[4]			
White	4.6		
Indian subcontinent	120		
Black–African	210		
Black–Caribbean	25		

*For variations with age and time since first arrival see text.

Table 2 Risk factors for tuberculosis.

Factor	Increased risk (times)
HIV-positivity	60–150
Immunosuppression (not corticosteroids alone)	10–20
Chronic renal failure	10
Recent immigration	8
Tumour necrosis factor-alpha antagonists	5
Diabetes	2

tuberculosis: there is a strong upper lobe predeliction, with infiltrates progressing to cavitation. Cavitation in tuberculosis correlates highly with sputum smear positivity. Less typical patterns are seen in HIV-positive people, as CD4 cell counts fall. A 'miliary' pattern is seen in only 1–2% of cases.

The diagnosis is confirmed by microscopy and culture of respiratory secretions for acid-alcohol-fast bacilli. Three separate morning sputums should be sent. If a patient is admitted to hospital, they should remain in a single side ward until the results are known. Smear positivity on one or more sputum samples means the patient should remain segregated until two weeks of treatment has been given.[7] If a patient is unable, or unwilling, to produce sputum, bronchoscopy with washings is a recognised alternative technique, but smear positivity on bronchial washings as opposed to spontaneously expectorated sputum is a less reliable predictor of infectivity.[7] A positive smear microscopy has a high probability of being a true positive. The only false positives are from opportunist non-tuberculous mycobacteria. Polymerase chain reaction tests are available for confirmation of species on microscopy or culture positive material if needed and are advised if a large contact tracing exercise (for example, in a school or hospital) is contemplated.[8] Awareness of the possibility of multidrug-resistant tuberculosis is also needed (see later). A minority of cases will be negative on microscopy but positive later on culture, and the decision to start treatment will be clinical.

Between 5% and 10% cases of respiratory tuberculosis are pleural effusions. Pleural effusion usually is a primary infection, developing within 12 months of initial infection and associated with strong tuberculin skin test positivity. On aspiration, the fluid is a lymphocyte-rich exudate, which is highly suggestive of tuberculosis. Blind pleural biopsy will show granulomas in 60% of cases, and a positive culture for *Mycobacterium tuberculosis* is obtained in 50% of cases, as few bacilli are present, but a marked lymphocytic inflammatory response is seen. A further 5–10% of cases of respiratory tuberculosis, almost exclusively in ethnic minority groups, have isolated mediastinal lymphadenopathy without any lung lesion. These cases also are associated with a strongly positive tuberculin skin test. Computed tomography scanning of the thorax may show central hypodensity in these nodes because of central caseous necrosis. Sputum usually is negative on microscopy and culture but occasionally can be microscopy positive, as hilar or paratracheal glands can discharge caseous material directly into the bronchial tree. Invasive biopsy for tissue (mediastinoscopy) is indicated only if the patient fails to improve after the initial two-month phase of anti-tuberculosis treatment.[9] This form of disease is even more common in children because of primary infection.

The much higher rates of tuberculosis in ethnic minority groups and the clinical patterns described above mean that certain situations should be regarded as tuberculosis until proved otherwise and investigated appropriately (Box 1).

Box 1 Clinical situations* in patients from ethnic minorities.

☐   Isolated mediastinal lymphadenopathy (plus positive tuberculin test)

☐   Pleural effusion (plus positive tuberculin test)

☐   Persistent cervical lymphadenopathy (>4 weeks)

☐   Monoarthritis, particularly if subacute

---

* Should be regarded as tuberculosis until proved otherwise and investigated as such.

Drug resistance is a problem in tuberculosis as in other bacterial infections. This is monitored continuously by the Health Protection Agency, and current levels of resistance to isoniazid are 7% overall, with a rate of multidrug-resistant tuberculosis of 0.8% of isolates.[2] Rates of drug resistance are higher in all ethnic minority groups, in people who are HIV-positive and, particularly, in people with a history of prior treatment, which can increase drug resistance by up to 10-fold. As more than two-thirds of cases of tuberculosis are now in people born abroad, some knowledge of global drug resistance patterns is needed. International surveys show that multidrug-resistant tuberculosis has a number of 'hotspots', in which the incidence is more than 5%.[10] These include Lithuania, Latvia and Estonia (which recently joined the European Union), Cote D'Ivoire, the Dominican Republic and some former Russian states, in which current and former prison inmates have high rates.[10] Rates of resistance to isoniazid are often >5% in people with no history of treatment but much higher in re-treatment cases. If a patient has geographical or personal risk factors for multidrug-resistant tuberculosis, such as a history of prior treatment, a polymerase chain reaction resistance probe for rifampicin resistance should be carried out on microscopy- or culture-positive material. Isolated rifampicin monoresistance is uncommon, and the finding of rifampicin resistance on such a probe is 95% predictive of multidrug resistance tuberculosis. In such cases, the patient should be segregated in a negative pressure room[8] and treated as having multidrug-resistant tuberculosis[7] until the results of full drug susceptibility tests are available.

The treatment of respiratory tuberculosis is highly evidence based, with data for pulmonary tuberculosis being Scottish Intercollegiate Guidelines Network category 1++.[11] Detailed advice on the treatment of tuberculosis was published by the Joint Tuberculosis Committee of the British Thoracic Society in 1998.[7] Updated guidelines on the treatment of tuberculosis are under preparation by the National Institute for Clinical Excellence and are expected in early 2006, but this is not likely to alter the advised treatment. Respiratory tuberculosis should be treated with two months of initial rifampicin, isoniazid, pyrazinamide and ethambutol, followed by a continuation phase of four months of rifampicin and isoniazid. Such treatment gives cure rates of 97–100% for fully sensitive organisms in randomised trials and clinical practice.[12] The treatment regimen needs to be adjusted and lengthened if there is significant drug resistance or drug reaction.[7] Before antituberculotic treatment begins, liver and renal function should be checked, as should visual acuity with a Snellen chart. Ethambutol is cleared renally, and the dose may need to be reduced or the drug substituted in patients with moderate or severe renal impairment. Up to 3% of people develop some drug reaction, often drug-induced hepatitis, and liver function may need to be monitored if pretreatment liver function is abnormal or the person is a carrier of hepatitis B or C.[7]

Tuberculosis is an infectious disease and should be notified to the proper officer – the Consultant in Public Health in England and Wales. Notification has two purposes: it allows contact tracing to be arranged[8] and provides data for continuous enhanced surveillance of tuberculosis locally and nationally.

REFERENCES

1   Dye C, Scheele S, Dolin P, Pathania V *et al.* Consensus statement. Global burden of tuberculosis: estimated incidence, prevalence, and mortality by country. WHO global surveillance and monitoring project. *JAMA* 1999;**282**:677–86.

2   Health Protection Agency. *Tuberculosis.* London: Health Protection Agency, 2005. www.hpa.org.uk (last accessed 5 September 2005).

3   Ormerod LP, Charlett A, Gilham C, Darbyshire JH *et al.* Geographical distribution of tuberculosis notifications in national surveys of England and Wales in 1988 and 1993: report of the Public Health Laboratory Service/British Thoracic Society/Department of Health Collaborative Group. *Thorax* 1998;**53**:176–81.

4   Medical Research Council Cardiothoracic Epidemiology Group. National survey of notifications of tuberculosis in England and Wales in 1988. *Thorax* 1992;**47**:770–5.

5   Rose AMC, Watson JM, Graham C, Nunn AJ *et al.* Tuberculosis at the end of the 20th century in England and Wales: results of a national survey in 1998. *Thorax* 2001;**56**:173–9.

6   Citron KM, Southern A, Dixon M. *Out of the shadow: detecting and treating tuberculosis amongst single homeless people.* London: Crisis, 1995.

7   Joint Tuberculosis Committee of the British Thoracic Society. Chemotherapy and management of tuberculosis in the United Kingdom: recommendations 1998. *Thorax* 1998; **53**:536–48.

8   Joint Tuberculosis Committee of the British Thoracic Society. Control and prevention of tuberculosis in the United Kingdom: code of practice 2000. *Thorax* 2000;**55**:887–901.

9   Farrow PR, Jones DA, Stanley PJ, Bailey JS *et al.* Thoracic lymphadenopathy in Asians resident in the United Kingdom: role of mediastinoscopy in the initial diagnosis. *Thorax* 1985;**40**: 121–4.

10 Espinal MA, Laszio A, Simonsen L, Boulahbal F *et al.* Global trends in resistance to antituberculosis drugs. World Health Organization–International Union Against Tuberculosis and Lung Disease Working Group on Anti-Tuberculosis Drug Resistance Surveillance. *N Engl J Med* 2001;**344**:1294–303.

11 Scottish Intercollegiate Guidelines Network. *SIGN 50: a guideline developers' handbook.* Edinburgh: Scottish Intercollegiate Guidelines Network, 2004. Available at:
   www..sign.ac.uk/guidelines/fulltext/50/section6.html (last accessed 22 August 2005.)

12 Ormerod LP. Chemotherapy of tuberculosis. *Eur Respir J* 1997;**4**:273–97.

Pulmonary arteriovenous malformations

Claire Shovlin

☐ INTRODUCTION

Most medical practitioners think that pulmonary arteriovenous malformations (PAVMs) have little relevance to their clinical practice. They are considered to be extremely rare, and, in the absence of dyspnoea or haemoptysis, serious pathology usually is assumed to be unlikely.

These assumptions are incorrect. Pulmonary arteriovenous malformations are thought to be rare because most patients remain undiagnosed; it is poorly recognised that the majority of individuals with PAVMs have no respiratory symptoms. Furthermore, in spite of minimal respiratory symptoms, patients with PAVMs need to be identified, because they are at high risk of early onset stroke and cerebral abscesses – complications that can be limited if the condition is treated, with embolization methods offering the safest treatment options.

☐ HOW COMMON ARE PULMONARY ARTERIOVENOUS MALFORMATIONS?

Data from the British Thoracic Society Orphan Lung Disease Register (BOLD) supports the contention that PAVMs are extremely rare, as fewer than 30 UK patients were registered between January 2001 and September 2004. However, there should be 3–4,000 individuals in the UK with PAVMs since:

☐ PAVMs affect at least 30% of patients with hereditary haemorrhagic telangiectasia (HHT, Osler-Weber-Rendu syndrome)[1,2]

☐ HHT affects one in 5–8,000 individuals.[3,4]

The lack of detection of PAVMs can be explained, in part, by the fact that HHT presents in many different guises to diverse medical practitioners.[5,6] Although HHT causes pulmonary and other visceral AVMs, the condition is recognised classically by familial nose bleeds, chronic gastrointestinal bleeding and the characteristic mucocutaneous telangiectasia that make these patients popular cases for medical examinations. As a result, many ear, nose and throat surgeons, dermatologists, gastroenterologists, and other specialists who review patients with HHT will be managing patients with PAVMs. Unless chest X-rays or respiratory investigations are performed, the specialist and patient are likely to be unaware that the patient has PAVMs because of the paucity of PAVM-associated signs and symptoms.

☐ HOW DO PAVMs PRESENT?

Data amalgamated from all case series reported between 1948 and 1998 showed that, although one-third of patients were cyanosed or clubbed, barely 50% of patients had any respiratory symptoms (Table 1). These data themselves are misleading, as symptoms at presentation were included if the patient admitted to them on direct questioning, or symptoms were recognised retrospectively after treatment of PAVMs. When symptoms that precipitated the diagnosis of PAVMs are considered, a very different picture emerges (Table 2). Respiratory symptoms led to the diagnosis of PAVMs in only 46/222 (21%) patients reviewed at Hammersmith Hospital between 1983 and 2005. Of these, 176 (79%) were diagnosed because of incidental investigations (chest imaging or detection of hypoxaemia) and, sadly, in 22 (10%) of these, investigations were instituted after a stroke or brain abscess.

Table 1 Symptoms, signs and complications of untreated PAVMs.

	Mean	**Range**	*n*
Signs			
Cyanosis	30%	9–73%	275
Clubbing	32%	6–68%	267
Respiratory symptoms			
Asymptomatic	49%	25–58%	260
Breathlessness	49%	27–71%	483
Chest pain	14%	6–18%	198
Haemoptysis	11%	4–18%	479
Embolic phenomenon			
Cerebral abscess	9%	0–25%	368
CVA or TIA	27%	11–55%	401

n = number of patients assessed for feature in 18 series reviewed in reference.[7]

☐ HOW CAN PAVMs BE TREATED?

Surgical resection of PAVMs has been performed for more than 60 years. Embolization generally has supplanted surgical procedures because of reduced periprocedural risks, parenchymal sparing in patients at risk of recurrent disease and the documented physiological benefits. During embolization, the feeding vessels to PAVMs are occluded by thrombus which organises either on thrombogenic fibres associated with carefully positioned metallic coils (Fig 1) or secondary to the stasis of blood by an occluding balloon.[8,9] Embolization has proven long-term physiological benefits (regression of the PAVM sac, reduction of right-to-left shunting and improvement in hypoxaemia), and we have recently demonstrated a reduction in the rate of cerebral complications (Shovlin and Jackson, unpublished data). In experienced centres, safety profiles are excellent. This has supported a trend towards earlier treatment of asymptomatic patients. Antibiotic prophylaxis before dental and surgical interventions is recommended to reduce the risk of embolic abscesses.

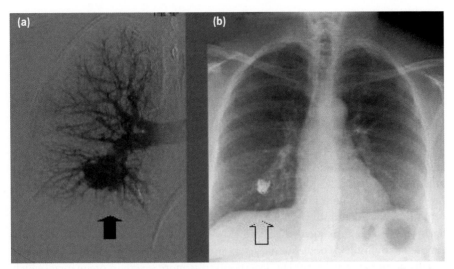

Fig 1 Pulmonary arteriovenous malformations: (a) pre-embolization pulmonary angiogram illustrating PAVMs (filled arrow) and (b) chest X ray four months after embolization illustrating nest of embolization coils (unfilled arrows) and regression of the PAVM sac.

☐ PAVMs: FEW RESPIRATORY SYMPTOMS BUT FREQUENT PARADOXICAL EMBOLIC STROKE: MECHANISMS AND RECENT DATA

Pulmonary arteriovenous malformations are thin-walled abnormal vessels that replace normal capillaries between the pulmonary arterial and venous circulations, often resulting in bulbous sac-like structures (see Fig 1). They provide a direct capillary-free communication between the pulmonary and systemic circulations (Fig 2), with three main clinical consequences:

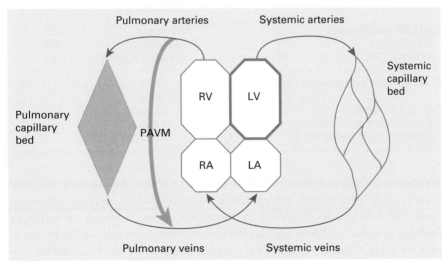

Fig 2 Anatomical site of pulmonary arteriovenous malformations. RV = right ventricle. LV = left ventricle. RA = right atrium. LA = left atrium.

☐   Pulmonary arterial blood that passes through these right-to-left shunts cannot be oxygenated, which leads to hypoxaemia.

☐   The fragile vessels may haemorrhage into a bronchus, the pulmonary parenchyma or the pleural cavity.

☐   The absence of a filtering capillary bed allows particulate matter to reach the systemic circulation, where it impacts in other capillary beds, causing clinical sequelae, particularly in the cerebral circulation.

Unexplained and often profound hypoxaemia is the hallmark of large PAVMs, and generally it is assumed that all patients with clinically significant PAVMs will be breathless. However, PAVM patients tolerate worsening hypoxaemia on exercise well, however, reflecting their low pulmonary vascular resistance and ability to generate a supranormal cardiac output, which may increase further on exercise.[10] Furthermore, haemoptysis is less frequent than might be expected, because the AVM walls are exposed to pulmonary not systemic artery pressure and, therefore, systolic pressures usually do not exceed 25 mmHg. Haemoptysis is more severe in pregnancy (which has led to recent maternal deaths in the UK[11]) or if the PAVM sac has a systemic arterial supply. Asymptomatic or small PAVMs generally are believed to pose a lower risk of cerebral complications, but no evidence has been presented to support this.

Recent data from Hammersmith series

Table 2 Features of Hammersmith PAVM population.

A: Reasons for diagnosis of PAVMs (n=222)

Respiratory symptoms	21%	**Incidental investigations**	24%
Breathless	13%	Imaging	18%
Haemoptysis	6%	Hypoxaemia	4%
Chest pain	4%	Clubbing, cyanosis	2%
Post CNS complications	10%	**HHT screen**	45%
Brain abscess	7%	Hammersmith	39%
Ischaemic CVA	3%	Referring hospitals	6%

B: Pre treatment assessment of PAVM severity

	mean	range	n
SaO$_2$ at rest, standing	91%	59–100%	192
Right-to-left shunt (% of cardiac output)	12.5%	1.4–40%	139
Diameter of largest feeding artery	4.9mm	< 2–12mm	133

A criticism of historical data presented in Table 1 is that the cases are weighted towards early symptomatic presentations, whereas modern imaging techniques mean that PAVMs are diagnosed in many patients as incidental or screening findings. In order to address whether the concerns about the risks of PAVMs are as valid for such patients, we conducted systematic reviews on the 292 patients with PAVMs who have been reviewed at the Hammersmith since 1983. Of these, 246 underwent pulmonary angiography in order to embolize PAVMs, with only one long-term adverse event: a persistent mild facial nerve palsy. Small PAVMs were seen in 165/214 (77%) of patients: 126 patients with residual disease following maximal embolization and 39 patients with PAVMs too small for embolization. Table 2 shows the demographics of these patients.

Although the physiological data confirm the presence of significant hypoxaemia and right-to-left shunts in most patients, this was not reflected by respiratory symptoms of sufficient severity to justify general investigation. Of the 176 patients with PAVMs who did not present with respiratory symptoms, one quarter had oxygen saturations less than 88% at rest and half less than 94%.

Complications of PAVMs in Hammersmith series

Strokes and cerebral abscesses affected a significant number of these patients (see Fig 3). Importantly, many of these occurred in relatively young patients and those with normal oxygenation, small right-to-left shunts and small PAVMs. Furthermore, most patients who developed strokes and abscesses had no pre-existing diagnosis of PAVMs or HHT, despite the presence of standing clinical signs and symptoms.

Three pregnancies in women with PAVMs were complicated by massive haemoptysis that required emergency embolization or early delivery: all three patients had normal pulmonary artery pressures and two had normal oxygenation. Growth of PAVMs was a usual feature of pregnancy, as previously described.[11]

These data highlight that, in modern practice, patients with undiagnosed PAVMs are being missed and are developing preventable complications.

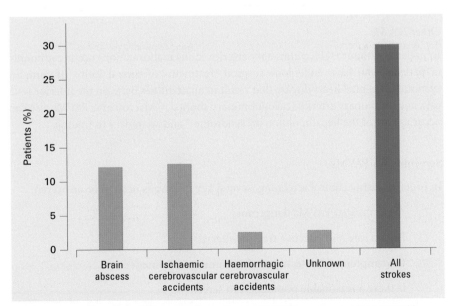

Fig 3 Incidence of stroke in 229 consecutive patients with PAVMs reviewed at Hammersmith Hospital during 1999–2005. The age range of patients with abscesses was 11–69 (mean 43) years and of patients with embolic cerebrovascular accidents was 22–68 (mean 49) years. Haemorrhagic cerebrovascular accidents from cerebral arteriovenous malformations were the result of underlying HHT.

☐ SCREENING CONSIDERATIONS FOR PAVMs

Where are the 'missing' 3,000 patients with pulmonary arteriovenous malformations?

Sporadic PAVMs

Although patients with PAVMs will pass through respiratory clinics, as discussed above, these patients account for a small fraction of the undiagnosed population. For patients without underlying HHT, the lack of respiratory symptoms implies that many will not be referred to respiratory doctors unless the diagnosis is picked up by incidental imaging. A significant proportion of patients with PAVMs will be reviewed when they present with a stroke or brain abscess. Although that event has already occurred, the importance of detecting and treating PAVMs lies in the prevention of further events for the patient.

PAVMs associated with HHT

The majority of people with PAVMs have underlying HHT. As a result, many will be reviewed by specialists who manage the other aspects of HHT, particularly ear, nose and throat surgeons (nose bleeds); dermatologists (skin telangiectasia); gastro-enterologists (chronic and acute upper and lower gastrointestinal haemorrhage); haematologists (for transfusions and management of iron-deficiency anaemia); or clinical geneticists. Consideration of a diagnosis of PAVMs here is important, not only for the patient, but also because it should raise the possibility that affected family members may be undiagnosed.

Other PAVMs

In patients without HHT, pulmonary arteriovenous malformations occur commonly in patients who have undergone surgical treatments of several forms of complex cyanotic congenital heart disease that result in anastemoses between the inferior vena cava and pulmonary arteries (cavopulmonary shunts).[12] Macroscopic PAVMs also can occur as part of the hepatopulmonary syndrome[13] and secondary to trauma.

Screening for PAVMs

In order to justify clinical screening, several key questions need to be answered:

- ☐ Are untreated PAVMs dangerous?
- ☐ Does a safe and effective treatment exist?
- ☐ Is asymptomatic detection and treatment warranted?
- ☐ Is there a reasonable population to screen?

The high frequency of PAVMs (30–50%) in the population with HHT suggests that these criteria would be met for the one in 5,000–8,000 members of the population who have HHT if financially viable. For patients already under review for other aspects of HHT, aspects of PAVM screening programmes are discussed in the next section.

Hereditary hemorrhagic telangiectasia

A disorder of late onset-penetrance

The crucial point that needs to be recognised is that most individuals with HHT do not know their diagnosis because (a) they have not yet developed symptoms or signs of concern or (b) the significance of their symptoms or symptoms in family members is not appreciated.

Data suggest that by the age of 16 years, 71% of people will have developed some sign of HHT; this rises to more than 90% by the age of 40 years.[6,14] These data imply that during child-bearing years, an apparently unaffected child of an HHT patient still has a 5–20% chance of carrying the HHT gene.

Often an innocuous condition

The severity of symptoms of HHT varies widely. Although features of HHT were recorded in 229 of our patients, only 83 (36%) of these had required specialist medical care for other aspects of HHT (Table 3).

Table 3 Frequency of HHT features.

Feature	Overall Frequency ^	Clinically significant frequency*
Nose bleeds	90%	34%†
Gastrointestinal bleeds	15%	
Pulmonary AVMs	30%	–
Skin and oral telangiectasia	80%	1%
Cerebral AVMs	10%	3.7%
Hepatic AVMs	20–30%	2.6%
Other	?	1%

^ Overall frequency of HHT features in published series.[6]
*Features of HHT requiring prior medical attention in 229 Hammersmith patients with PAVMs
†32% of this population were on iron supplements and 9.6% required transfusions.

Diagnostic criteria

To permit a high level of clinical suspicion without leading to overdiagnosis, recent international consensus diagnostic criteria were developed on the basis of the four criteria of spontaneous recurrent nosebleeds, mucocutaneous telangiectasia, visceral involvement and an affected first-degree relative.[15] These define 'definite HHT', in which three criteria are present, 'suspected HHT', in which two criteria are present (most commonly family history and nose bleeds) or 'unlikely HHT', in which one criterion is present, such as spontaneous nose bleeds without a family history or a first-degree relative of a patient with HHT with no signs of the disease. An important issue for families (and doctors) is that no child of a patient with HHT can be informed they do not have HHT unless they have had a genetic test.

As most patients with HHT do not know their diagnosis, if the patient has a feature that may reflect underlying HHT, the most important clinical question is 'Do you, or does anyone in your family, have nosebleeds?'

☐ PRINCIPLES OF PAVM SCREENING IN PATIENTS WITH HHT

Screening methods are based on non-invasive methods that image the PAVMs (thoracic radiography and computed tomography scanning) or detect the right-to-left shunt (hypoxaemia on room air and 100% oxygen rebreathing, radionucleide perfusion scans or contrast echocardiography). Currently, discussions are taking place about the optimal methods of screening in specialist centres and, in particular, screening for small PAVMs.

The key principles are that:

☐ Simple investigations (such as finger oximetry and chest X-rays) will detect many PAVMs but often are non-specific (single specificity is about 15%) and cannot be used to rule out the diagnosis (sensitivity ≤90%).

☐ Confirmation of right-to-left shunting by 100% oxygen rebreathing methods or nuclear medicine perfusion scans may be helpful but carries practical difficulties in performance and interpretation in many centres and, again, has inadequate sensitivity to exclude PAVMs.

☐ Contrast echocardiography is emerging as a favoured screening method by many centres because of the lack of radiation exposure and apparently high sensitivities.[16] Further imaging is needed in patients with positive results, however, and availability is limited.

☐ Thoracic computed tomography scans without contrast have at least similar sensitivity to contrast echocardiography,[17] are widely available, are fast to perform (as no intravenous access is needed) and, in a single test, allow distinction of lesions amenable to embolization or that need medical management. These features, improved scanner resolution, reduced radiation exposure and time considerations have led us to favour this as the screening method if chest X-rays do not show an obvious PAVM.

☐ At our centre, due to considerations of radiation exposure, resource use, time and cost, pulmonary angiography is only performed at the time of planned embolization.

The optimal timing and intervals between screenings for PAVMs are not clear, as data on the natural history of PAVMs are limited. These data suggest that most pulmonary arteriovenous malformations develop at the time of puberty (earlier presentations generally are symptomatic), and we therefore only screen asymptomatic people after they have reached adult height – for women, ideally before pregnancy. We currently are evaluating long-term growth patterns in order to develop an evidence base for further screens later in life.

☐ MOLECULAR BASIS OF PAVMS ASSOCIATED WITH HHT

Hereditary hemorrhagic telangiectasia is inherited as an autosomal dominant trait, and HHT-associated PAVMs can develop as the result of a mutation in one of at least four different HHT genes. *HHT1* and *HHT2* have been recognised for more than a decade as being the result of mutations in *endoglin*[18] and *ALK-1*,[19] respectively. In addition, mutations in *Smad4/MADH4*, which cause a juvenile polyposis/HHT overlap syndrome,[20] and a new *HHT3* gene locus[21] have been described recently – both associated with PAVMs.

The three identified HHT genes encode proteins that mediate signalling by the transforming growth factor-beta (TGF-β) superfamily. These peptide growth factors include TGF-βs, activins and the bone morphogenetic proteins and affect cellular growth and differentiation through signal transduction cascades from transmembrane receptor complexes.[22] Endoglin and ALK-1 display tissue-restricted expression patterns, and recent studies have begun to delineate the molecular basis of their roles in mediating TGF-β signalling in vascular endothelial cells (Fig 4).

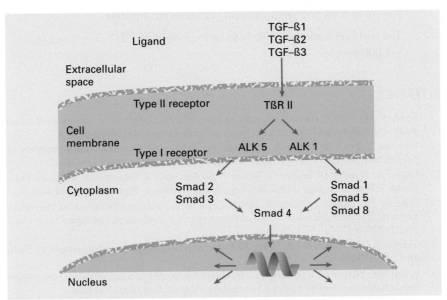

Fig 4 Transforming growth factor-β signalling pathways in endothelial cells. Ligands of transforming growth factor-β initiate downstream signalling, primarily through heteromeric complexes of type I and II transmembrane receptors that phosphorylate cytoplasmic Smad proteins. In most cell types, TGF-β1 signals through the ubiquitously expressed receptors, TβRII and ALK5 (also known as TβRI). Endothelial cells also express a second TGF-β type I receptor, ALK1. Reproduced from Ref 21 with permission from the BMJ Publishing Group.

Transforming growth factor-β1 signals transduced through the two type I receptors expressed in endothelial cells, ALK5 and ALK1, have opposing effects. For example, proliferation and migration of endothelial cells are inhibited by signalling through ALK5, whereas ALK1 signals stimulate both processes and functionally antagonise ALK5-induced signalling.[23] Endoglin – a co-receptor for the TGF-β superfamily – binds to TβRII[24] and ALK-1 and modulates ALK1- and ALK5-dependent TGF-β1 signalling pathways. In endothelial cells, endoglin promotes signalling through the endothelial cell-specific ALK1[25] but downregulates ALK5-dependent TGF-β1-induced responses.[25] How mutations in *Smad4*, which encodes a ubiquitous common partner Smad, can specifically modulate these pathways in endothelial cells and how mutations in the HHT genes lead to the generation of abnormal vascular structures in man and mouse remains unclear.

□ SUMMARY

- □ Most individuals with PAVMs are asymptomatic but at risk of early strokes, brain abscesses and pregnancy-related complications.

- □ Most individuals with PAVMs have underlying HHT, often, again, with minimal symptoms. Between 30% and 50% of patients with HHT have PAVMs.

- □ Screening tools and safe treatment regimens are available.

- □ The cost implications are likely to be important, as HHT affects one in 5–8,000 people.

REFERENCES

1   Kjeldsen AD, Vase P, Green A. Hereditary hemorrhagic telangiectasia: a population-based study of prevalence and mortality in Danish patients. *J Intern Med* 1999;**245**:31–9.

2   Haitjema T, Disch F, Overtoom TT, Westermann CJ *et al*. Screening family members of patients with hereditary haemorrhagic telangiectasia. *Am J Med* 1995;**99**:519–24.

3   Bideau A, Plauchu H, Brunet G, Robert J. Epidemiological investigation of Rendu-Osler disease in France: its geographical distribution and prevalence. *Population* 1989;**44**:3–22.

4   Dakeishi M, Shioya T, Wada Y, Shindo T *et al*. Genetic epidemiology of hereditary haemorrhagic telangiectasia in a local community in the northern part of Japan. *Hum Mutat* 2002;**19**:140–8.

5   Guttmacher AE, Marchuk DA, White RI Jr. Hereditary hemorrhagic telangiectasia. *N Engl J Med* 1995;**333**:918–24.

6   Begbie ME, Wallace GM, Shovlin CL. Hereditary haemorrhagic telangiectasia (Osler-Weber-Rendu syndrome): a view from the 21st century. *Postgrad Med J* 2003;**79**:18–24.

7   Shovlin CL, Letarte M. Hereditary haemorrhagic telangiectasia and pulmonary arteriovenous malformations: issues in clinical management and review of pathogenic mechanisms. *Thorax* 1999;**54**:714–29.

8   White RI Jr, Lynch-Nyhan A, Terry P, Buescher PC *et al*. Pulmonary arteriovenous malformations: techniques and long-term outcome of embolotherapy. *Radiology* 1988;**169**:663–9.

9   Gupta P, Mordin C, Curtiss J, Hughes JM *et al*. PAVMs: pulmonary arteriovenous malformations: effect of embolization on right-to-left shunt, hypoxemia, and exercise tolerance in 66 patients. *AJR Am J Roentgenol* 2002;**179**:347–55.

10 Whyte MK, Hughes JM, Jackson JE, Peters AM *et al*. Cardiopulmonary response to exercise in patients with intrapulmonary vascular shunts. *J Appl Physiol* 1993;**75**:321–8

11 Shovlin CL, Winstock AR, Peters AM, Jackson JE *et al*. Medical complications of pregnancy in hereditary haemorrhagic telangiectasia. *QJM* 1995;**88**:879–87.

12 Kopf GS, Laks H, Stansel HC, Hellenbrand WE *et al*. Thirty-year follow-up of superior vena cava-pulmonary artery (Glenn) shunts. *J Thorac Cardiovasc Surg* 1990;**100**:662–70.

13 Schraufnagel DE, Kay JM. Structure and pathologic changes in the lung vasculature in chronic liver disease. *Clin Chest Med* 1996;**17**:1–15.

14 Plauchu H, de Chadarévian JP, Bideau A, Robert JM. Age-related profile of hereditary hemorrhagic telangiectasia in an epidemiologically recruited population. *Am J Med Genet* 1989;**32**:291–7.

15 Shovlin CL, Guttmacher AE, Buscarini E, Faughnan ME *et al.* Diagnostic criteria for hereditary haemorrhagic telangiectasia (Rendu-Osler-Weber syndrome). *Am J Med Genet* 2000;**91**:66–7.

16 Cottin V, Plauchu H, Bayle JY, Barthelet M *et al.* Pulmonary arteriovenous malformations in patients with hereditary hemorrhagic telangiectasia. *Am J Respir Crit Care Med* 2004; **169**:994–1000.

17 Remy J, Remy-Jardin M, Wattinne L, Deffontaines C. Pulmonary arteriovenous malformations: evaluation with CT of the chest before and after treatment. *Radiology* 1992;**182**:809–16.

18 McAllister KA, Grogg KM, Johnson DW, Gallione CJ *et al.* Endoglin, a TGF-beta binding protein of endothelial cells, is the gene for hereditary haemorrhagic telangiectasia type 1. *Nat Genet* 1994;**8**:345–51.

19 Johnson DW, Berg JN, Baldwin MA, Gallione CJ *et al.* Mutations in the activin receptor-like kinase 1 gene in hereditary haemorrhagic telangiectasia type 2. *Nat Genet* 1996;**13**:189–95.

20 Gallione CJ, Repetto GM, Legius E, Rustgi AK *et al.* A combined syndrome of juvenile polyposis and hereditary haemorrhagic telangiectasia is associated with mutations in MADH4 (SMAD4). *Lancet* 2004;**363**:852–9.

21 Cole SG, Begbie ME, Wallace GM, Shovlin CL. A new locus for hereditary haemorrhagic telangiactasia (HHT3) maps to chromosome 5. *J Med Genet* 2005;**42**:577–82.

22 Heldin CH, Miyazono K, ten Dijke P. TGF-beta signalling from cell membrane to nucleus through SMAD proteins. *Nature* 1997;**390**:465–71.

23 Goumans MJ, Valdimarsdottir G, Itoh S, Lebrin F *et al.* Activin receptor-like kinase (ALK)1 is an antagonistic mediator of lateral TGFbeta/ALK5 signaling. *Mol Cell* 2003;**12**:817–28.

24 Barbara NP, Wrana JL, Letarte M. Endoglin is an accessory protein that interacts with the signaling receptor complex of multiple members of the transforming growth factor-beta superfamily. *J Biol Chem* 1999;**274**:584–94.

25 Lebrin F, Goumans MJ, Jonker L, Carvalho RL *et al.* Endoglin promotes endothelial cell proliferation and TGF-beta/ALK1 signal transduction. *EMBO J* 2004;**23**:4018–28.

☐ RESPIRATORY SELF ASSESSMENT QUESTIONS

Advances in therapy of asthma

1   With respect to immunoglobulin E and asthma:
   (a) Immunoglobulin E is involved in asthma by activating mast cells when cross-linked by allergen
   (b) Immunoglobulin E is involved in asthma only in allergic but not non-allergic (intrinsic) asthma
   (c) Total immunoglobulin E is a useful screen for allergy
   (d) Immunoglobulin E is involved in asthma can focus antigens for presentation to T cells by dendritic cells
   (e) Immunoglobulin E activation is prevented by steroid therapy

2   Anti-immunoglobulin E therapy in asthma
   (a) Improves lung function
   (b) Reduces exacerbation rates
   (c) Will obviate the need for inhaled steroid therapy
   (d) Has been shown to be cost-effective
   (e) Carries a risk of anaphylaxis

3   The following anti-cytokine therapies have been effective in phase I/II studies in asthma
   (a) Anti-interleukin (IL) 4
   (b) Anti-IL-5
   (c) Anti-tumour necrosis factor alpha
   (d) Anti-IL-13
   (e) Anti-IL-1

4   Allergen immunotherapy:
   (a) Is widely used to treat asthma in the United States
   (b) Is safe for primary care use for allergic asthma
   (c) May be improved by use of short allergen-derived peptides
   (d) May be combined with anti-immunoglobulin E treatment
   (e) Can prevent development of asthma

5   Systematic assessment of patients with severe asthma
   (a) Reveals that 30% do not take prescribed treatments
   (b) Identifies misdiagnosis in 10% of cases
   (c) Identifies psychiatric disease in up to 30% of cases
   (d) Suggests variable underlying patterns of inflammation
   (e) Can delineate which patients will benefit from anti-immunoglobulin E treatment

Respiratory tuberculosis

1   With respect to tuberculosis:
    (a) The white ethnic group has a rate of tuberculosis >40 per 100,000 per year
    (b) The ethnic group from the Indian subcontinent has a rate of tuberculosis >100 per 100,000 per year
    (c) The Black-African ethnic group has a rate of tuberculosis >200 per 100,000 per year
    (d) The risk factor that most increases the risk of tuberculosis is coinfection with HIV
    (e) Treatment with anti-tumour necrosis factor alpha increases the risk of tuberculosis 20-fold

2   With respect to tuberculosis:
    (a) Activity of tuberculosis can be ascertained from a chest X-ray
    (a) Cavitation on a chest X-ray in a patient with tuberculosis is associated strongly with positive sputum microscopy
    (b) The chest X-ray pattern in patients with tuberculosis remains typical as the CD4 count falls in patient coinfected with HIV
    (c) Isolated mediastinal lymphadenopathy occurs in >20% of people with respiratory tuberculosis
    (d) Central hypodensity is seen commonly in computed tomography images in patients with tuberculosis and mediastinal lymph nodes

3   With respect to tuberculosis:
    (a) Patients suspected of having pulmonary tuberculosis should be isolated in a single room until sputum microscopy results are known
    (b) Bronchoscopy with washings is an appropriate technique in patients with suspected tuberculosis who are unable to produce sputum
    (c) Acid-fast bacilli seen on sputum microscopy are always *Mycobacterium tuberculosis*
    (d) A positive rifampicin resistance probe in a case of *M. tuberculosis* disease should lead to the patient being isolated in a negative pressure room
    (e) Tuberculosis is not a notifiable disease

4   With respect to tuberculosis:
    (a) The current rate of isoniazid resistance in tuberculosis in England and Wales is 7%
    (b) The current rate of multidrug-resistant tuberculosis in England and Wales is >5%
    (c) The Baltic states have high (>5%) rates of multidrug-resistant tuberculosis
    (d) A history of previous treatment for tuberculosis significantly increases the risk of drug resistance
    (e) Isolated rifampicin resistance is common in patients infected with *M. tuberculosis*

Pulmonary arteriovenous malformations

1   Pulmonary arteriovenous malformations (PAVMs):
    (a) Affect approximately 250 people in the United Kingdom
    (b) Usually are associated with Osler-Weber-Rendu syndrome
    (c) Usually present with dyspnoea or haemoptysis
    (d) Commonly cause brain abscesses and paradoxical embolic stroke
    (e) Can cause maternal death during pregnancy

2   The diagnosis of PAVMs can be excluded by:
    (a) The absence of respiratory symptoms
    (b) The absence of a personal or family history of Osler-Weber-Rendu syndrome
    (c) A normal chest X-ray
    (d) Normal blood gases
    (e) The combination of all of the above

3   Appropriate management for an asymptomatic but hypoxaemic patient with a moderately sized PAVM could include:
    (a) No treatment
    (b) Surgical resection
    (c) Embolization therapy
    (d) Antibiotic prophylaxis for dental and surgical procedures
    (e) Oxygen at home

4   Hereditary haemorrhagic telangiectasia (Osler-Weber-Rendu syndrome):
    (a) Affects one in 5–8,000 people
    (b) Usually is diagnosed during childhood
    (c) Requires a positive family history to secure the diagnosis
    (d) Results in PAVMs in up to 20% of affected people
    (e) Usually requires specialist medical intervention for nose bleeds, gastrointestinal bleeding and anaemia

Croonian Lecture

Molecular mousetraps, α_1-antitrypsin deficiency and the serpinopathies

David A Lomas

☐ INTRODUCTION

Point mutations in members of the serine proteinase inhibitor or serpin superfamily cause them to change shape, polymerise and be deposited in the tissues. This process is best seen in mutants of α_1-antitrypsin within hepatocytes to cause periodic acid-Schiff (PAS) positive inclusions and cirrhosis. An identical process underlies the PAS positive inclusions of mutants of neuroserpin within neurones to cause a dementia that we have called familial encephalopathy with neuroserpin inclusion bodies (FENIB). In both cases, there is a direct correlation between the molecular instability, the rate of intracellular polymer formation and the severity of disease. This process of polymerisation also explains the failure to secrete mutants of other members of the serpin superfamily – antithrombin, C1 inhibitor and α_1-antichymotrypsin – to cause thrombosis, angio-oedema and emphysema, respectively. In view of the common mechanism underlying these conditions, we have grouped them together as the serpinopathies.

☐ THE SERINE PROTEINASE INHIBITOR OR SERPIN SUPERFAMILY

The serine proteinase inhibitors or serpins are important inhibitors of a wide range of proteolytic cascades. Members of this family include α_1-antitrypsin, C1 inhibitor, antithrombin and plasminogen activator inhibitor-1 which play important roles in the control of proteinases involved in the inflammatory, complement, coagulation and fibrinolytic pathways, respectively.[1] The superfamily is defined by more than 30% sequence homology with the archetypal member α_1-antitrypsin and conservation of tertiary structure. This structure is composed of three β-sheets (A–C) and an exposed mobile reactive loop (Fig 1a).[2–8] The reactive loop presents a peptide sequence as a pseudosubstrate for the target proteinase. After docking, the enzyme cleaves the P1–P1' peptide bond of the serpin[9] and the proteinase is inactivated by a dramatic conformational transition that swings it 70 Å from the upper to the lower pole of the protein in association with the insertion of the reactive loop as an extra strand (s4A) in β-sheet A (Fig 1a).[10–14] The altered conformation of α_1-antitrypsin bound to its target enzyme is then recognised by hepatic receptors and cleared from the circulation.[15–17] This remarkable conformational transition can be likened to the function of a mousetrap and is central to the inhibitory activity of the serpins. However, as with most sophisticated mechanisms, the mobile domains

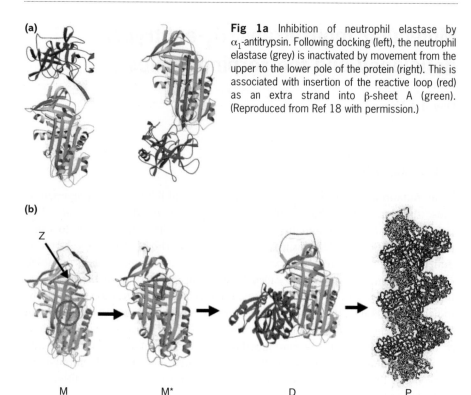

(a)

Fig 1a Inhibition of neutrophil elastase by α_1-antitrypsin. Following docking (left), the neutrophil elastase (grey) is inactivated by movement from the upper to the lower pole of the protein (right). This is associated with insertion of the reactive loop (red) as an extra strand into β-sheet A (green). (Reproduced from Ref 18 with permission.)

(b)

Z

M   M*   D   P

Fig 1b The structure of α_1-antitrypsin is centred on β-sheet A (green) and the mobile reactive centre loop (red). Polymer formation results from the Z variant of α_1-antitrypsin (Glu342Lys at P_{17}; arrowed) or mutations in the shutter domain (blue circle) that open β-sheet A to favour partial loop insertion and the formation of an unstable intermediate (M*). The patent β-sheet A can accept the loop of another molecule to form a dimer (D) which then extends into polymers (P). The individual molecules of α_1-antitrypsin within the polymer, although identical, are coloured red, yellow and blue for clarity. (Adapted from Ref 77 with permission from National Academy of Sciences, USA.)

are vulnerable to dysfunction. In the case of the serpins, mutations cause aberrant conformational transitions that result in the retention of the serpin within the cell of synthesis. This gives rise to clinical conditions that result from either:

(i) protein overload and death of the cell in which the serpin is synthesised (toxic gain of function) such as Z α_1-antitrypsin related cirrhosis and the dementia familial encephalopathy with neuroserpin inclusion bodies (FENIB), or

(ii) plasma deficiency (loss of function) such as deficiency of plasma antithrombin, C1-inhibitor or α_1-antichymotrypsin. These can be manifest as diseases as diverse as thrombosis, angio-oedema and emphysema respectively.

We have shown that there is a common mechanism underlying these conditions and so have grouped them together as a new class of disease, the serpinopathies.[18–20]

☐ POLYMERISATION OF MUTANTS OF α_1-ANTITRYPSIN CAUSES CIRRHOSIS AND PLASMA DEFICIENCY

Alpha-1-antitrypsin is an acute phase glycoprotein that is synthesised and secreted by the liver. The primary role of α_1-antitrypsin is to inhibit the enzyme neutrophil elastase. Most individuals carry two normal M alleles that result in plasma concentrations of 1.5–3.5 g/l. The most important deficiency mutation is the Z allele (Glu342Lys). Approximately 4% of Northern Europeans are heterozygous for the Z allele (PI*MZ) with approximately 1 in 2,000 being homozygotes (PI*Z). The Z allele results in the retention of synthesised α_1-antitrypsin within the endoplasmic reticulum of hepatocytes. The accumulation of abnormal protein starts *in utero*[21] and is characterised by the formation of diastase-resistant, periodic acid-Schiff positive inclusions of α_1-antitrypsin in the periportal cells[22,23] (Fig 2). Seventy-three

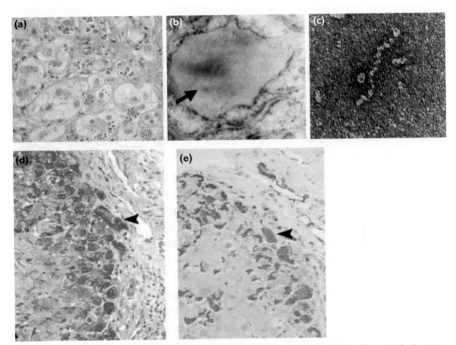

Fig 2 Z α_1-antitrypsin is retained within hepatocytes as intracellular inclusions. These inclusions are PAS positive and diastase resistant (2a) and are associated with neonatal hepatitis and hepatocellular carcinoma. (2b) Electron micrograph of an hepatocyte from the liver of a patient with Z α_1-antitrypsin deficiency shows the accumulation of α_1-antitrypsin within the rough endoplasmic reticulum. These inclusions are composed of chains of α_1-antitrypsin polymers shown here from the plasma of a Siiyama α_1-antitrypsin homozygote (2c). More recently, polymers have been identified within PAS positive inclusions with a monoclonal anti-α_1-antitrypsin polymer antibody[30,36] (2d and e). Immunohistochemistry of liver from an individual with Z α_1-antitrypsin deficiency showing staining with an anti-α_1-antitrypsin polyclonal antibody (2d) and a monoclonal anti-α_1-antitrypsin polymer antibody (2e). It is these intracellular inclusions of polymers that are associated with neonatal hepatitis and hepatocellular carcinoma. Fig 2a reproduced from Ref 96 with permission from the Biochemical Society. Fig 2b reproduced from Ref 29 with permission. Fig 2c reproduced from Ref 44 with permission from the American Society for Biochemistry and Molecular Biology. Figs 2d and e reproduced from Ref 36 with permission from Wiley-Liss, Inc.

per cent of Z α_1-antitrypsin homozygote infants have a raised serum alanine aminotransferase in the first year of life but in only 15% of children is it still abnormal by 12 years of age.[24-27] Similarly, serum bilirubin is raised in 11% of PI*Z infants in the first 2–4 months but falls to normal by six months of age. One in 10 infants develops cholestatic jaundice and 6% develop clinical evidence of liver disease without jaundice. These symptoms usually resolve by the second year of life but approximately 15% of patients with cholestatic jaundice progress to juvenile cirrhosis. The overall risk of death from liver disease in PI*Z children during childhood is 2–3%, with boys being at greater risk than girls. All adults with the Z allele of α_1-antitrypsin have slowly progressive hepatic damage that is often subclinical and only evident as a minor degree of portal fibrosis. However, up to 50% of Z α_1-antitrypsin homozygotes present with clinically evident cirrhosis and occasionally with hepatocellular carcinoma.[28] The lack of circulating plasma α_1-antitrypsin leaves the lungs exposed to enzymatic damage that is thought to underlie the adult onset emphysema (see later).

We have shown that the Z variant of α_1-antitrypsin is retained within hepatocytes as it causes a unique conformational transition and protein–protein interaction. The mutation distorts the relationship between the reactive centre loop and β-sheet A (Fig 1b). The consequent perturbation in structure allows the reactive centre loop of one α_1-antitrypsin molecule to lock into the A sheet of a second to form a dimer which then extends to form chains of loop-sheet polymers.[29-34] These polymers accumulate within the endoplasmic reticulum of hepatocytes to form the PAS positive inclusions that are the hallmark of Z α_1-antitrypsin liver disease.[29,35,36] Although many α_1-antitrypsin deficiency variants have been described, only two other mutants of α_1-antitrypsin have similarly been associated with profound plasma deficiency and hepatic inclusions: α_1-antitrypsin Siiyama (Ser53Phe)[37,38] and Mmalton[39] (deletion of phenylalanine at position 52, also known as Mnichinan[40] and Mcagliari[41]). Both of these mutants are in the shutter domain underlying the bifurcation of strands 3 and 5 of β-sheet A (Fig 1b). The mutations disrupt a hydrogen bond network that is based on 334His and bridges strands 3 and 5 of the A sheet,[42] causing it to part to allow the formation of folding intermediates[43] and loop-sheet polymers *in vivo.*[44,45]

Polymerisation also underlies the mild plasma deficiency of other variants that perturb the shutter domain: S (Glu264Val) and I (Arg39Cys) α_1-antitrypsin.[46,47] These point mutations cause less disruption to β-sheet A than does the Z variant. Thus, the rates of polymer formation are much slower than that of Z α_1-antitrypsin[31] and this results in less retention of protein within hepatocytes, milder plasma deficiency, and the lack of a clinical phenotype. However, if a mild, slowly polymerising I or S variant of α_1-antitrypsin is inherited with a rapidly polymerising Z variant, then the two can interact to form heteropolymers within hepatocytes leading to inclusions and finally cirrhosis.[47-49] Thus, the severity of retention of mutants of α_1-antitrypsin within hepatocytes can be explained by the rate of polymer formation. Those mutants that cause the most rapid polymerisation cause the most retention of α_1-antitrypsin within the liver. This in turn correlates with the greatest risk of liver damage and cirrhosis, and the most severe plasma deficiency.

☐ POLYMERISATION OF Z α_1-ANTITRYPSIN AND EMPHYSEMA

Emphysema was noted in some of the first individuals who were reported to have an absence of the alpha-1 band on serum protein electrophoresis.[50] It was confirmed by family studies[51] and is now the only genetic factor that is widely accepted to predispose smokers to emphysema. The respiratory disease associated with α_1-antitrypsin deficiency usually presents with increasing dyspnoea with cor pulmonale and polycythaemia occurring late in the course of the disease. Chest radiographs typically show bilateral basal emphysema with paucity and pruning of the basal pulmonary vessels. Upper lobe vascularisation is relatively normal. Ventilation perfusion radioisotope scans and angiography also show abnormalities with a lower zone distribution.[52] Lung function tests are typical for emphysema with a reduced ratio of forced expiratory volume in 1 second to forced vital capacity (FEV_1/FVC), gas trapping (raised ratio of residual volume to total lung capacity) and low gas transfer factor. The onset of respiratory disease can be delayed to the sixth decade in never-smokers with PI*Z α_1-antitrypsin deficiency, and these individuals often have a normal lifespan.[53]

Emphysema associated with plasma deficiency of a_1-antitrypsin is widely believed to be due to the reduction in plasma levels of α_1-antitrypsin to 10–15% of normal. This in turn markedly reduces the α_1-antitrypsin that is available to protect the lungs against proteolytic attack by the enzyme neutrophil elastase.[54] The situation is exacerbated as the Z mutation reduces the association rate between α_1-antitrypsin and neutrophil elastase approximately five-fold.[55-58] Thus the α_1-antitrypsin available within the lung is not as effective as the normal M protein. The combination of α_1-antitrypsin deficiency, reduction in efficacy of the α_1-antitrypsin molecule and cigarette smoke can have a devastating effect on lung function,[59,60] probably by allowing the unopposed action of proteolytic enzymes. The inhibitory activity of Z α_1-antitrypsin can be further reduced as the Z mutation favours the spontaneous formation of α_1-antitrypsin loop-sheet polymers within the lung.[61] This conformational transition inactivates α_1-antitrypsin as a proteinase inhibitor, thereby further reducing the already depleted levels of α_1-antitrypsin that are available to protect the alveoli. Moreover, the conversion of α_1-antitrypsin from a monomer to a polymer converts it to a chemoattractant for human neutrophils.[62,63] The magnitude of the effect is similar to that of the chemoattractant C5a and present over a range of physiological concentrations (EC_{50} 4.5 $\pm$ 2 µg/ml). Polymers also induce neutrophil shape change and stimulate myeloperoxidase release and neutrophil adhesion.[62] The chemotactic properties of polymers were confirmed by one group[63] but refuted by another.[64] More recently, we have used a monoclonal antibody to demonstrate polymers in emphysematous tissue associated with Z α_1-antitrypsin deficiency (Fig 3a) but not in emphysema in individuals with normal levels of α_1-antitrypsin (Fig 3b). Neutrophils co-localised with polymers in the alveoli (Fig 3c). The pro-inflammatory properties of polymers were further confirmed by the demonstration that they caused a neutrophil influx when instilled into the lungs of mice.[65] Therefore, the chemoattractant properties of polymers may explain the excess number of neutrophils in bronchoalveolar lavage[66] and in tissue

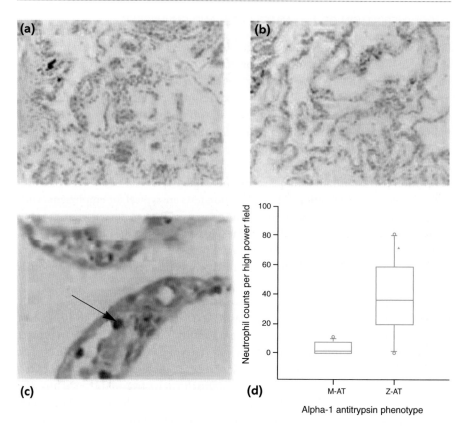

Fig 3 Polymers of α_1-antitrypsin can be detected in the emphysematous regions of the lungs from individuals with Z α_1-antitrypsin deficiency (a) brown staining, but not in regions of emphysema from M α_1-antitrypsin controls (b). The polymers co-localise with neutrophils in alveolar tissue (c); neutrophils in red and arrowed, polymers in brown. The chemoattractant properties of polymers are likely to be an important factor in the recruitment of excess neutrophils to the lungs of Z, rather than M α_1-antitrypsin homozygotes with emphysema (d). (Reproduced from Ref 65 with permission from the American Society for Investigative Pathology.)

sections of lung parenchyma (Fig 3d) from individuals with Z α_1-antitrypsin deficiency. Moreover, polymers may contribute to the excess inflammation that is apparent even in individuals with Z α_1-antitrypsin deficiency with very early lung disease[67] and may drive the progressive inflammation that continues even after cessation of smoking. Any pro-inflammatory effect of polymers is likely to be exacerbated by inflammatory cytokines, cleaved or complexed α_1-antitrypsin,[68] elastin degradation products[69] and cigarette smoke, which themselves cause neutrophil recruitment. Thus our understanding of the biological properties of α_1-antitrypsin provides novel pathways for the pathogenesis of emphysema in individuals who are homozygous for the Z mutation (Fig 4).

For many years the emphysema associated with Z α_1-antitrypsin deficiency has been a paradigm for emphysema seen in smokers who have normal levels of α_1-antitrypsin. However, this is clearly an oversimplification as emphysema

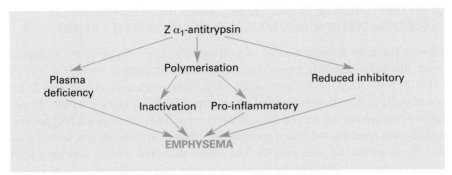

Fig 4 Proposed model for the pathogenesis of emphysema in patients with Z α_1-antitrypsin deficiency. The plasma deficiency and reduced inhibitory activity of Z α_1-antitrypsin may be exacerbated by the polymerisation of α_1-antitrypsin within the lungs. Polymerisation inactivates α_1-antitrypsin thereby further reducing the antiproteinase screen. Alpha$_1$-antitrypsin polymers may also act as a pro-inflammatory stimulus to attract and activate neutrophils thereby further increasing tissue damage. (Modified from Ref 19.)

associated with Z α_1-antitrypsin deficiency has a different distribution (lower rather than upper lobe), different pathology (panlobular rather than centrilobular emphysema), the presence of pro-inflammatory lung polymers[61–63,65] and different patterns of gene expression.[70] It seems likely that more differences will become apparent as we dissect the pathways of inflammation and tissue damage in individuals with α_1-antitrypsin deficiency.

☐ POLYMERISATION OF MUTANTS OF ANTITHROMBIN, C1 INHIBITOR, α_1-ANTICHYMOTRYPSIN AND HEPARIN CO-FACTOR II CAUSES LIVER RETENTION AND PLASMA DEFICIENCY

The phenomenon of loop-sheet polymerisation is not restricted to α_1-antitrypsin and has now been reported in mutants of other members of the serpin superfamily to cause disease. Naturally occurring mutations have been described in the shutter (Fig 1b) and other domains of the plasma proteins C1-inhibitor (Phe52Ser, Pro54Leu, Ala349Thr, Val366Met; Phe370Ser, Pro391Ser),[71,72] antithrombin (Pro54Thr, Asn158Asp, Phe229Leu)[73,74] and α_1-antichymotrypsin (Leu55Pro, Pro229Ala).[75–77] These mutations destabilise the serpin architecture to allow the formation of inactive reactive loop-β-sheet polymers that are also retained within hepatocytes. The associated plasma deficiency results in uncontrolled activation of proteolytic cascades and angio-oedema, thrombosis and chronic obstructive pulmonary disease respectively (see reviews[18–20]). More recently, a mutation in heparin co-factor II (Glu428Lys) has been associated with plasma deficiency, but as yet this has not been shown to cause disease.[78] The mutation is of particular interest as it is the same as the Z allele that causes polymerisation and deficiency of α_1-antitrypsin. We have shown that this same mutation also causes temperature-dependent polymerisation and inactivation of the *Drosophila* serpin, necrotic.[79]

☐ POLYMERISATION OF NEUROSERPIN CAUSES THE DEMENTIA FAMILIAL ENCEPHALOPATHY WITH NEUROSERPIN INCLUSION BODIES (FENIB)

Perhaps the most striking finding of polymer-associated disease is the inclusion body dementia, familial encephalopathy with neuroserpin inclusion bodies (FENIB).[80–82] This is an autosomal dominant dementia characterised by eosinophilic neuronal inclusions of neuroserpin (Collins' bodies) in the deeper layers of the cerebral cortex and the substantia nigra. The inclusions are PAS positive and diastase resistant and bear a striking resemblance to those of Z α_1-antitrypsin that form within the liver (Fig 2). The observation that FENIB was associated with a mutation Ser49Pro in the neuroserpin gene that was homologous to one in α_1-antitrypsin that causes cirrhosis (Ser53Phe)[44] strongly indicated a common molecular mechanism. This was confirmed by the finding that the neuronal inclusion bodies of FENIB were formed by entangled polymers of neuroserpin with identical morphology to those isolated from hepatocytes from an individual with Z α_1-antitrypsin related cirrhosis.[81]

Other families have now been identified with FENIB. These have allowed comparison of the severity of the mutation (as predicted by molecular modelling), the number of inclusions and the age of onset of dementia (Table 1). Affected

Table 1 Correlation between the rate of polymerisation of mutants of neuroserpin, the number of inclusions and the severity of the associated dementia (based on data from Refs 81, 83–85, 87). There is a striking genotype-phenotype correlation that is explicable by the rate of polymer formation and hence the number and size of intracellular inclusions (shown in red).

Mutation	Histology of inclusions at post-mortem	Rate of polymerisation	Age of onset of symptoms	Clinical manifestations
Ser49Pro		+	48	Dementia, temor, seizures in terminal stages
Ser52Arg		++	24	Myoclonus, status epilepticus, dementia
His338Arg	N/A	+++	15	Myoclonic seizures, dementia, tremor, dysarthria
Gly392Glu		++++	13	Myoclonus, status epilepticus, dementia, chorea

members in the original family with Ser49Pro neuroserpin (neuroserpin Syracuse) had diffuse small intraneuronal inclusions of neuroserpin with an onset of dementia between the ages of 45 and 60 years.[80–82] A second family, with a conformationally more severe mutation (neuroserpin Portland; Ser52Arg), had larger inclusions and an onset of dementia in early adulthood, whilst a third family, with yet another mutation (His338Arg), had even more inclusions and the onset of dementia in adolescence. The most striking example was the family with the most 'polymerogenic' mutation of neuroserpin, Gly392Glu. This replacement of a consistently conserved residue in the shutter region resulted in large inclusions with affected family members dying by age 20 years.[83]

The role of polymerisation in disease is supported in our demonstration that recombinant Ser49Pro neuroserpin has a greatly accelerated rate of polymerisation when compared to the wild type protein,[84–86] and that Ser52Arg, which causes a more severe clinical phenotype, polymerises even more rapidly.[85] The cellular handling of neuroserpin has been assessed by transiently transfecting COS cells with wildtype neuroserpin and mutants of neuroserpin that cause FENIB (Fig 5). The most striking feature of the cell model is the retention of Syracuse (Ser49Pro) and

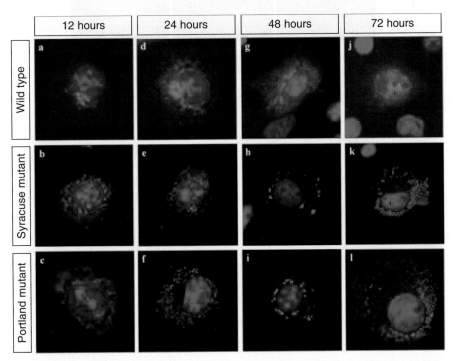

Fig 5a Mutant Syracuse and Portland neuroserpin aggregate within COS-7 transfected cells. a-l: Immunocytochemistry with an anti-neuroserpin antibody showing the distribution of wildtype (a, d, g, j), Syracuse (b, e, h, k) and Portland (c, f, i, l) neuroserpin in COS-7 transfected cells. The nucleus appears blue due to DNA staining with DAPI. Over a three-day period, wild type neuroserpin shows a normal endoplasmic reticulum staining pattern whereas the neuroserpin mutants form distinct protein aggregates after 24 hours of expression that persist for the three days of the experiment.

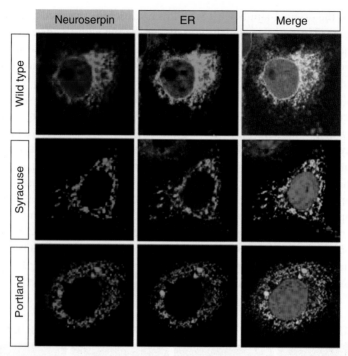

Fig 5b Intracellular localization of wildtype, Syracuse and Portland neuroserpin in COS-7 transfected cells. Confocal microscopy of cells cultured for 24 h after transfection and stained for neuroserpin (labelled with Texas red) and an ER-resident protein, calreticulin (labelled with fluorescein). The merged image shows that the mutant protein is retained within the endoplasmic reticulum. The nucleus appears blue due to DNA staining with DAPI. (Figures reproduced from Ref 87 with permission from the American Society for Biochemistry and Molecular Biology.)

Portland (Ser52Arg) neuroserpin as intracellular aggregates composed of polymers of mutant neuroserpin, similar to the loop-sheet polymers of mutant neuroserpin that can be isolated from the brains of individuals affected by FENIB.[87] Once again, Portland (Ser52Arg) neuroserpin accumulates more rapidly than the Syracuse (Ser49Pro) mutant, in keeping with the more severe clinical phenotype. Thus FENIB shows a clear genotype–phenotype correlation, with the severity of disease correlating closely with the propensity of the mutated neuroserpin to form polymers (Table 1).

☐ NOVEL STRATEGIES TO PREVENT POLYMER FORMATION AND DISEASE

Our understanding of the serpinopathies has allowed the development of new strategies to attenuate polymerisation and so treat the associated disease. We have identified a hydrophobic pocket in α_1-antitrypsin that is bounded by strand 2A and helices D and E.[5,88] The cavity is patent in the native protein but is filled as β-sheet A accepts an exogenous reactive loop peptide during polymerisation.[5] The introduction of bulky residues into this pocket retards the polymerisation of M α_1-antitrypsin and increases the secretion of Z α_1-antitrypsin from a *Xenopus* oocyte expression system.[89] We are currently screening data bases for lead compounds that can bind to this cavity, stabilise β-sheet A and so ameliorate polymer formation.

An alternative approach is to block the aberrant reactive loop-β-sheet A linkage that underlies polymerisation. We have shown previously that the polymerisation of Z α_1-antitrypsin can be blocked by annealing of reactive loop peptides to β-sheet A.[29,90] However, such peptides were too long (11–13 amino acids in length) to be lead compounds for blocking mimetics and were non-specific, being able to bind to other members of the serpin superfamily.[90–92] More recently, we have designed a 6-mer peptide that specifically anneals to Z α_1-antitrypsin alone and blocks polymerisation.[93–95] The aim now is to convert these peptides into small drugs that can be used *in vivo*.

ACKNOWLEDGEMENTS

This work was supported by the Medical Research Council (UK), the Wellcome Trust (UK) and Papworth NHS Trust.

REFERENCES

1   Silverman GA, Bird PI, Carrell RW, Church FC *et al.* The serpins are an expanding superfamily of structurally similar but functionally diverse proteins. Evolution, novel functions, mechanism of inhibition and a revised nomenclature. *J Biol Chem* 2001;276:33293–6.

2   Elliott PR, Lomas DA, Carrell RW, Abrahams J-P. Inhibitory conformation of the reactive loop of α_1-antitrypsin. *Nat Struct Biol* 1996;3:676–81.

3   Ryu S-E, Choi H-J, Kwon K-S, Lee KN, Yu M-H. The native strains in the hydrophobic core and flexible reactive loop of a serine protease inhibitor: crystal structure of an uncleaved α_1-antitrypsin at 2.7Å. *Structure* 1996;4:1181–92.

4   Elliott PR, Abrahams J-P, Lomas DA. Wildtype α_1-antitrypsin is in the canonical inhibitory conformation. *J Mol Biol* 1998;275:419–25.

5   Elliott PR, Pei XY, Dafforn TR, Lomas DA. Topography of a 2.0Å structure of α_1-antitrypsin reveals targets for rational drug design to prevent conformational disease. *Protein Science* 2000; 9:1274–81.

6   Kim S-J, Woo J-R, Seo EJ, Yu M-H, Ryu S-E. A 2.1Å resolution structure of an uncleaved α_1-antitrypsin shows variability of the reactive centre and other loops. *J Mol Biol* 2001; 306:109–19.

7   Jin L, Abrahams J-P, Skinner R, Petitou M *et al.* The anticoagulant activation of antithrombin by heparin. *Proc Natl Acad Sci USA* 1997;94:14683–8.

8   Li J, Wang Z, Canagarajah B, Jiang H *et al.* The structure of active serpin 1K from *Manduca sexta. Structure* 1999;7:103–9.

9   Wilczynska M, Fa M; Ohlsson P-I, Ny T. The inhibition mechanism of serpins. Evidence that the mobile reactive centre loop is cleaved in the native protease-inhibitor complex. *J Biol Chem* 1995;270:29652–5.

10 Wilczynska M, Fa M, Karolin J, Ohlsson P-I *et al.* Structural insights into serpin-protease complexes reveal the inhibitory mechanism of serpins. *Nat Struc Biol* 1997;4:354–7.

11 Stratikos E, Gettins PGW. Major proteinase movement upon stable serpin-proteinase complex formation. *Proc Natl Acad Sci* 1997;4:453–8.

12 Stratikos E, Gettins PGW. Mapping the serpin-proteinase complex using single cysteine variants of α_1-antitrypsin inhibitor Pittsburgh. *J Biol Chem* 1998;273:15582–9.

13   Stratikos E, Gettins PGW. Formation of the covalent serpin-proteinase complex involves translocation of the proteinase by more than 70Å and full insertion of the reactive centre loop into β-sheet A. *Proc Natl Acad Sci USA* 1999;**96**:4808–13.

14   Huntington JA, Read RJ, Carrell RW. Structure of a serpin-protease complex shows inhibition by deformation. *Nature* 2000;**407**:923–6.

15   Mast AE, Enghild JJ, Pizzo SV, Salvesen G. Analysis of the plasma elimination kinetics and conformational stabilities of native, proteinase-complexed, and reactive site cleaved serpins: comparison of α_1-proteinase inhibitor, α_1-antichymotrypsin, antithrombin III, α_2-antiplasmin, angiotensinogen, and ovalbumin. *Biochemistry* 1991;**30**:1723–30.

16   Nykjær A, Petersen CM, Møller B, Jensen PH *et al.* Purified α_2-macroglobulin receptor/LDL receptor-related protein binds urokinase*plasminogen activator inhibitor type-1 complex. Evidence that the α_2-macroglobulin receptor mediates cellular degradation of urokinase receptor-bound complexes. *J Biol Chem* 1992;**267**:14543–6.

17   Andreasen PA, Sottrup-Jensen L, Kjøller L, Nykjær A *et al.* Receptor-mediated endocytosis of plasminogen activators and activator/inhibitor complexes. *FEBS Lett* 1994; **338**:239–45.

18   Lomas DA, Carrell RW. Serpinopathies and the conformational dementias. *Nat Rev Genet* 2002;**3**:759–68.

19   Lomas DA, Mahadeva R. Alpha-1-antitrypsin polymerisation and the serpinopathies: pathobiology and prospects for therapy. *J Clin Invest* 2002;**110**:1585–90.

20   Carrell RW, Lomas DA. Alpha$_1$-antitrypsin deficiency: a model for conformational diseases. *N Engl J Med* 2002;**346**:45–53.

21   Malone M, Mieli-Vergani G, Mowat AP, Portmann B. The fetal liver in PiZZ alpha-1-antitrypsin deficiency: a report of 5 cases. *Pediatric Pathology* 1989;**9**:623–31.

22   Sharp HL, Bridges RA, Krivit W, Freier EF. Cirrhosis associated with alpha-1-antitrypsin deficiency: a previously unrecognised inherited disorder. *J Lab Clin Med* 1969;**73**:934–9.

23   Eriksson S, Larsson C. Purification and partial characterization of PAS-positive inclusion bodies from the liver in alpha$_1$-antitrypsin deficiency. *N Eng J Med* 1975;**292**:176–80.

24   Sveger T. Liver disease in alpha$_1$-antitrypsin deficiency detected by screening of 200,000 infants. *N Engl J Med* 1976;**294**:1316–21.

25   Sveger T. α_1-antitrypsin deficiency in early childhood. *Pediatrics* 1978; **62**:22–25.

26   Sveger T. The natural history of liver disease in α_1-antitrypsin deficient children. *Acta Paed Scand* 1988;**77**:847–51.

27   Sveger T, Eriksson S. The liver in adolescents with α_1-antitrypsin deficiency. *Hepatology* 1995;**22**:514–17.

28   Eriksson S, Carlson J, Velez R. Risk of cirrhosis and primary liver cancer in alpha$_1$-antitrypsin deficiency. *N Engl J Med* 1986;**314**:736–9.

29   Lomas DA, Evans DL, Finch JT, Carrell RW. The mechanism of Z α_1-antitrypsin accumulation in the liver. *Nature* 1992;**357**:605–7.

30   Janciauskiene S, Dominaitiene R, Sternby NH, Piitulainen E, Eriksson S. Detection of circulating and endothelial cell polymers of Z and wildtype alpha$_1$-antitrypsin by a monoclonal antibody. *J Biol Chem* 2002;**277**:26540–6.

31   Dafforn TR, Mahadeva R, Elliott PR, Sivasothy P, Lomas DA. A kinetic mechanism for the polymerisation of α_1-antitrypsin. *J Biol Chem* 1999;**274**:9548-55.

32   Sivasothy P, Dafforn TR, Gettins PGW, Lomas DA. Pathogenic α_1-antitrypsin polymers are formed by reactive loop-β-sheet A linkage. *J Biol Chem* 2000;**275**:33663–8.

33   James EL, Bottomley SP. The mechanism of α_1-antitrypsin polymerization probed by fluorescence spectroscopy. *Arch Biochem Biophys* 1998;**356**:296–300.

34   Purkayastha P, Klemke JW, Lavender S, Oyola R *et al.* α_1-antitrypsin polymerisation: A fluorescence correlation spectroscopic study. *Biochemistry* 2004;In press.

35   Wu Y, Swulius MT, Moremen KW, Sifers RN. Elucidation of the molecular logic by which misfolded α_1-antitrypsin is preferentially*selected for degradation. *Proc Natl Acad Sci USA* 2003;**100**:8229–34.

36   Janciauskiene S, Eriksson S, Callea F, Mallya M *et al.* Differential detection of PAS-positive

inclusions formed by the Z, Siiyama and Mmalton variants of α_1-antitrypsin. *Hepatology* 2004;**40**:1203–10.

37 Seyama K, Nukiwa T, Takabe K, Takahashi H *et al.* Siiyama (serine 53 (TCC) to phenylalanine 53 (TTC)). A new α_1-antitrypsin-deficient variant with mutation on a predicted conserved residue of the serpin backbone. *J Biol Chem* 1991;**266**:12627–32.

38 Seyama K, Nukiwa T, Souma S, Shimizu K, Kira S. α_1-antitrypsin-deficient variant Siiyama (Ser[53][TCC] to Phe[53][TTC]) is prevalent in Japan. Status of α_1-antitrysin deficiency in Japan. *Am Rev Respir Dis* 1995;**152**:2119–26.

39 Roberts EA, Cox DW, Medline A, Wanless IR. Occurrence of alpha-1-antitrypsin deficiency in 155 patients with alcoholic liver disease. *Am J Clin Pathol* 1984;**82**:424–7.

40 Matsunaga E, Shiokawa S, Nakamura H, Maruyama T *et al.* Molecular analysis of the gene of the α_1-antitrypsin deficiency variant, Mnichinan. *Am J Hum Genet* 1990;**46**:602–12.

41 Sergi C, Consalez GC, Fabbretti G, Brisigotti M *et al.* Immunohistochemical and genetic characterization of the M Cagliari α-1-antitrypsin molecule (M-like α-1-antitrypsin deficiency). *Lab Invest* 1994;**70**:130–3.

42 Zhou A, Stein PE, Huntington JA, Carrell RW. Serpin polymerisation is prevented by a hydrogen bond network that is centered on His-334 and stabilized by glycereol. *J Biol Chem* 2003;**278**:15116–122.

43 Kang HA, Lee KN, Yu M-H. Folding and stability of the Z and Siiyama genetic variants of human α_1-antitrypsin. *J Biol Chem* 1997;**272**: 510–16.

44 Lomas DA, Finch JT, Seyama K, Nukiwa T, Carrell RW. α_1-antitrypsin S$_{iiyama}$ (Ser[53]→Phe); further evidence for intracellular loop-sheet polymerisation. *J Biol Chem* 1993;**268**:15333–5.

45 Lomas DA, Elliott PR, Sidhar SK, Foreman RC *et al.* Alpha$_1$-antitrypsin Mmalton ([52]Phe deleted) forms loop-sheet polymers *in vivo*: evidence for the C sheet mechanism of polymerisation. *J Biol Chem* 1995; **270**:16864–70.

46 Elliott PR, Stein PE, Bilton D, Carrell RW, Lomas DA. Structural explanation for the dysfunction of S α_1-antitrypsin. *Nat Struct Biol* 1996;**3**:910–11.

47 Mahadeva R, Chang W-SW, Dafforn TR, Oakley DJ *et al.* Heteropolymerisation of S, I and Z α_1-antitrypsin and liver cirrhosis. *J Clin Invest* 1999;**103**:999–1006.

48 Cruz M, Molina JA, Pedrola D, Muñoz-López F. Cirrhosis and heterozygous α_1-antitrypsin deficiency in a 4 year old girl. *Helv Paediatr Acta* 1975;**30**:501–7.

49 Campra JL, Craig JR, Peters RL, Reynolds TB. Cirrhosis associated with partial deficiency of alpha-1-antitrypsin in an adult. *Ann Intern Med* 1973;**78**:233–8.

50 Laurell C-B, Eriksson S. The electrophoretic α_1-globulin pattern of serum in α_1-antitrypsin deficiency. *Scand J Clin Lab Invest* 1963;**15**: 132–40.

51 Eriksson S. Studies in α_1-antitrypsin deficiency. *Acta Med Scand* 1965; suppl.432:1–85.

52 Stein PD, Leu JD, Welsh MH, Guenter CA. Pathophysiology of the pulmonary circulation in emphysema associated with alpha-1 antitrypsin deficiency. *Circulation* 1971;**43**:227–39.

53 Seersholm N, Kok-Jensen A. Clinical features and prognosis of life time non-smokers with severe α_1-antitrypsin deficiency. *Thorax* 1998;**53**:265–8.

54 Wewers MD, Casolaro MA, Sellers SE, Swayze SC *et al.* Replacement therapy for alpha$_1$-antitrypsin deficiency associated with emphysema. *N Engl J Med* 1987;**316**:1055–62.

55 Ogushi F, Fells GA, Hubbard RC, Straus SD, Crystal RG. Z-type α_1-antitrypsin is less competent than M1-type α_1-antitrypsin as an inhibitor of neutrophil elastase. *J Clin Invest* 1987;**80**:1366–74.

56 Guzdek A, Potempa J, Dubin A, Travis J. Comparative properties of human α-1-proteinase inhibitor glycosylation variants. *FEBS Lett* 1990;**272**:125–7.

57 Lomas DA, Evans DL, Stone SR, Chang W-SW, Carrell RW. Effect of the Z mutation on the physical and inhibitory properties of α_1-antitrypsin. *Biochemistry* 1993;**32**:500–8.

58 Llewellyn-Jones CG, Lomas DA, Carrell RW, Stockley RA. The effect of the Z mutation on the ability of α_1-antitrypsin to prevent neutrophil mediated tissue damage. *Biochim Biophys Acta* 1994;**1227**:155–60.

59 Larsson C. Natural history and life expectancy in severe alpha$_1$-antitrypsin deficiency, PiZ. *Acta Med Scand* 1978;**204**:345–51.

60 Janus ED, Phillips NT, Carrell RW. Smoking, lung function, and α_1-antitrypsin deficiency. *Lancet* 1985;**i**:152–4.

61 Elliott PR, Bilton D, Lomas DA. Lung polymers in Z α_1-antitrypsin related emphysema. *Am J Respir Cell Mol Biol* 1998;**18**:670–74.

62 Parmar JS, Mahadeva R, Reed BJ, Farahi N *et al.* Polymers of α_1-antitrypsin are chemotactic for human neutrophils: a new paradigm for the pathogenesis of emphysema. *Am J Respir Cell Mol Biol* 2002;**26**:723–30.

63 Mulgrew AT, Taggart CC, Lawless MW, Greene CM *et al.* Z α_1-antitrypsin polymerizes in the lung and acts as a neutrophil chemoattractant. *Chest* 2004;**125**:1952–7.

64 Janciauskiene S, Zelvyte I, Jansson L, Stevens T. Divergent effects of α_1-antitrypsin on neutrophil activation, *in vitro. Biochem Biophys Res Commun* 2004;**315**:288–96.

65 Mahadeva R, Atkinson C, Li Z, Stewart S *et al.* Polymers of Z α_1-antitrypsin co-localise with neutrophils in emphysematous alveoli and are chemotactic *in vivo. Am J Pathol* 2005;**166**: 377–86.

66 Morrison HM, Kramps JA, Burnett D, Stockley RA. Lung lavage fluid from patients with α_1-proteinase inhibitor deficiency or chronic obstructive bronchitis: anti-elastase function and cell profile. *Clinical Science* 1987;**72**:373–81.

67 Rouhani F, Paone G, Smith NK, Krein P *et al.* Lung neutrophil burden correlates with increased pro-inflammatory cytokines and decreased lung function in individuals with α_1-antitrypsin deficiency. *Chest* 2000:250S–251S.

68 Banda MJ, Rice AG, Griffin GL, Senior RM. The inhibitory complex of human α_1-proteinase inhibitor and human leukocyte elastase is a neutrophil chemoattractant. *J Exp Med* 1988; **167**:1608–15.

69 Senior RM, Griffin GL, Mecham RP. Chemotactic activity of elastin derived peptides. *J Clin Invest* 1980;**66**:859–62.

70 Golpon HA, Coldren CD, Zamora MR, Cosgrove G *et al.* Emphysema lung tissue gene expression profiling. *Am J Respir Cell Mol Biol* 2004; **31**:595–600.

71 Aulak KS, Eldering E, Hack CE, Lubbers YP *et al.* A hinge region mutation in C1-inhibitor (Ala$^{436}\rightarrow$Thr) results in nonsubstrate-like behavior and in polymerization of the molecule. *J Biol Chem* 1993;**268**:18088–94.

72 Eldering E, Verpy E, Roem D, Meo T, Tosi M. COOH-terminal substitutions in the serpin C1 inhibitor that cause loop overinsertion and subsequent multimerization. *J Biol Chem* 1995;**270**:2579–87.

73 Bruce D, Perry DJ, Borg J-Y, Carrell RW, Wardell MR. Thromboembolic disease due to thermolabile conformational changes of antithrombin Rouen VI (187 Asn$\rightarrow$Asp). *J Clin Invest* 1994;**94**:2265–74.

74 Picard V, Dautzenberg M-D, Villoutreix BO, Orliaguet G *et al.* Antithrombin Phe229Leu: a new homozygous variant leading to spontaneous antithrombin polymerisation in vivo associated with severe childhood thrombosis. *Blood* 2003;**102**:919–25.

75 Faber J-P, Poller W, Olek K, Bauman U *et al.* The molecular basis of α_1-antichymotrypsin deficiency in a heterozygote with liver and lung disease. *J Hepatology* 1993;**18**:313–21.

76 Poller W, Faber J-P, Weidinger S, Tief K *et al.* A leucine-to-proline substitution causes a defective α_1-antichymotrypsin allele associated with familial obstructive lung disease. *Genomics* 1993;**17**:740–3.

77 Gooptu B, Hazes B, Chang W-SW, Daffron TR *et al.* Inactive conformation of the serpin α_1-antichymotrypsin indicates two stage insertion of the reactive loop; implications for inhibitory function and conformational disease. *Proc Natl Acad Sci USA* 2000;**97**:67–72.

78 Corral J, Aznar J, Gonzalez-Conejero R, del Rey ML *et al.* Homozygous deficiency of heparin cofactor II: relevance of P17 glutamate residue in serpins, relationship with conformational diseases, and role in thrombosis. *Circulation* 2004;**110**:1303–7.

79   Green C, Brown G, Dafforn TR, Morley T *et al.* Mutations in the *Drosophila* serpin: Necrotic mirror disease-associated mutations of human serpins. *Development* 2003;**130**:1473–8.

80   Davis RL, Holohan PD, Shrimpton AE, Tatum AH *et al.* Familial encephalopathy with neuroserpin inclusion bodies (FENIB). *Am J Pathol* 1999;**155**:1901–13.

81   Davis RL, Shrimpton AE, Holohan PD, Bradshaw C *et al.* Familial dementia caused by polymerisation of mutant neuroserpin. *Nature* 1999;**401**:376–9.

82   Bradshaw CB, Davis RL, Shrimpton AE, Holohan PD *et al.* Cognitive deficits associated with a recently reported familial neurodegenerative disease. *Arch Neurol* 2001;**58**:1429–34.

83   Davis RL, Shrimpton AE, Carrell RW, Lomas DA *et al.* Association between conformational mutations in neuroserpin and onset and severity of dementia. *Lancet* 2002;**359**:2242–7.

84   Belorgey D, Crowther DC, Mahadeva R, Lomas DA. Mutant neuro-serpin (Ser49Pro) that causes the familial dementia FENIB is a poor proteinase inhibitor and readily forms polymers *in vitro. J Biol Chem* 2002;**277**:17367–73.

85   Belorgey D, Sharp LK, Crowther DC, Onda M *et al.* Neuroserpin Portland (Ser52Arg) is trapped as an inactive intermediate that rapidly forms polymers: implications for the epilepsy seen in the dementia FENIB. *Eur J Biochem* 2004;**271**:3360–7.

86   Onda M, Belorgey D, Sharp LK, Lomas DA. Latent S49P neuroserpin spontaneously forms polymers: identification of a novel pathway of polymerization and implications for the dementia FENIB. *J Biol Chem* 2005;**280**:13735–41.

87   Miranda E, Römisch K, Lomas DA. Mutants of neuroserpin that cause dementia accumulate as polymers within the endoplasmic reticulum. *J Biol Chem* 2004;**279**:28283–91.

88   Lee C, Maeng J-S, Kocher J-P, Lee B, Yu M-H. Cavities of α_1-antitrypsin that play structural and functional roles. *Prot Sci* 2001;**10**:1446–53.

89   Parfrey H, Mahadeva R, Ravenhill NA, Zhou A *et al.* Targeting a surface cavity of α_1-antitrypsin to prevent conformational disease. *J Biol Chem* 2003;**278**:33060–66.

90   Skinner R, Chang W-SW, Jin L, Pei X *et al.* Implications for function and therapy of a 2.9Å structure of binary-complexed antithrombin. *J Mol Biol* 1998;**283**:9–14.

91   Fitton HL, Pike RN, Carrell RW, Chang W-SW. Mechanisms of antithrombin polymerisation and heparin activation probed by insertion of synthetic reactive loop peptides. *Biol Chem* 1997;**378**:1059–63.

92   Chang W-SW, Wardell MR, Lomas DA, Carrell RW. Probing serpin reactive loop conformations by proteolytic cleavage. *Biochem J* 1996;**314**:647–53.

93   Mahadeva R, Dafforn TR, Carrell RW, Lomas DA. Six-mer peptide selectively anneals to a pathogenic serpin conformation and blocks polymerisation: implications for the prevention of Z α_1-antitrypsin related cirrhosis. *J Biol Chem* 2002;**277**:6771–4.

94   Parfrey H, Dafforn TR, Belorgey D, Lomas DA, Mahadeva R. Inhibiting polymerisation: new therapeutic strategies for Z α_1-antitrypsin related emphysema. *Am J Respir Cell Mol Biol* 2004; **31**:133–9.

95   Zhou A, Stein PE, Huntington JA, Sivasothy P *et al.* How small peptides block and reverse serpin polymerization. *J Mol Biol* 2004;**342**:931–41.

96   Lomas DA, Belorgey D, Mallya M, Miranda E *et al.* Molecular mousetraps and the serpinopathies. *Biochem Soc Trans* 2005;**33** (**part 2**);321–30.

Lumleian Lecture

Gut feeling – the secret of satiety?

Steve R Bloom, Katie Wynne and Owais Chaudhri

□ INTRODUCTION

The worsening global epidemic of obesity has increased the urgency of research aimed at understanding the mechanisms of appetite regulation. An important aspect of the complex pathways involved in modulating energy intake is the interaction between hormonal signals of energy status released from the gut in response to a meal, and appetite centres in the brain and brainstem. In particular, the gut peptides cholecystokinin, peptide YY, glucagon-like peptide 1, oxyntomodulin and pancreatic polypeptide have been implicated in signaling satiety post-prandially. The ultimate goal of work in this field is the development of effective treatments for obesity, and manipulation of these gut–brain axes offers potentially useful strategies for the conquest of this significant cause of morbidity and mortality and future burden on healthcare systems worldwide.

The World Health Organization estimates that over a billion adults are currently overweight worldwide, and the increasing prevalence of obesity in younger generations points to a worsening of this epidemic in the future, resulting in an inevitable strain on healthcare systems. Obesity is causally associated with cardiovascular disease, non-insulin dependent diabetes mellitus, obstructive pulmonary disease and certain cancers, a disease burden which currently costs the National Health Service over half a billion pounds every year. Although even modest weight loss can reduce the morbidity and mortality associated with diabetes and cardiovascular disease, public health campaigns to improve diet and promote exercise have not prevented the nation's weight from increasing exponentially, and initiatives aimed at prevention are hampered somewhat by charges of excessive 'nannying'.

While drugs such as orlistat and sibutramine are moderately effective in the short-term, with some authors suggesting that 50–80% of patients achieve greater than 5% weight loss,[1] their effects are relatively short-lived and their usefulness is limited by side effects. More durable weight loss has been achieved through gastrointestinal surgery, but resource limitations and complications restrict its use to motivated patients suffering from morbid obesity. The mechanism by which surgery effects its weight loss is thought to involve a permanent loss of appetite,[2] and this appetite loss may be secondary to a change in the signals of energy balance released from the gut. Over the last decade, our understanding of these signals has advanced substantially. The regulation of appetite and food intake is dependent on complex interactions between higher cognitive centres, more primitive areas of the brain and the periphery, and the gut–endocrine system plays an important role in inducing and maintaining the feeling of satiety. Although signals involved in energy homeostasis have, in evolutionary terms, developed to maintain body weight, interactions between the environment and genetic factors can result in obesity. Manipulation of the gut–brain endocrine axis to overcome this failure of homeostasis may provide a new approach in the design of anti-obesity drugs.

☐ THE GUT AND SATIETY

Gut peptides are released in response to a meal and these hormones optimise the digestive process and signal a change in energy status that influences both physiology and behaviour. Previous work has identified the gut hormones cholecystokinin, peptide YY (PYY), glucagon-like peptide 1 (GLP-1), oxyntomodulin and pancreatic polypeptide as factors which influence post-prandial satiety. The main appetite-related sites of action of these peptides are certain key areas of the hypothalamus (such as the arcuate and the dorso-medial nuclei), the brainstem (and in particular, the nucleus of the solitary tract), and the vagus nerve. The interrelationships between the nervous system, the seat of appetite, and the endocrine intermediaries deployed by the gastro-intestinal tract, the site of nutrient absorption, are complex. However, an understanding of these interactions, the main aspects of which are illustrated in Fig 1, is a necessary precursor to the successful development of viable therapies.

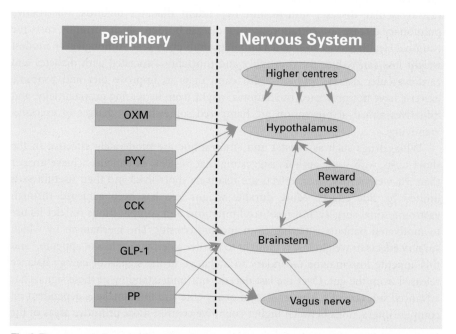

Fig 1 The neuronal sites of action of gut hormones associated with induction and maintenance of a feeling of satiety. CCK = cholecystokinin; GLP-1 = glucagon-like peptide 1; OXM = oxyntomodulin; PP = pancreatic polypeptide; PYY = peptide YY.

Cholecystokinin

Cholecystokinin (CCK) is rapidly released from the gastrointestinal tract post-prandially and plasma levels remain elevated for up to 5 hours. Although it is widely distributed within the gastrointestinal tract, the majority is found in cells of the upper small intestine. The stimulatory effect of CCK on gall bladder contraction, pancreatic enzyme release and intestinal motility is well established, as is its inhibitory effect on gastric emptying, but CCK was also the first gut hormone to be implicated in satiety, as it was found to reduce food intake when administered to rodents.[3] Its acute effects in man are similar: an intravenous infusion of the terminal octapeptide reduces both meal size and meal duration.[3]

The usefulness of CCK as a therapeutic agent is, however, likely to be limited by its short half-life; it is ineffective when given more than 30 minutes before a meal and repeated administration does not alter body weight in rats, for although food intake is reduced, meal frequency increases, and so overall intake is unchanged. In fact, when given to rats as a continuous intra-peritoneal infusion, the anorectic effect is lost after 24 hours.[4]

Although the therapeutic potential of CCK may seem less than promising, there is evidence that CCK might influence body weight over a more prolonged timescale, perhaps by interacting with long-term signals of adiposity. Studies of specific receptor agonists suggest that the CCK_A receptor mediates the effects of CCK on appetite; chronic administration of CCK_A receptor antagonists or anti-CCK antibodies accelerates weight gain in rodents, though without evidence of significant hyperphagia,[5] whereas the Otsuka Long-Evans Tokushima fatty (OLETF) rat, which lacks CCK_A receptors, is both hyperphagic and obese.[6] These effects of CCK on body weight may be the result of an interaction with leptin, as peripheral administration of CCK potentiates the central effect of leptin on body weight.[4]

The CCK_A receptor is present on the vagus nerve, enteric neurones, the brainstem and the dorso-medial nucleus of the hypothalamus (DMH), and there is evidence that the role of CCK in regulating appetite occurs via both the brainstem and hypothalamus. Peripheral administration of CCK induces localised synthesis of c-fos, a marker of neuronal activation, in brainstem areas, and release of CCK at low concentrations from the gut modulates vagus nerve activity, which then relays satiety signals to the brainstem.[4] CCK may signal nutritional status via the hypothalamus by crossing the blood–brain barrier and acting on receptors expressed in the DMH, where it reduces the level of a potent orexigenic peptide, neuropeptide Y (NPY).[7]

Peptide YY

Gut endocrine cells, particularly those from the distal intestine, release peptide YY $(PYY)_{1-36}$ and a shortened form, PYY_{3-36}, post-prandially. PYY levels rise to a plateau 1–2 hours post-ingestion in proportion to the calories ingested, and remain elevated for up to 6 hours. Amongst its actions, PYY increases ileal absorption, slows gastric emptying and delays gall bladder and pancreatic secretions. The truncated form, PYY_{3-36}, created by cleavage of the N-terminal residues by dipeptidyl peptidase IV, is thought to be the biologically active species and has been reported to decrease food intake in rodents[8,9] and primates,[10] and reduce food intake and promote satiety in man, an effect which persists even after plasma PYY levels have returned to baseline.[8]

Chronic administration of PYY to rodents results in reduced weight gain[8] and PYY levels are raised in man in conditions associated with weight loss, such as tropical sprue, inflammatory bowel disease, and post-gastrointestinal surgery for obesity. Conversely, fasting PYY levels are suppressed in obese subjects[11] and overweight subjects have a relative deficiency of post-prandial PYY release associated with reduced satiety,[12] although they retain sensitivity to the anorectic effect of exogenous PYY_{3-36}.[11] PYY_{3-36} may therefore be a pathogenic factor in their weight gain. With better definition of its effects on body weight in man, PYY_{3-36} might then constitute a good candidate target for an anti-obesity therapy.

PYY_{3-36} crosses the blood–brain barrier freely by non-saturable mechanisms, and the peripheral administration of PYY_{3-36} results in an induction of c-fos in the arcuate nucleus of the hypothalamus in rodents. It has been proposed that here, circulating PYY_{3-36} affects energy homeostasis by acting directly on Y_2 receptors, and in particular, those expressed on NPY neurones.[13] These receptors occur on the pre-synaptic membrane and are thought to inhibit neurotransmitter release. PYY_{3-36} reduces levels of NPY and also increases signalling through anorectic melanocortin neurones.[8] There remains some debate in the literature, however, as to the precise nature of the interaction with these latter neurones and there is some evidence that the melanocortin pathway may not be obligatory for the actions of PYY_{3-36}.[9] Despite this, PYY_{3-36} is noted to be ineffective in Y_2 receptor null mice, inferring that NPY signalling is essential.[8] It is also worthy of comment that several investigators have had difficulty in reliably reproducing the anorectic effects of PYY_{3-36} in rodents. This may be secondary to the confounding effects of stress, which can in itself cause a reduction in food intake[9] via actions on the arcuate nucleus.

Glucagon-like peptide

The glucagon-like peptides are products of the pre-proglucagon gene, which is widely expressed in the pancreas, small intestine and nucleus of the solitary tract in the brainstem.[14] Post-translational cleavage of proglucagon by prohormone convertase 1 and 2 results in the generation of glucagon-like peptides 1 and 2 (GLP-1 and GLP-2) and oxyntomodulin in the intestine and brain, whereas glucagon is the primary product in pancreatic tissue (Fig 2).

Gut endocrine cells release GLP-1 after a meal, and GLP-1 then augments post-prandial insulin release, inhibits glucagon release and delays gastric emptying.[4] This integrative role in post-prandial digestion is accompanied by an inhibitory effect of GLP-1 on food intake. Several studies have demonstrated a reduction in food intake and increase in satiety after an intravenous infusion of GLP-1 in healthy subjects, obese subjects, and diabetic patients. Although the effect on food intake seems small when the dosing of GLP-1 mimics post-prandial concentrations of the hormone, a recent meta-analysis of GLP-1 administration has concluded that a dose-dependent reduction in food intake does occur.[15]

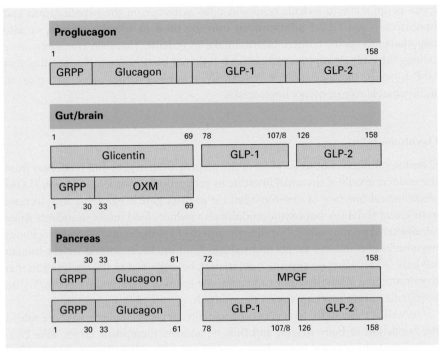

Fig 2 The major cleavage products of proglucagon in the gut and brain, and in the pancreas. GLP-1 = glucagon-like peptide 1; GLP-2 = glucagon-like peptide 2; GRPP = glicentin-related pancreatic peptide; MPGF = major proglucagon fragment; OXM = oxyntomodulin. Numbers refer to amino acid residues.

Circulating GLP-1 levels and post-prandial GLP-1 release are reduced in obese individuals, and if low GLP-1 contributes to the pathogenesis of obesity, it is not unreasonable to suggest that exogenous GLP-1 might restore satiety and result in weight loss. Injections of subcutaneous GLP-1 administered prior to eating have been found to produce a small, but significant, weight loss in healthy obese subjects over 5 days of treatment. An effect on body weight has also been demonstrated, as a secondary end-point, in studies of the incretin effect in diabetic patients: a 6-week continuous infusion of GLP-1 resulted in improved glycaemic control and a 2 kg reduction in body weight.[17] The implications for the management of type 2 diabetic patients are obvious. Translating these findings into clinical practice will prove a challenge, but not an insurmountable one. One of the disadvantages of GLP-1 as a potential therapy is its short half-life, as it is rapidly broken down by dipeptidyl peptidase IV. Resistant analogues of the hormone and orally active dipeptidyl peptidase IV inhibitors are currently in various stages of development. The Food and Drug Administration recently approved the GLP-1 receptor agonist (and incretin mimetic) exenatide for use as an adjunct to conventional oral therapy in type 2 diabetic patients.

GLP-1 exerts its effects via the GLP-1 receptor, which is present in the nucleus of the solitary tract in the brainstem and the hypothalamus,[3] and GLP-1 may exert its effect on food intake through signalling pathways in both these areas. Indeed, GLP-1 given peripherally to rodents results in c-fos activation in the hypothalamus and brainstem,[18] and GLP-1 administered into the third or fourth ventricle, or into hypothalamic nuclei, reduces calorie intake in rodents. However, transgenic mice lacking the GLP-1 receptor are diabetic, but do not become obese,[18] suggesting that GLP-1, while therapeutically a potentially rewarding target, does not play an indispensable role in energy homeostasis.

Oxyntomodulin

Oxyntomodulin is another product of the preproglucagon gene and is released from the endocrine cells of the small intestine in proportion to nutrient ingestion.[19] One physiological function of oxyntomodulin is to delay gastric emptying and decrease gastric acid secretion, but oxyntomodulin also reduces food intake in rodents when administered peripherally[19,20] or directly into the hypothalamus,[19,21] and exogenous oxyntomodulin induces satiety and reduces food intake in normal-weight human subjects.[22] This effect on appetite may, in part, be explained by the observation that oxyntomodulin administration suppresses the levels of endogenous ghrelin,[20,22] an orexigenic hormone released from the stomach.

As well as these short-term effects on appetite, oxyntomodulin may play a role in the regulation of body weight, and thus be another therapeutic target. Like PYY, oxyntomodulin is raised in conditions associated with weight loss such as tropical sprue, and after jejunoileal bypass surgery. Repeated administration of oxyntomodulin to rodents over seven days reduces body-weight gain and adiposity,[20] and this effect may partly be due to an increase in energy expenditure, as well as a reduction in food intake.[23] It remains to be seen whether oxyntomodulin could represent an effective anti-obesity therapy. However, preliminary results from our laboratory have shown that subcutaneous oxyntomodulin, self-administered pre-prandially three times daily for four weeks by overweight subjects, results in a reduction in food intake and a loss of more than 2% of body weight.

A better understanding of the mechanism of action of oxyntomodulin may shed light on its role as a potential treatment for obesity, but here, again, the current literature raises more questions than it answers. It has been suggested that oxyntomodulin exerts its anorectic effect by signalling through the GLP-1 receptor, as it is ineffective in GLP-1 receptor knockout mice.[24] Moreover, the administration of a GLP-1 receptor antagonist (exendin$_{9-39}$) into the cerebral ventricles inhibits the anorectic actions of both centrally administered GLP-1 and oxyntomodulin.[21,25] However, there is some evidence that oxyntomodulin may also signal appetite via an unidentified receptor. The effect of peripherally administered oxyntomodulin is blocked by exendin$_{9-39}$ administered directly into certain areas of the hypothalamus, but the effect of peripheral GLP-1 is retained despite antagonism of hypothalamic receptors in these areas.[20] Furthermore, human and rodent studies show that GLP-1 and oxyntomodulin both potently reduce food intake, even though the affinity of oxyntomodulin for the GLP-1 receptor is two orders of magnitude lower than that of GLP-1. It is thus possible that oxyntomodulin signals through an alternative pathway that has not been elucidated.

Pancreatic polypeptide

Pancreatic polypeptide (PP) is mainly secreted by cells situated at the periphery of the pancreatic islets, but is also released by the exocrine pancreas and distal gut. Post-prandially, PP is secreted in a biphasic manner in proportion to food intake, and plasma levels remain elevated for up to 6 hours. Peripheral PP administration reduces food intake in lean and genetically obese mice, and also reduces food intake when given as an intravenous infusion in man.[26]

Evidence that PP signalling might have a role in the development of obesity takes the form of demonstrably low endogenous PP levels in obese subjects and a reduced second-phase release after a meal. Reduced basal and blunted post-prandial PP release is also noted in patients with the Prader-Willi syndrome, characterised by hyperphagia and obesity.[26] As expected, circulating PP levels are higher in very lean individuals, such as anorexic subjects. Interestingly, levels of PP are reduced after gastric surgery for obesity, but increased after jejuno-ileal bypass surgery for obesity. Thus, PP might contribute to the loss of appetite and weight that occurs after bypass of the small intestine. However, the relationship between PP and body weight remains controversial and some investigators have shown similar levels in lean and obese patients with stable body weight.[27] A recent prospective study in Pima Indians demonstrated that high fasting baseline levels of PP were positively correlated with weight change, whereas a high post-prandial PP release was negatively correlated with weight change over the subsequent years of follow-up.[28]

There is evidence that artificially increasing PP levels reduces body weight. Mice over-expressing PP to supraphysiological levels are lean and hypophagic with reduced gastric emptying. Repeated administration of PP to genetically obese mice results in reduced insulin resistance and hyperlipidaemia, increased energy expenditure, hypophagia and reduced weight gain.[29] Although PP could represent a possible therapeutic target for the treatment of obesity, the current lack of clarity regarding its effect on appetite and body weight in obese humans diminishes its potential in the absence of more data. Whilst PP administration has resulted in desirable effects on food intake when infused twice daily in subjects with Prader-Willi syndrome,[30] these patients do not provide an ideal model of non-syndromic obesity, and the effectiveness of PP in the vast majority of obese patients remains to be determined.

PP shares significant sequence homology with PYY and both are members of a PP-fold family of peptides which have a 'U-shaped' tertiary structure.[26] This family of peptides bind to a group of G-protein-coupled receptors, classified as Y_1–Y_5.[31] PP has the highest affinity for Y_4 and Y_5 receptors, which are present in both the arcuate nucleus and brainstem. However, evidence suggests several types of Y receptor may be involved in the feeding response to PP. Some of the influence of circulating PP on appetite may be mediated via the vagal pathway to the brainstem.

☐ THE BRAIN AND SATIETY

Once a meal is ingested, satiety hormones are released from the gut in a coordinated manner and contribute both to effective digestion and a feeling of fullness. As described above, central circuits in the brain integrate these satiety signals, along with important signals of long-term energy status, such as leptin and insulin, in order to produce a coordinated response to the change in nutritional status.

The hypothalamus and brainstem are important regions regulating energy homeostasis, and the arcuate nucleus of the hypothalamus has recently been identified as a region vital for the reception and integration of signals from the periphery. This nucleus is situated at the base of the hypothalamus, and is exposed to the circulation as it is close to the median eminence – a region lacking a complete blood–brain barrier. Peripheral signals of satiety interact with receptors expressed on the arcuate nucleus, and thus alter neuropeptide release from two neuronal populations within the hypothalamus. One population of neurones co-expresses the orexigenic neuropeptides agouti-related peptide (AgRP) and NPY; the other population releases cocaine and amphetamine-regulated transcript (CART) and propiomelanocortin, which inhibit feeding[4] (Fig 3). Propiomelanocortin is a precursor protein which gives rise to a-melanocyte stimulating hormone, an important anorexic neuropeptide which forms part of the melanocortin system, and is antagonised by AgRP. Both of these neuronal populations in the arcuate nucleus project to the paraventricular nucleus and other nuclei involved in energy regulation within the hypothalamus.[4]

The hypothalamus integrates input from the brainstem and corticolimbic regions concerned with sensations of reward. Extensive reciprocal connections exist

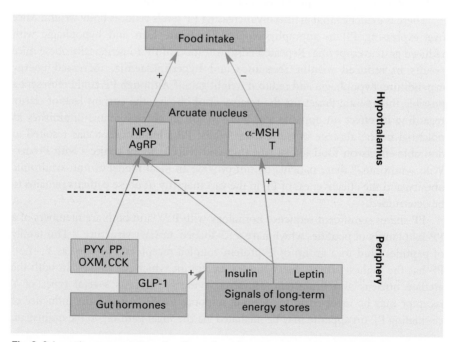

Fig 3 Schematic representation of actions of gut hormones and long-term adiposity signals on neuronal populations in the arcuate nucleus. a-MSH = alpha-melanocyte stimulating hormone; AgRP = Agouti-related peptide; CART = cocaine and amphetamine-regulated transcript; CCK = cholecystokinin; GLP-1 = glucagon-like protein 1; NPY = neuropeptide Y; OXM = oxyntomodulin; PP = pancreatic polypeptide; PYY = peptide YY. + signifies net stimulation; – signifies net inhibition.

between the hypothalamus and brainstem, particularly the nucleus of the solitary tract.[4] Like the arcuate nucleus of the hypothalamus, the brainstem is well placed to receive circulating signals, being close to an area with an incomplete blood–brain barrier – the area postrema. In addition, the brainstem receives vagal input from the gastrointestinal tract and afferents from the glossopharyngeal nerve. Projections from the nucleus accumbens to hypothalamic structures such as the arcuate nucleus, paraventricular nucleus and lateral hypothalamic nucleus may also influence the homeostatic mechanisms controlling food intake.[4]

Defects in neuropeptide circuits can deregulate energy homeostasis, resulting in obesity. For instance, up to 5% of severely obese patients have mutations in their melanocortin 4 receptor. However, in most obese individuals there is no single gene defect and although genetic factors certainly predispose to obesity, environmental factors are powerful influences which can override homeostatic mechanisms. Eating palatable food is a pleasurable experience which activates a diffuse network of reward centres, connected by mu-opioid signalling. Structures such as the amygdala and nucleus accumbens are thought to process the feeling of desire for palatable and calorie-dense food.[32] Interaction between the ingestion of palatable food, the activation of reward centres such as the amygdala and nucleus accumbens and subsequent alteration of hypothalamic neuropeptide circuits may be an important mechanism of disordered energy homeostasis.

□ FUTURE DIRECTION

Obesity is a disease which adversely affects the cardiovascular system, alters pulmonary function, disorders the immune system, and alters the endocrine system, resulting in morbidity and mortality. The normal homeostatic mechanisms which operate to tightly regulate the balance between energy intake and energy expenditure break down in obesity and this may, in part, be a reflection of a relative deficiency of satiety signals such as PYY, GLP-1 and PP. Manipulation of gastrointestinal hormones therefore holds out the prospect of an effective and well-tolerated treatment for obesity. Drugs targeting appetite-signalling neuropeptides in the brain, downstream of gut hormones, also affect other central nervous system functions which use the same receptors. Agents based on the gut hormones themselves would have the advantage of targeting specific appetite circuits within the brain, and may indeed be the secret to satiety.

□ ACKNOWLEDGEMENTS

Dr K Wynne and Dr O Chaudhri are supported by the Wellcome Trust.

REFERENCES

1   Finer N. Pharmacotherapy of obesity. *Best Pract Res Clin Endocrinol Metab* 2002;**16**(4):717–42.
2   Atkinson RL, Brent EL. Appetite suppressant activity in plasma of rats after intestinal bypass surgery. *Am J Physiol* 1982;**243**(1):R60–R64.

3   Wynne K, Stanley S, Bloom S. The gut and regulation of body weight. *J Clin Endocrinol Metab* 2004;**89**(6):2576–82.

4   Neary NM, Goldstone AP, Bloom SR. Appetite regulation: from the gut to the hypothalamus. *Clin Endocrinol (Oxf)* 2004;**60**(2):153–60.

5   Meereis-Schwanke K, Klonowski-Stumpe H, Herberg L, Niederau C. Long-term effects of CCK-agonist and -antagonist on food intake and body weight in Zucker lean and obese rats. *Peptides* 1998;**19**(2):291–9.

6   Schwartz GJ, Whitney A, Skoglund C, Castonguay TW, Moran TH. Decreased responsiveness to dietary fat in Otsuka Long-Evans Tokushima fatty rats lacking CCK-A receptors. *Am J Physiol* 1999;**277**(4 Pt 2):R1144–R1151.

7   Bi S, Ladeneeim EE, Schwartz C, Castonquay TW, Moran TH. Decreased responsiveness to dietary fat in Otsuka Long-Evans Tokushima fatty rats lacking CCK-A receptors. *Am J Physiol Regul Integr Com Physiol* 2001;**281**(1):R254–60.

8   Batterham RL, Cowley MA, Small CJ, Herzog H *et al.* Gut hormone PYY(3-36) physiologically inhibits food intake. *Nature* 2002; **418**(6898):650–4.

9   Halatchev IG, Ellacott KL, Fan W, Cone RD. Peptide YY3-36 inhibits food intake in mice through a melanocortin-4 receptor-independent mechanism. *Endocrinology* 2004;**145**(6): 2585–90.

10   Moran TH, Smedh U, Kinzig KP, Scott KA *et al.* Peptide YY (3–36) inhibits gastric emptying and produces acute reductions in food intake in rhesus monkeys. *Am J Physiol Regul Integr Comp Physiol* 2005;**288**(2):R384–8.

11   Batterham RL, Cohen MA, Ellis SM, Le Roux CW *et al.* Inhibition of food intake in obese subjects by peptide YY3-36. *N Engl J Med* 2003;**349**(10):941–8.

12   Le Roux CW, Aylwyn SJB, Batterham RL, Wynne K *et al.* PYY deficiency may reinforce obesity. *Gut* 2004. Abstract.

13   Broberger C, Landry M, Wong H, Walsh JN, Hokfelt T. Subtypes Y1 and Y2 of the neuro-peptide Y receptor are respectively expressed in pro-opiomelanocortin- and neuropeptide-Y-containing neurons of the rat hypothalamic arcuate nucleus. *Neuroendocrinology* 1997;**66**(6): 393–408.

14   Tang-Christensen M, Vrang N, Larsen PJ. Glucagon-like peptide containing pathways in the regulation of feeding behaviour. *Int J Obes Relat Metab Disord* 2001;**25**(Suppl 5):S42–S47.

15   Verdich C, Flint A, Gutzwiller JP, Naslund E *et al.* A meta-analysis of the effect of glucagon-like peptide-1 (7–36) amide on *ad libitum* energy intake in humans. *J Clin Endocrinol Metab* 2001;**86**(9):4382–9.

16   Naslund E, King N, Mansten S, Adner N *et al.* Prandial subcutaneous injections of glucagon-like peptide-1 cause weight loss in obese human subjects. *Br J Nutr* 2004;**91**(3):439–46.

17   Zander M, Madsbad S, Madsen JL, Holst JJ. Effect of 6-week course of glucagon-like peptide 1 on glycaemic control, insulin sensitivity, and beta-cell function in type 2 diabetes: a parallel-group study. *Lancet* 2002;**359**(9309):824–30.

18   Scrocchi LA, Brown TJ, MaClusky N, Brubaker PL *et al.* Glucose intolerance but normal satiety in mice with a null mutation in the glucagon-like peptide 1 receptor gene. *Nat Med* 1996; **2**(11):1254–8.

19   Ghatei MA, Uttenthal LO, Christofides ND, Bryant MG, Bloom SR. Molecular forms of human enteroglucagon in tissue and plasma: plasma responses to nutrient stimuli in health and in disorders of the upper gastrointestinal tract. *J Clin Endocrinol Metab* 1983;**57**(3): 488–95.

20   Dakin CL, Small CJ, Batterham RL, Neary NM *et al.* Peripheral oxyntomodulin reduces food intake and body weight gain in rats. *Endocrinology* 2004;**145**(6):2687–95.

21   Dakin CL, Gunn I, Small CJ, Edwards CM *et al.* Oxyntomodulin inhibits food intake in the rat. *Endocrinology* 2001;**142**(10):4244–50.

22   Cohen MA, Ellis SM, Le Roux CW, Batterham RL *et al.* Oxyntomodulin suppresses appetite and reduces food intake in humans. *J Clin Endocrinol Metab* 2003;**88**(10):4696–701.

23   Dakin CL, Small CJ, Park AJ, Seth A *et al.* Repeated ICV administration of oxyntomodulin causes a greater reduction in body weight gain than in pair-fed rats. *Am J Physiol Endocrinol Metab* 2002;**283**(6): E1173–E1177.

24 Baggio LL, Huang Q, Brown TJ, Drucker DJ. Oxyntomodulin and glucagon-like peptide-1 differentially regulate murine food intake and energy expenditure. *Gastroenterology* 2004; **127**(2):546–8.

25 Turton MD, O'Shea D, Gunn I, Beak SA *et al*. A role for glucagons-like peptide-1 in the central regulation of feeding. *Nature* 1996;**379**(6560): 69–72.

26 Druce MR, Small CJ, Bloom SR. Minireview: gut peptides regulating satiety. *Endocrinology* 2004;**145**(6):2660–5.

27 Jorde R, Burhol PG. Fasting and postprandial plasma pancreatic polypeptide (PP) levels in obesity. *Int J Obes* 1984;**8**(5):393–7.

28 Koska J, Delparigi A, de Court, Weyer C, Tataranni PA. Pancreatic polypeptide is involved in the regulation of body weight in Pima Indian male subjects. *Diabetes* 2004;**53**(12):3091–6.

29 Asakawa A, Inui A, Yuzuriha H, Ueno N *et al*. Characterization of the effects of pancreatic polypeptide in the regulation of energy balance. *Gastroenterology* 2003;**124**(5):1325–36.

30 Berntson GG, Zipf WB, O'Dorisio TM, Hoffman JA, Chance RE. Pancreatic polypeptide infusions reduce food intake in Prader-Willi syndrome. *Peptides* 1993;**14**(3):497–503.

31 Larhammar D. Structural diversity of receptors for neuropeptide Y, peptide YY and pancreatic polypeptide. *Regul Pept* 1996;**65**(3):165–74.

32 Berridge KC, Robinson TE. Parsing reward. *Trends Neurosci* 2003; **26**(9):507–13.

Answers to self assessment questions

☐ THE EAR IN GENERAL MEDICINE

Ear

1a True	2a True	3a True	4a True
b True	b True	b True	b True
c False	c False	c False	c False
d True	d False	d True	d True
e True	e True	e False	e True

☐ GASTROENTEROLOGY

Coeliac disease

1a False	2a False	3a True	4a True
b True	b True	b True	b True
c True	c True	c False	c False
d True	d True	d True	d True
	e False	e True	e True

☐ DERMATOLOGY

Psoriasis

1a False	2a True	3a True	4a False
b True	b True	b False	b False
c False	c False	c True	c True
d True	d False	d True	d True
e True	e False	e True	e True

Photosensitivity disorders

1a True	2a False	3a False	4a False	5a False
b True	b True	b True	b True	b True
c True	c False	c True	c True	c True
d False	d True	d True	d False	d False
e False	e True	e False	e True	e False

☐ OBESITY

Psychosocial burden of obesity in children

1a True	2a True	3a False
b True	b True	b False

c True c False c True
d False d True d False
e True e False e False

☐ IMMUNOSUPPRESSION

Immunosuppressive drugs in renal transplantation

1a True	2a True	3a True
b True	b False	b False
c False	c True	c True
d False	d True	d False
e False	e False	e False

Biological agents

1a True	2a False	3a True	4a False
b False	b True	b False	b True
c False	c True	c False	c True
d False	d False	d False	d True
e False	e True	e True	e False

Unwanted sequelae of immunosuppression

1a False	2a True	3a True
b True	b True	b False
c False	c False	c False
d False	d True	d True
e True	e False	e True

☐ VASCULAR RISK FACTORS

Prevention of atherosclerosis in diabetes

1a False	2a False	3a True	4a False	5a True
b True	b True	b True	b True	b True
c True	c True	c False	c False	c False
d True	d True	d True	d True	d True
e True	e False	e False	e True	e True

Vascular dysfunction in atherosclerosis: importance of lifetime management

1a True	2a False	3a True
b True	b True	b True
c True	c True	c True
d True	d False	d False
e True		e False

☐ CARDIOLOGY

Genetics of cardiomyopathy

1a False	2a True	3a False	4a False	5a False
b True	b False	b True	b True	b False
c False	c True	c True	c False	c True
d True	d True	d True	d False	d False
e False	e False	e True	e True	e False

Pulmonary hypertension

1a False	2a False	3a False
b True	b False	b False
c False	c True	c True
d False	d False	d True
e True	e False	e True

☐ ADVANCES IN CARDIOVASCULAR IMAGING

Magnetic resonance imaging

1a False	2a True	3a True	4a True
b True	b True	b True	b True
c False	c True	c False	c True
d False	d True	d True	d False
e False	e True	e True	e True

☐ RHEUMATOLOGY

Rheumatoid arthritis

1a False	2a False	3a True
b False	b False	b False
c True	c False	c True
d False	d True	d False
e False	e True	e False

Seronegative spondyloarthopathies

1a True	2a False	3a False	4a False	5a False
b True	b True	b True	b False	b True
c True	c False	c False	c True	c False
d True	d False	d False	d True	d False
e True	e True	e True	e True	e False

Fibromyalgia

1a False	2a True	3a False	4a False	5a True
b False	b False	b False	b True	b True
c False	c False	c True	c False	c False
d True	d True	d False	d True	d False
e True	e True	e True	e False	e True

☐ ENDOCRINOLOGY

Vitamin D deficiency

1a True	2a False	3a False	4a True	5a True
b False	b True	b False	b False	b True
c True	c True	c True	c True	c True
d False	d False	d False	d False	d True
e False	e True	e True	e True	e False

Genetics of endocrine cancer syndromes

1a False	2a False	3a False
b False	b False	b True
c True	c True	c True
d False	d True	d True
e False	e False	e False

Molecular genetics goes to the diabetic clinic

1a True	2a True	3a False
b False	b True	b False
c False	c False	c True
d False	d False	d True
e True	e False	e True

☐ TRANSPLANTATION

Stem cells

1a False	2a False	3a False
b True	b True	b False
c False	c False	c False
d False	d False	d True
e False	e False	e False

☐ RENAL

Management of chronic kidney disease: population-based approach

1a True	2a False	3a False
b False	b True	b True
c False	c True	c False
d False	d True	d False
e True	e False	e True

Inherited renal diseases

1a True	2a False	3a True	4a True	5a True
b True	b False	b True	b False	b True
c True	c True	c True	c False	c False
d False	d False	d True	d False	d True
e False	e True	e True	e True	e True

☐ NEUROLOGY

Update in multiple sclerosis

1a True	2a True	3a False	4a True
b False	b False	b True	b False
c False	c False	c False	c False
d True	d True	d True	d False
e True	e True	e True	e False

Advances in headache management

1a False	2a False	3a True
b False	b False	b False
c False	c True	c False
d True	d False	d True

☐ HEPATOLOGY

Advances in viral hepatitis

1a False	2a False	3a False	4a False
b False	b False	b False	b True
c False	c True	c False	c False
d True	d False	d True	d False
e False	e False	e False	e False

Primary biliary cirrhosis

1a False	2a False	3a True	4a False
b False	b True	b False	b True
c True	c True	c False	c False
d True	d True	d False	d True
e False	e False	e True	e False

☐ RESPIRATORY

Advances in therapy of asthma

1a True	2a False	3a False	4a True	5a True
b False	b True	b False	b False	b True
c False	c False	c True	c True	c True
d True	d False	d False	d True	d True
e False	e False	e False	e True	e False

Respiratory tuberculosis

1a False	2a False	3a True	4a True
b True	b True	b True	b False
c True	c False	c False	c True
d True	d False	d True	d True
e False	e False	e False	e False

Pulmonary arteriovenous malformations

1a False	2a False	3a False	4a True
b True	b False	b True	b False
c False	c False	c True	c False
d True	d False	d True	d False
e True	e False	e False	e False